TUBE FEEDING
Practical Guidelines and Nursing Protocols

Peggi Guenter, PhD, RN, CNSN
Editor-in-Chief
Nutrition in Clinical Practice
American Society for Parenteral and Enteral Nutrition
Silver Spring, Maryland

Marcia Silkroski, RD, CNSD
Consulting Nutritionist
Nutrition Advantage
Chester Springs, Pennsylvania

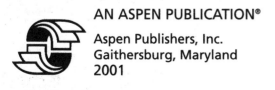

AN ASPEN PUBLICATION®

Aspen Publishers, Inc.
Gaithersburg, Maryland
2001

The author has made every effort to ensure the accuracy of the information herein. However, appropriate information sources should be consulted, especially for new or unfamiliar procedures. It is the responsibility of every practitioner to evaluate the appropriateness of a particular opinion in the context of actual clinical situations and with due considerations to new developments. The author, editors, and the publisher cannot be held responsible for any typographical or other errors found in this book.

The brand-name products mentioned in this book are for informational purposes only and not intended as an advertisement. Most of these products have been used directly and satisfactorily by the authors. No endorsement should be assumed (or was meant) for products mentioned, nor criticism for products omitted.

Library of Congress Cataloging-in-Publication Data

Guenter, P. (Peggi)
Tube feeding : practical guidelines and nursing protocols / Peggi Guenter, Marcia Silkroski.
p. ; cm.
Includes bibliographical references and index.
ISBN 0-8342-1939-5
1. Tube feeding.   2. Nursing.   3. Nursing care plans.   I. Silkroski, Marcia.   II. Title.
[DNLM: 1. Enteral Nutrition—nursing.   2. Enteral Nutrition—adverse effects.   3. Nursing Assessment. WY 100 .G927t 2001]
RM225 G84 2001
615.8'54—dc21
00-067405

Orders: (800) 638-8437
Customer Service: (800) 234-1660

About Aspen Publishers • For more than 40 years, Aspen has been a leading professional publisher in a variety of disciplines. Aspen's vast information resources are available in both print and electronic formats. We are committed to providing the highest quality information available in the most appropriate format for our customers. Visit Aspen's Internet site for more information resources, directories, articles, and a searchable version of Aspen's full catalog, including the most recent publications: **www.aspenpublishers.com**

Aspen Publishers, Inc. • The hallmark of quality in publishing
Member of the worldwide Wolters Kluwer group.

Editorial Services: Timothy Sniffin
Library of Congress Catalog Card Number: 00-067405
ISBN: 0-8342-1939-5

Printed in the United States of America

1 2 3 4 5

Dedication

This book is dedicated to the kids in our lives—

Michael, Stephen, Sydney, Marissa, and Adam.

They keep life fun.

Contents

Contributors

Peggi Guenter, PhD, RN, CNSN
Editor-in-Chief
Nutrition in Clinical Practice
American Society for Parenteral and Enteral Nutrition
Silver Spring, Maryland

Michelle Harrington, RD, CSP, CNSD
Pediatric Dietitian
Children's Hospital of Philadelphia
Philadelphia, Pennsylvania

Beth Lyman, RN, MSN
Nutrition Support Nurse
The Children's Mercy Hospitals and Clinics
Kansas City, Missouri

Marcia Silkroski, RD, CNSD
Consulting Nutritionist
Nutrition Advantage
Chester Springs, Pennsylvania

Foreword

Enteral nutrition is defined as the delivery of liquid formula diets either by tube or mouth into the gastrointestinal tract. It is the preferred feeding method for those patients with normally functioning gastrointestinal tracts and the inability to ingest adequate nutrients solely by mouth. Although it has been used for more than a hundred years, enteral nutrition only recently has been shown to be efficacious and safe in selected groups of patients.

Significant advances and changes occurred in the nutritional care of hospitalized and home patients during the past 30 years. During the 1970s, there was tremendous emphasis on objectively assessing nutritional status. This was followed by studies identifying those malnourished patients who were at increased risk for adverse clinical outcomes. At that time, the ability to give most nutrients by vein (total parenteral nutrition) became widespread. Initial hopes and speculations for the efficacy of parenteral nutrition were diminished when later prospective randomized controlled clinical trials failed to confirm its efficacy. Subsequent studies revealed that parenteral feeding was indicated only in a small percentage—less than 5%—of malnourished hospitalized patients. The 1980s heralded the gradual decrease in the usage of parenteral nutrition while recognition that the gastrointestinal tract could be used safely for feeding increased. Improved and more complete liquid formula diets and safer access techniques led to the increased usage of enteral nutrition in the 1990s. This practice has continued on to the present.

Enteral nutrition is the preferred nutritional therapy for malnourished patients in whom the gastrointestinal tract can be used safely. Depending upon patient demographics, up to 15% of hospitalized patients may be potential candidates for this feeding method. The patients with the best response to enteral nutrition include those with trauma, central nervous system illnesses, critical illness, and major upper gastrointestinal surgery. Examples of patients in whom the gastrointestinal tract cannot be used safely include those with major gastrointestinal bleeding, marked abdominal distention, intestinal obstruction, and peritonitis.

Despite being safer and considerably less expensive than parenteral feeding, enteral nutrition is more labor-intensive. Attention to detail is the *sine qua non* of delivery of enteral feeding. Nurses and dietitians, frequently at the bedside, are best able to administer this nutritional therapy safely. The importance of experienced personnel in the delivery of enteral nutrition is underscored by the prevention of complications such as diarrhea and aspiration. When administered with the guidance of established protocols, these complications can be significantly reduced and, in many instances, prevented. Thus, a textbook on this topic, primarily oriented to nurses and their colleagues, is especially relevant.

Tube Feeding: Practical Guidelines and Nursing Protocols emphasizes those tasks in need of specialized nursing skills. Information is provided not only to identify those patients in need of enteral nutrition, but to ensure that the therapy is delivered properly and safely. Topics of special interest to nurses include the administration of medications, drug nutrient interactions, and the prevention and treatment of complications. A significant component of the book addresses specialized needs for the long-term and home care patient. This is especially important in view of current trends in the delivery of health care. Finally, the means and needs to establish quality assurance programs, clinical pathways, and their financial implications are well described.

Who should read this book? It is intended to be read primarily by clinical nurses, nurse practitioners, educators, and case managers. Additionally, clinical dietitians will discover new and important information contained herein. Finally, it should be a resource for every hospital and home care facility that administers tube feeding and enteral nutrition.

In summary, enteral nutrition by tube is the preferred method of feeding for malnourished patients who are unable to ingest adequate nutrients by mouth. It is safer and less expensive than intravenous feeding. Enteral nutrition is associated with potential complications that can only be prevented by appropriate knowledge and training. *Tube Feeding* provides this knowledge and the rationale for training expertise. I recommend it with great enthusiasm.

John L. Rombeau, MD
Professor of Surgery
Hospital of the University of Pennsylvania
Philadelphia, Pennsylvania

Preface

Since the beginning of their profession, nurses have recognized the importance of food in the process of healing. Florence Nightingale in 1859 stated: "Every careful observer of the sick will agree in this that thousands of patients are annually starved in the midst of plenty, from want of attention to the ways which alone make it possible for them to take food."[1]

According to Medicare statistics, in the US there are 16,995 total nursing facilities with 1,813,665 total nursing facility beds, and many of these patients require tube feeding. More patients are receiving care in critical care units, the home, and alternative settings than ever before. This care is most often given, supervised, and/or managed by nurses. Many staff nurses are administering tube feeding therapy and delivering patient education without the benefit of practical resources and problem-solving tools. It has often been expected that all nurses will know exactly how to give tube feeding, considered a simple, "low tech" therapy.

Over the past 20 years, tube feeding has become more widely used and more complicated, and basic nursing education on the topic has not grown accordingly. Generally, nursing texts lack in-depth information about administering enteral therapy. This book should serve as a comprehensive practical primer on tube feeding for nurses in a variety of health care settings. This includes staff nurses, nursing administrators, consulting nurses, case managers, nurse educators, and graduate-level nursing students in acute care, long-term care, and home care. This book will serve as a resource for nurses who deliver tube feedings as only a small part of their clinical practice along with nurse educators who instruct other nurses about this topic. Case managers can utilize this information to better refer their patients to appropriate care facilities. Nurses who work for insurance companies may benefit from this information in order to approve therapies for reimbursement. Having the practical information in this book for all nurses will help prevent tube feeding–related complications, thus becoming a cost-effective tool in clinical practice. Included are definitions, Internet resources, troubleshooting guides, problem-solving strategies, decision algorithms, documentation concepts, illustrations, photographs, patient education materials, specific tables such as medication lists, and how-to protocols to give readers a variety of information at their fingertips.

Our wish is that this book will help all nurses in their practice, which in turn will help tube-fed patients to achieve their optimal outcomes.

---

1. Nightingale F. *Notes on Nursing*. London: Harrison & Sons; 1859:36.

Acknowledgments

We wish to thank our families for their patience, our colleagues for their content review, our contributing authors for their pediatric expertise, and especially Dr. John L. Rombeau for his eloquent book foreword and for the knowledge he has shared with us over the years.

Nutrition Screening and Assessment

MARCIA SILKROSKI

INTRODUCTION

Assessing an individual's nutritional status is the most important step in determining nutrient needs and requirements. A careful assessment gives a starting point from which to work and helps to define patient goals. In the hospital setting, a nutrition assessment is often performed by a Registered Dietitian (RD). However, the tools in this chapter are designed to assist nurses and other clinicians to conduct a nutrition assessment for their patients. This chapter also offers a realistic acknowledgement and appreciation of the time and effort that are expended in reaching goals and ultimately achieving positive outcomes for patients.

The assessment of a tube-fed patient is often a collaborative effort conducted by an interdisciplinary group of professional staff and support personnel. Often this group approach utilizes a nutrition support team (NST). This team may include any of the following:

- Registered Dietitian
- Nurse
- Pharmacist
- Physician
- Medical Specialists
- Physical Therapist
- Respiratory Therapist
- Social Worker
- Students/Fellows/Residents
- Dietetic Technician

Dedicated secretarial and billing staff can also be an integral part of the team, especially related to patient recordkeeping and other data collection. Certification exams in the area of nutrition support exist for nurses, dietitians, physicians, and pharmacists. For more information on guidelines, standards of practice, and certification exams, consult the resources listed at the end of this chapter.

MALNUTRITION

The primary reason for a nutrition assessment is to determine if malnutrition is present or if the patient is at risk for developing malnutrition. Charles Butterworth published a landmark study in 1974 titled *The Skeleton in the Hospital Closet.*[1] This study was the first to outline the incidence and degree of malnutrition in the hospitalized patient. It outlined 14 undesirable practices affecting the nutritional health of hospitalized patients. Among the undesirable practices Butterworth mentions, failure to record height and weight is number one. He also cites failure to observe a patient's intake, withholding meals due to tests, use of tube feedings in inadequate amounts, failure to recognize increased nutritional needs during times of injury or (metabolic) illness, and poor communication among staff as factors influencing a patient's nutritional status. More than 25 years later, we have many of the same "skeletons" and a whole host of new ones rattling in our facility closets. Several studies have shown that the presence of malnutrition among hospitalized patients remains lofty and can be as high as 48% of all admissions.[2,3]

Malnutrition can be classified into several subgroups. *Marasmus* is characterized by an energy deficit resulting in decreased body weight, overall decrease in body fat reserves, low somatic stores, normal or slightly diminished visceral protein stores, and a depressed immune status. It is normally the result of poor calorie intake over long periods. *Kwashiorkor* is defined as malnutrition because of a protein deficiency over a shorter period (i.e., weeks). A patient with kwashiorkor presents with a loss of body weight and moderate to severe depletion of visceral protein stores; however, body fat and somatic protein stores are often normal.[4] True kwashiorkor is rarely, if ever, seen in the hospitalized setting. It is more commonly found in underdeveloped countries. Perhaps the most prevalent type of malnutrition witnessed in the acute setting and among the elderly is *protein-energy malnutrition* (PEM). PEM is characterized by weight loss and poor protein status as a result of poor nutritional intake over a long period of time. Finally, a combined form of *marasmic-kwashiorkor* state occurs when a chronically starved patient is burdened with a metabolic insult. This form of malnutrition is characterized by a protein and energy deficit resulting in loss of both somatic and visceral proteins, body fat, and total body weight.[4–8]

The reason malnutrition is cause for concern is multi-factorial. First, malnutrition interferes with a patient's normal treatment for medical or surgical problems. A patient with normal protein and energy stores will recover from an injury or illness much faster than a patient who is admitted with a moderate or severe degree of wasting.[9] Malnutrition combined with acute injury can contribute to increased length of stay, and increased risk for morbidity and mortality. Whether the malnutrition is preexisting or iatrogenic, failure to properly address this problem will likely increase health care costs.

NUTRITION SCREENING

Most hospitals have heeded the mandate by the Joint Commission on Accreditation for Healthcare Organizations requiring all patients to be screened for nutritional status, to avoid the pitfall of letting a patient "slip through the cracks." It is often a very simple tool, including just a few basic questions to determine the patient's likelihood of developing a problem. Questions about recent nutritional intake, usual and current weight, any recent weight changes, and/or special dietary practices are common. Patients are screened for any diagnoses that are known to affect nutritional status, such as GI disorders, diabetes, trauma, organ failure, or stroke. Checking for chewing and swallowing problems, nausea, recent vomiting, and fatigue is also part of a thorough screening.[10] Exhibit 1–1 is an example of a nutrition screening tool.[11]

If it is surmised that the patient is at risk or has actual malnutrition, it is prudent to notify the RD and/or the NST, in order to follow up with a more complete nutritional assessment or to implement treatment.

Exhibit 1–1 Admission nutrition screening tool

A. Diagnosis
   If the patient has at least ONE of the following diagnoses, circle and proceed to section E to consider the patient AT NUTRITIONAL RISK and stop here.
   Anorexia nervosa/bulimia nervosa
   Malabsorption (celiac sprue, ulcerative colitis, Crohn's disease, short bowel syndrome)
   Multiple trauma (closed-head injury, penetrating trauma, multiple fractures)
   Decubitus ulcers
   Major gastrointestinal surgery within the past year
   Cachexia (temporal wasting, muscle wasting, cancer, cardiac)
   Coma
   Diabetes
   End-stage liver disease
   End-stage renal disease
   Nonhealing wounds

B. Nutrition intake history
   If the patient has at least ONE of the following symptoms, circle and proceed to section E to consider the patient AT NUTRITIONAL RISK and stop here.
   Diarrhea (>500 mL × 2 days)
   Vomiting (>5 days)
   Reduced intake (<1/2 normal intake for >5 days)

C. Ideal body weight standards
   Compare the patient's current weight for height to the ideal body weight chart on the back of this form.
   If at <80% of ideal body weight, proceed to section E to consider the patient AT NUTRITIONAL RISK and stop here.

D. Weight history
   Any recent unplanned weight loss?   No _____   Yes _____   Amount (lbs or kg) _____

   If yes, within the past _____ weeks or _____ months

   Current weight (lbs or kg) _____

   Usual weight (lbs or kg) _____

   Height (ft, in or cm) _____

   Find percentage of weight lost:
   $$\frac{\text{usual wt} - \text{current wt}}{\text{usual wt}} \times 100 = \underline{\hspace{1cm}} \% \text{ wt loss}$$

   Compare the % wt loss with the chart values and circle appropriate value

Length of time	Significant (%)	Severe (%)
1 week	1–2	>2
2–3 weeks	2–3	>3
1 month	4–5	>5
3 months	7–8	>8
5+ months	10	>10

   If the patient has experienced a significant or severe weight loss, proceed to section E and consider the patient AT NUTRITIONAL RISK

E. Nurse assessment
   Using the above criteria, what is this patient's nutritional risk? (check one)
   _____ LOW NUTRITIONAL RISK
   _____ AT NUTRITIONAL RISK

In addition to the screening data, a nutritional assessment includes more detailed information such as anthropometric measurements, biochemical data, clinical findings, and, finally, the development of a nutrition prescription. A thorough nutrition assessment contains information obtained directly from the patient, or indirectly via caregivers. Subjective data such as usual intake, food allergies, or intolerance of food, use of herbs or alternative therapies, etc., is helpful in assessing the patient's current status. Due to time constraints, diagnostic tests, and procedures, a lengthy interview with the patient may be difficult to conduct. Therefore, the clinician should strive to be efficient with time in order to obtain needed information without making the patient feel rushed or the process impersonal.

Observing for signs of malnutrition during the interview can reveal volumes to the observer. Examine hair and skin for abnormal rashes and dryness, lips and gums for bleeding or cracked areas, nails for splitting or poor blood flow, and the overall appearance for muscle wasting, edema, or bony protrusions.[12] Review the medical record for clinical findings made by other clinicians. See Table 1–1 for more detail on the physical assessment.

SUBJECTIVE GLOBAL ASSESSMENT

Exhibit 1–2 shows the features of the Subjective Global Assessment (SGA) as designed by Detsky et al. This tool is considered one of the most complete and easy to use. Used after proper training, it has been shown to give reproducible results by multiple clinical specialties. The final ratings are summarized into three categories: well nourished; moderately or suspected of being malnourished; and severely malnourished.[13,14]

DIET HISTORY[10,15]

In alert patients, obtaining a diet history can be very useful to the clinician. Some of the most commonly used methods of obtaining a history will be reviewed.

24-Hour Recall

The 24-hour recall involves questioning patients about their intake over the past 24-hour period. In the alert and healthy population, this method is quick and easy; however, it is not often useful in a critically ill patient. Often, patients are sick prior to admission and their 24-hour recall is not reflective of a usual intake. Patients may also be unable to communicate within the early stages of an admission.

Food Frequency Model

This usual picture of intake is derived from the patient's responses to questions about types and amounts of foods normally consumed per week. It is a standard list of foods typically eaten, and may not be representative of every patient's

Table 1–1 Physical assessment of the malnourished patient[12–16]

System	Signs of Malnutrition/ Nutrition Deficiencies	Possible Nutritional Causes	Examples of Differential Diagnosis
General survey	Altered weight for height	Marasmus, kwashiorkor	Endocrine disorders, osteogenic disorders, menopausal disorders secondary to decreased estrogen, anorexia, cachexia, occult malignancy, alcohol abuse, mental health problems
Vital signs	Decreased baseline temperature	Protein deficiency	Hypothyroidism, lupus, heart block
Skin	Pallor	Iron or folic acid deficiency	Skin pigmentation disorders, diseases of the bone marrow, hemorrhage, phenylketonuria, arsenic ingestion, corticosteroids
	Dermatitis	EFA deficiency, zinc deficiency, niacin deficiency, riboflavin deficiency	Hypersensitivity reactions, connective tissue disease, thermal/sun/chemical burns, Addison's disease
	Petechiae, ecchymosis	Vitamin C (ascorbic acid) deficiency, vitamin K deficiency	Liver disease, anticoagulants, trauma, platelet disorders, hematologic disorders
	Decreased healing	Zinc, vitamin C, protein deficiency	Diabetes, use of steroids, AIDS, malignancy
	Anascara (general edema with accumulation of serum in connective tissue)	Kwashiorkor	Kidney disease, CHF, liver disease
	Rough, dry, scaly (xerosis, general dryness)	Vitamin A deficiency, essential fatty acid deficiency	Hypothyroidism, seasonal climate changes, dermatitis, hygiene, uremia, psoriasis
Nails	Brittle, ridged, erosive ridges or grooves, thin concave (bilateral), spoon-shaped nails (koilonychia)	Iron deficiency	COPD, heart disease, aortic stenosis
Head and Hair	Thinning, easily pluckable, lackluster, comes out in clumps	Protein deficiency	Hypothyroidism, chemotherapy, psoriasis, color treatment of hair, infection, heredity
Mouth	Cheilosis	Vitamin B_2 (riboflavin), niacin, iron, and pyridoxine deficiency	AIDS, Kaposi's sarcoma, ill-fitting dentures, oral candidiasis, climate
	Reddened mouth, lips, and tongue	Vitamin B_3 (niacin) deficiency	Anaphylactic reaction, carbon monoxide poisoning

Table 1–1 *continued*

System	Signs of Malnutrition/ Nutrition Deficiencies	Possible Nutritional Causes	Examples of Differential Diagnosis
	Swollen, bleeding gingavae	Vitamin C (ascorbic acid) deficiency	Thrombocytopenia, poly-cythemia vera, chronic overdose of Dilantin, poor hygiene, lym-phoma, pyorrhea, trauma, aging
	Glossitis	Folic acid deficiency	Crohn's disease, infectious diseases
	Loose teeth	Vitamin C deficiency	Trauma, syphilis, aging, Marfan syndrome, poor dental care
	Angular stomatis	Niacin, iron, and pyridox-ine deficiency	Poorly fitted dentures, herpes, syphilis
	Papilla atrophy	Vitamin B$_3$ (niacin) defi-ciency, iron, folate, B$_{12}$ deficiency	Radiation therapy, smok-ing, chronic use of alcohol
	Shrinking mucous membrane	Vitamin A deficiency	Aging, rheumatoid arthri-tis, pyorrhea
Eyes	Dry, rough, swollen con-junctiva, reddened eye-lids; clouded cornea; lusterless, thickened, softening, and ulcera-tion of cornea	Vitamin A deficiency	Cataracts, trauma, herpetic corneitis, Sjogren's syndrome
	Angular blepharitis	Vitamin B$_2$ (riboflavin) deficiency	Infection, foreign objects
	Mild conjunctivitis	Vitamin B$_2$ (riboflavin) deficiency	Measles, infection of conjunctiva, HTN
	Hemorrhage in conjunctiva	Vitamin C (ascorbic acid) deficiency	Malignant hypertension, trauma, diabetes
Neck	Enlarged thyroid	Iodine deficiency	Cancer, cold nodules, infections, cysts, hyper-thyroidism, allergies
	Parotid enlargement	Iodine deficiency	Hyperparathyroidism, infection, allergies
Abdomen	Hepatomegaly (spleen enlargement usually not nutritionally caused)	Protein deficiency (kwashiorkor)	Neoplastic diseases, cirrhosis, infections, hematologic disorders, AIDS, megaloblastic anemia
Musculoskeletal	Muscle wasting, calf ten-derness, bone and joint tenderness	Calorie and protein defi-ciency, thiamine de-ficiency, ascorbic acid deficiency, vitamin D deficiency, calcium de-ficiency, phosphorus deficiency, vitamin B$_{12}$ deficiency	Muscular dystrophy, deep vein thrombosis, arthri-tis (Lyme disease, Reiter's syndrome), malignancy, paralysis, renal dysfunction, liver dysfunction, trauma, osteomalacia, hyper-parathyroidism
	Motor weakness	Thiamine deficiency	Multiple sclerosis, menin-gitis, CVA, Parkinson's disease, ataxia, periph-eral neuropathy

continues

Table 1–1 *continued*

System	Signs of Malnutrition/ Nutrition Deficiencies	Possible Nutritional Causes	Examples of Differential Diagnosis
	Muscle wasting, edema, calf tenderness, decreased position and vibration sense, decreased tendon, reflex and slowed relaxation phase	Thiamine deficiency	CVA, Parkinson's disease, ataxia, psychiatric disease, deep vein thrombosis, peripheral neuropathy
	Rickets, bowlegs, knock-knees, beading of ribs (rachitic rosary)	Vitamin D deficiency	Congenital heart disease, hyperparathyroidism disease, renal dysfunction, liver dysfunction
Neurological	Decreased vibration sense and knee and ankle reflexes, confusion, hyperirritability	Protein deficiency, vitamin B_{12} deficiency, thiamine deficiency	Meningitis, peripheral neuropathy, trauma
	Dementia, encephalopathy	Vitamin B_{12} deficiency, thiamine deficiency	Aging per se, psychiatric disease

normal diet. It also does not effectively cover portion sizes/amounts to allow assessment of calorie consumption.

Usual Intake

The usual intake method involves questioning the patients about how they typically eat on an average day. It tends to gather more accurate information about how a patient eats on a regular basis. This is a quick and simple method, and often it is easy to obtain normal portion sizes consumed. However, the interviewer should be skilled at obtaining information about meals, snacks, portion sizes, and "extras" in order to get an accurate account of the diet.

Calorie Counts

Recording a patient's actual intake over a period of time is very useful if oral intake is hard to quantify through other methods. Calorie counts are generally recorded for 3 to 7 days. Documentation of percent eaten versus foods served should be written in the patient's chart. This gives a basis to determine actual calories consumed and helps to set goals related to improving intake, if needed. For an example of a calorie count, refer to Exhibit 8–6 in Chapter 8, Transitional Feeding.

ANTHROPOMETRICS

Anthropometrics are physical measurements that reflect body composition and development. *Anthros* means human and *metric* means measuring.[16] Among the

Exhibit 1–2 Features of subjective global assessment (SGA)

(Select appropriate category with a checkmark,
or enter numerical value where indicated by "#.")

A. History
  1. Weight change
     Overall loss in past 6 months: amount = # _____ kg; % loss = # _____.
     Change in past 2 weeks: _____ increase,
                               _____ no change,
                               _____ decrease.
  2. Dietary intake change (relative to normal)
     _____ No change
     _____ Change   _____ duration = # _____ weeks.
                 _____ type: _____ suboptimal solid diet, _____ full liquid diet
                                _____ hypocaloric liquids,   _____ starvation.
  3. Gastrointestinal symptoms (that persisted for >2 weeks)
     _____ none, _____ nausea, _____ vomiting, _____ diarrhea, _____ anorexia.
  4. Functional capacity
     _____ No dysfunction (e.g., full capacity),
     _____ Dysfunction _____ duration = # _____ weeks.
                 _____ type: _____ working suboptimally,
                                _____ ambulatory,
                                _____ bedridden.
  5. Disease and its relation to nutritional requirements
     Primary diagnosis (specify) _____
     Metabolic demand (stress): _____ no stress,   _____ low stress,
                                 _____ moderate stress, _____ high stress.
B. Physical (for each trait specify: 0 = normal, 1+ = mild, 2+ = moderate, 3+ = severe).
  # _____ loss of subcutaneous fat (triceps, chest)
  # _____ muscle wasting (quadriceps, deltoids)
  # _____ ankle edema
  # _____ sacral edema
  # _____ ascites
C. SGA rating (select one)
  _____ A = well nourished
  _____ B = moderately (or suspected of being) malnourished
  _____ C = severely malnourished

---

most common of these measurements are height and weight, but fat-fold and lean-tissue measurements are also included in the anthropometric measures. A variety of techniques can be used to assess these areas depending on the patient's clinical condition and ease of obtaining data. Anthropometrics can be used for both initial assessment as a baseline and then periodically thereafter to measure change over time.

OBTAINING AN ACCURATE HEIGHT

Often, obtaining a patient's height is overlooked and undervalued in the institutionalized environment. In most calculations to predict energy requirements, and for predicting an ideal weight, height is an essential data element. Asking patients to recall their height is usually ineffective. Most adults overestimate their height.[17] Humans tend to lose 1 inch every 20 years after the age of 35 or 40. The following methods outline several ways to obtain height.

TRADITIONAL METHOD

Height can be obtained traditionally by having the patient stand erect and bare-footed with heels together, back straight, hands resting comfortably at the sides. By using a rod or beam balance, or by placing a straight edge such as a ruler on top of the patient's head to the wall behind, mark that point and then take that measurement with a tape measure (see Figure 1–1).[15,18,19] Many scales conveniently offer the ability to obtain height by resting a rod on the patient's head.

KNEE HEIGHT METHOD

For patients unable to stand, knee-height estimations are calculated after obtaining a measurement from the bottom of the heel to the anterior surface of the

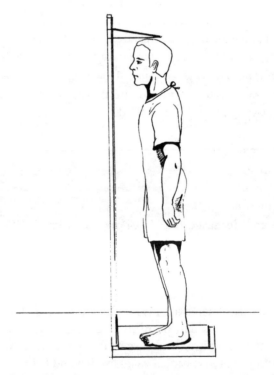

Figure 1–1 Traditional height measurement. Place measuring rod on crown of head.

thigh at the knee. The knee must be bent at a 90-degree angle to obtain this measurement. It is recommended that two or more measurements be obtained to improve accuracy.[15,18,19] See Figure 1–2 for an example of how to measure knee height.

The following is the calculation associated with obtaining the knee height measurement:

Males: Ht (cm) = 64.19 − [0.04 × age in years] + [2.02 × knee ht (cm)]

Females: Ht (cm) = 84.88 − [0.24 × age in years] + [1.83 × knee ht (cm)]

WINGSPAN METHOD

The "wingspan" method is obtained using a tape measure. Keeping the arm straight and at a 90-degree angle from the body, measure from the tip of the middle finger to the midpoint of the sternum. This number is then doubled to learn the patient's estimated height (see Figure 1–3).[15]

(a)

(b)

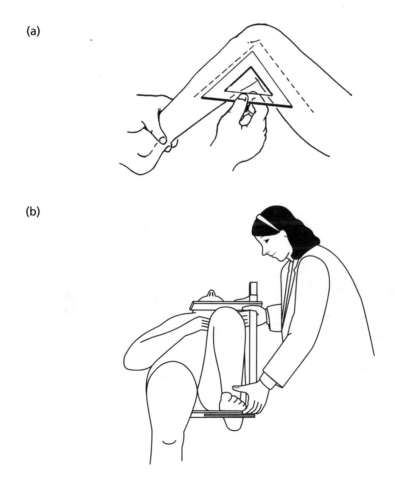

Figure 1–2 Knee-height measurement by positioning knee at a 90-degree angle (a) and using calipers to calculate (b).

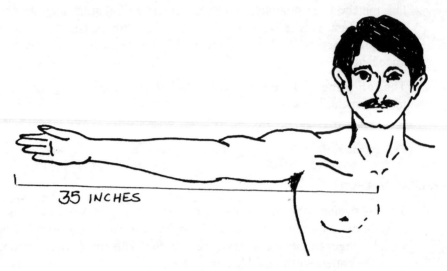

35 INCHES

Figure 1–3 Wingspan Method. Measure 35 inches from midpoint of sternum to tip of middle finger. The full wingspan is 70 inches and estimated height is 70 inches or 5'10".

RECUMBENT METHOD

Lastly, the recumbent measurement is obtained in a supine patient who is as straight as possible. The points at the top of the head and the heels of the feet are marked and the distance between them is measured to obtain the estimated height (see Figure 1–4).

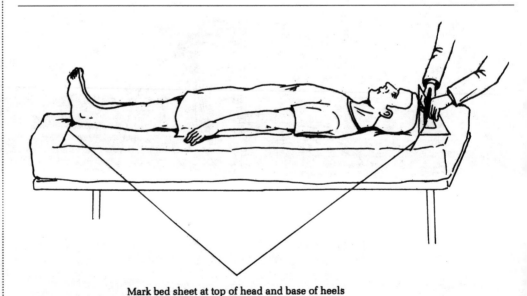

Mark bed sheet at top of head and base of heels

Figure 1–4 Recumbent height measurement

This method is used often for pediatric patients and for patients who are bedridden.[15,18–20] Both the wingspan and the recumbent methods have obvious room for error, especially if a patient has contractures, so it may be prudent to take 3 or 4 measurements and average them for greater accuracy.

OBTAINING AN ACCURATE FRAME SIZE

Often included in a patient's nutrition assessment is the clinician's estimation of frame size. Frame size is useful because it can significantly alter the amount of nutrients required. Two methods commonly used for estimating frame size follow.

WRIST CIRCUMFERENCE

For a quick and easy measurement, using a flexible tape, measure from the distal styloid process of the ulna. Repeat the process 3 times and record the mean (see Figure 1–5).[15,19,21]

Elbow Breadth

A more accurate measure of body frame size is the elbow breadth. This is obtained by measuring the patient's right arm extended forward, forearm bent

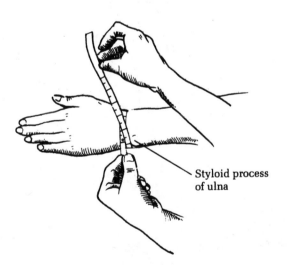

Styloid process of ulna

$$\text{Frame size} = \frac{\text{Ht (cm)}}{\text{Wrist Circumference (cm)}}$$

Key:	Small	Medium	Large
Males	>10.4	10.4–9.6	<9.6
Females	>10.9	10.9–9.9	<9.9

Figure 1–5 Wrist circumference measurement

upward at a 90-degree angle. Fingers should be pointing upward, with the inside of the wrist turned toward the patient. It is usually obtained with the patient standing erect, but it can also be obtained in a sitting or lying position for bedridden patients. Using a tape measure or a ruler, measure the distance between the medial and lateral epicondyles (see Figures 1–6 and 1–7). Frame size is then surmised by values according to age and sex. Table 1–2 represents values for a medium frame. Any value lower than the given range is considered a small frame, and conversely any value higher than the given range is considered a large frame.[15,19,22–24]

OBTAINING AN ACCURATE WEIGHT

Obtaining an admission weight on a hospitalized patient is important for the initial nutritional assessment. Of course, follow-up weights are equally important for tracking a patient's course of treatment. Weight can be measured with a medical scale, a bed scale, or a wheelchair scale. It is important that the scale is calibrated to zero before weighing the individual. To reduce the problem of user error, it is reasonable to document what the patient is wearing (e.g., shoes, heavy jacket, hospital gown); or what, besides the patient, was weighed (e.g., bedsheets, wheelchair).[19,25] Another way to improve accuracy is to ensure that the patient is weighed consistently over the course of his or her stay.

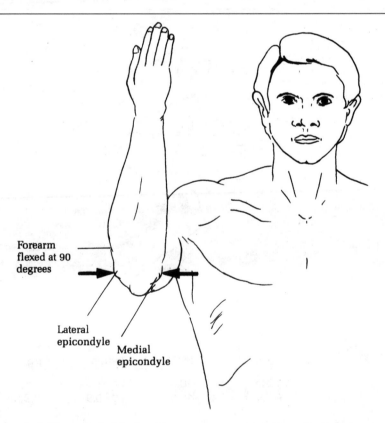

Forearm
flexed at 90
degrees

Lateral
epicondyle
Medial
epicondyle

Figure 1–6 Elbow breadth site

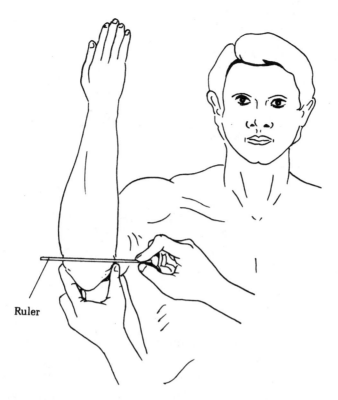

Ruler

Figure 1–7 Elbow breadth measurement

Desirable Body Weight/Ideal Body Weight

If feasible, it is helpful to obtain usual weight in order to estimate calorie needs and, if appropriate, a reasonable rate of repletion. Remember to be sensitive, as weight can be a touchy area for patients—even sick patients. Keep in mind that a patient may not fully understand why you need to have this information. The word "usual" can easily be misinterpreted to mean "ideal," so be aware of this as well when asking a patient this very important question. Always quantify the time frame you are asking about—e.g., How much did you weigh last year at this time? 6 months ago? 3 months ago? Is that usual for you? What is usual?

An ideal weight can be predicted using several methods, all of which have limitations.

Hamwi Method[15]

> Males: 106 lbs for the first 5 ft; 6 lbs for each inch over 5 ft

> Females: 100 lbs for the first 5 ft; 5 lbs for each inch over 5 ft

The end result is then adjusted for frame size adding 10% for a large frame and subtracting 10% for a small frame using the wrist measurement described earlier.

One problem with this calculation is that a patient must be over 5 feet in order

Table 1–2 Frame size according to height

Men			
HEIGHT (In 1-inch Heels)	**ELBOW BREADTH** (Inches)	**HEIGHT** (In 2.5-cm Heels)	**ELBOW BREADTH** (Centimeters)
5'2"–5'3"	2½"–2⅞"	158–161	6.4–7.2
5'4"–5'7"	2⅝"–2⅞"	162–171	6.7–7.4
5'8"–5'11"	2¾"–3"	172–181	6.9–7.6
6'0"–6'3"	2¾"–3⅛"	182–191	7.1–7.8
6'4"	2⅞"–3¼"	192–193	7.4–8.1

Women			
HEIGHT (In 1-inch Heels)	**ELBOW BREADTH** (Inches)	**HEIGHT** (In 2.5-cm Heels)	**ELBOW BREADTH** (Centimeters)
4'10"–4'11"	2¼"–2½"	148–151	5.6–6.4
5'0"–5'3"	2¼"–2½"	152–161	5.8–6.5
5'4"–5'7"	2⅜"–2⅝"	162–171	5.9–6.6
5'8"–5'11"	2⅜"–2⅝"	172–181	6.1–6.8
6'0"	2½"–2¾"	182–183	6.2–6.9

to use it. To estimate weight on smaller patients, the formula can be altered by dividing the first number (either 100 or 106 depending on the sex) by 60 inches (5 feet) and then multiplied by the patient's actual height to get a rough estimate. For example, if a woman was 4' 10" tall, divide 100 by 60 to get 1.66 and then multiply that number by 58" to get 96.6 pounds. The number can then be adjusted for frame size. If this patient had a large frame, one could estimate an additional 10% and place her ideal weight range between 97 and 106 pounds.

Metropolitan Life Insurance Tables

Another method to determine ideal body weight in clinical practice is the Metropolitan Life Insurance Tables (see Table 1–3). These were first developed in 1959 and most recently revised in 1983. The 1983 tables are criticized as having several "flaws" that limit their use. For instance, the subjects used for the tables were weighed with clothing intact and the weight of the clothing was estimated. They also represent an insured population and therefore may not represent a good cross-section of the total population. Subjects were not actually measured for frame size. After the data were collected, the lightest 25% of the total were deemed small frame and the heaviest 25% large frame. Data were obtained from healthy adults and may not apply to hospitalized or elderly patients.[15,24,26]

Percent Ideal Body Weight

Actual body weight shown as a percentage of ideal weight is commonly seen in nutrition assessment and helps to quantify degree of malnutrition/overnutrition if present.

Table 1–3 Metropolitan Life Insurance tables to assess ideal body weight*

| Men (in shoes, 1-in heels) | | | | | Women (in shoes, 1-in heels) | | | | |
Height (ft)	(in)	Small Frame	Medium Frame	Large Frame	Height (ft)	(in)	Small Frame	Medium Frame	Large Frame
5	2	128–134	131–141	138–150	4	10	102–111	109–121	118–131
5	3	130–136	133–143	140–153	4	11	103–113	111–123	120–134
5	4	132–138	135–145	142–156	5	0	104–115	113–126	122–137
5	5	134–140	137–148	144–160	5	1	106–118	115–129	125–140
5	6	136–142	139–151	146–164	5	2	108–121	118–132	128–143
5	7	138–145	142–154	149–168	5	3	111–124	121–135	131–147
5	8	140–148	145–157	152–172	5	4	114–127	124–138	134–151
5	9	142–151	148–160	155–176	5	5	117–130	127–141	137–155
5	10	144–154	151–163	158–180	5	6	120–133	130–144	140–159
5	11	146–157	154–166	161–184	5	7	123–136	133–147	143–163
6	0	149–160	157–170	164–188	5	8	126–139	136–150	146–167
6	1	160–164	160–174	168–192	5	9	129–142	139–153	149–170
6	2	155–168	164–178	172–197	5	10	132–145	142–156	152–173
6	3	158–172	167–182	176–202	5	11	135–148	145–159	155–176
6	4	162–176	171–187	181–207	6	0	138–151	148–162	158–179

*Weight according to frame (ages 25 to 59) for men wearing indoor clothing 5 lb, shoes with 1-in heels; for women, indoor clothing weighing 3 lb, shoes with 1-in heels.

$$\% \text{ ideal weight} = \frac{\text{Actual weight}}{\text{Ideal body weight}} \times 100$$

Morbidly Obese	>200%
Obese	>130%
Overweight	110–120%
Mild Malnutrition	80–90%
Moderate Malnutrition	70–79%
Severe Malnutrition	<69%

Percent Usual Weight

Percent usual weight is also commonly found in the assessment and is often a more reliable factor than the ideal or desirable percentage to represent severity of malnutrition.

$$\% \text{ ideal weight} = \frac{\text{Actual weight}}{\text{Usual body weight}} \times 100$$

Mild Malnutrition	85–90%
Moderate Malnutrition	75–84%
Severe Malnutrition	<74%

Significant Weight Change

Finally, percent weight change represents the significance of weight loss over a specific period of time. Blackburn developed the following equation and reference chart to determine a significant change in weight.[27]

$$\% \text{ Weight Loss} = \frac{\text{Usual body weight} - \text{Actual body weight}}{\text{Usual body weight}} \times 100$$

Significant weight loss	Severe weight loss
1–2% in 1 week	>2% in 1 week
5% in 1 month	>5% in 1 month
7.5% in 3 months	>7.5% in 3 months
10% in 6 months	>10% in 6 months

BODY MASS INDEX

The body mass index or BMI is usually reserved for the well population; however, it may be used in hospitalized patients. The value is a single standard derived mathematically by a patient's height and weight. Figure 1–8 is a chart of silhouettes with a corresponding BMI number under each figure for quick reference[28]; however, calculation as follows should be used for determining a patient's BMI value.

$$\text{BMI} = \frac{\text{weight (kg)}}{\text{height (m squared)}}$$

Weight in pounds is converted to kilograms through dividing by 2.2. Height in inches is converted to meters through dividing by 39.37 and then squared for the BMI equation.

Using pounds and inches, the formula for BMI is:

$$\text{BMI} = \frac{\text{weight (lb)}}{\text{height (in)squared}} \times 705$$

Translation of result:

Underweight:	BMI <20
Healthy Weight:	BMI 20 to 25
Overweight:	BMI 25 to 30
Obese:	BMI >30

A value above or below the 20 to 25 range is associated with higher incidence of morbidity and mortality. While this is a rapid way to ascertain a person's body size, it is still not indicative of where fat is located or how much of the weight is fat.[16,29]

Women

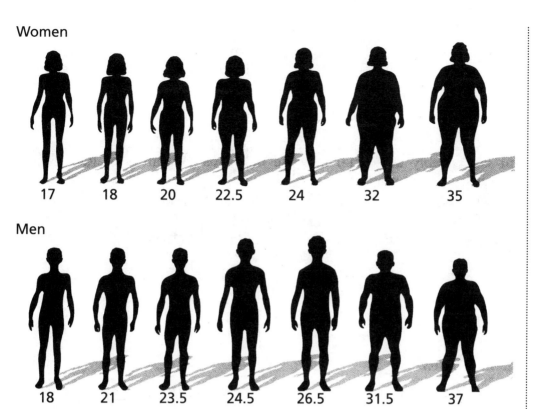

17	18	20	22.5	24	32	35

Men

18	21	23.5	24.5	26.5	31.5	37

Figure 1–8 Silhouettes chart for body mass index

ADJUSTED BODY WEIGHT FOR OBESITY

For very obese patients (greater than 120% of ideal body weight), an estimation can be determined using an adjusted body weight.[30]

Females: [(Actual Body Weight in kg − Ideal Body Weight in kg) × 0.25] + Ideal Body Weight

Males: [(Actual Body Weight in kg − Ideal Body Weight in kg) × 0.38] + Ideal Body Weight

The theory behind this equation is that 25% and 38% of excess weight is metabolically active for females and males respectively.

AMPUTATIONS

If a patient has amputations, it may be necessary to rely on a patient's previous height and adjust for the difference when calculating nutrient requirements. A calculation exists to adjust for body weight using a segmented body chart,[31] as shown in Figure 1–9.

$$\text{Body weight} = \frac{\text{Measured Weight}}{100 - \% \text{ of amputation}} \times 100$$

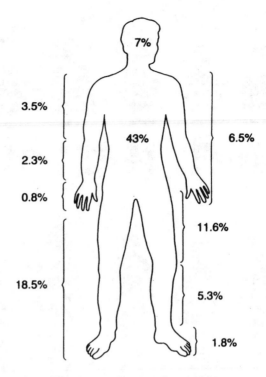

Figure 1–9 Percent of total body weight contributed by segmental body parts

SKINFOLD MEASUREMENTS

Using skinfold calipers (see Figure 1–10), one can determine the subcutaneous fat and total body fat of a patient. Common measurements obtained are triceps skinfold (TSF), arm muscle circumference (AMC), and midarm muscle circumference (MAMC). Review of this data is useful in monitoring long-term patients, using them as their own standard. The practicalities of obtaining skinfold measurements limit their use. The one or several persons obtaining the measurement limit accuracy because it is very difficult to duplicate the exact site at which to measure subcutaneous fat. The measurement techniques employed by clinicians are crude and training is rarely done, so inaccuracy is common. Skinfold measurements are usually reserved for the ambitious researcher studying large populations rather than the individual hospitalized patient.[32,33] There are a few circumstances where they may prove useful, such as with patients who have a chronic condition and are frequently hospitalized, or with long-term care or home care patients (see Chapter 10 for more on home care and alternate site care).

WAIST TO HIP RATIO

An easily obtained value is the waist to hip ratio. Dividing the waist circumference by the hip circumference derives the value. A ratio of 0.8 or greater for women or 0.95 or greater for men is considered undesirable in terms of health

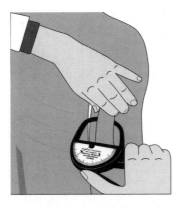

Figure 1–10 Triceps skinfold measurement using skinfold calipers

risk.[34] This measurement is used more often in the wellness setting rather than the hospital setting.

A FINAL WORD ON BODY COMPOSITION

Other methods for determining body composition exist but are beyond the scope of this chapter. Briefly mentioned, methods such as near-infrared interactance measures total body fat; bioelectrical impedance and whole body density measure total body fat and fat free mass; whole body conductivity measures fat-free mass; neutron activation measures lean body mass; and total body potassium measures body cell mass.[21,33,35] In short, these methods are not necessarily useful tools in the clinical setting but do have a more vital role in the research arena.

BIOCHEMICAL DATA

Anthropometric data, clinical findings, and review of patient data are all helpful when conducting an assessment, but biochemical data are equally important to the clinician. Combined with other tools, serum values help to compose a more distinct picture. As with other aspects of the assessment, it is important to view all data rather than relying on one factor.

Table 1–4 summarizes the next 4 serum proteins referred to in this text.[36]

ALBUMIN

The gold standard for determining visceral protein status in hospitalized patients has long been serum albumin. Although it is arguably not the best indicator of repletion because it changes so slowly, it is still one of the most often requested laboratory values to help evaluate a patient's baseline protein status. It has a half-life of approximately 20 days, and functions as a carrier protein for other nutrients in the blood stream. Due to this long half-life, it is a better indi-

Table 1-4 Serum proteins used to assess nutritional status*

Serum Protein	Biosynthetic Site	Normal Value (range)	Half-life/ Body Pool Size	Function	Advantages	Disadvantages	Factors Resulting in Increased Values	Factors Resulting in Decreased Values
Albumin	Hepatocytes	3.5 to 5.0 g/dL	~20 d/ 4.5 g/kg	Maintains plasma oncotic pressure, carrier for small molecules (Zn, Mg, Ca)	Easily measured; readily available, good prognostic index of clinical outcome, inexpensive	Large body pool; responds slowly to changes in nutritional status	Dehydration, anabolic steroids, insulin	Overhydration, edema, renal insufficiency, nephrotic syndrome, poor intake, impaired digestion, burns, congestive heart failure, cirrhosis, thyroid/ adrenal/pituitary removal
Transferrin	Hepatocytes	200 to 400 mg/dL	8 to 10 d/ <100 mg/kg	Binds iron in plasma and transports to bone	Smaller body pool, more sensitive to changes in nutritional status	Calculated from total iron-binding capacity not as accurate as direct measurement	Iron deficiency, pregnancy, hypoxia, chronic blood loss, estrogens	Chronic infection, cirrhosis, iron overdose, enteropathies, nephrotic syndrome, burns, cortisone, testosterone
Prealbumin (transthyretin)	Hepatocytes	10 to 40 mg/dL	2 to 3 d/ 10 mg/kg	Binds T3 and to a lesser extent T4; carrier for retinol-binding protein	Small body pool, responds quickly to changes in nutritional status	Depends on availability of kcal and protein; sensitive to nonnutritional factors	Renal dysfunction	Cirrhosis, hepatitis, stress, inflammation, surgery, hyperthyroidism, cystic fibrosis
Retinol-binding protein	Hepatocytes	2.7 to 7.6 mg/dL	~12 h/ 2 mg/kg	Transports vitamin A in plasma; binds noncovalently to prealbumin	Highly sensitive to changes in nutritional status	Sensitive to nonnutritional factors, protein and energy deprivation	Renal dysfunction, vitamin A supplementation	Same as prealbumin; also vitamin A deficiency

*These proteins are affected by hydration, use of growth hormone, and severe hepatocellular dysfunction.

cator of chronic protein depletion as opposed to an acute protein deficit.[4,8,36] The following are levels associated with morbidity and mortality:

- Mild Depletion   2.8 to 3.5 g/dL
- Moderate Depletion 2.1 to 2.7 g/dL
- Severe Depletion   <2.1 g/dL

In addition to malnutrition, serum albumin can be depressed due to metabolic stress, liver disease, infection, nephrotic syndrome, postoperative states, and in cases of fluid overload (edema, ascites, overhydration, syndrome of inappropriate anti-diuretic hormone).[37]

PREALBUMIN

Another commonly used laboratory value for determining visceral protein status is thyroxine binding prealbumin or transthyretin. Commonly referred to as prealbumin, it has a half-life of 2 to 3 days, rendering it especially useful in the critical care setting for monitoring acute changes to nutrition status. It functions as a carrier protein for retinol-binding protein and as a transport for thyroxine.[38–41] The ranges for prealbumin are:

- Mild Depletion   10 to 15 mg/dL
- Moderate Depletion 5 to 10 mg/dL
- Severe Depletion   <5 mg/dL

Prealbumin is not reliable post-surgery, or in the face of acute catabolic states, liver disease, infection, steroid use, chronic renal failure, or for patients on dialysis.[39]

RETINOL BINDING PROTEIN

Retinol binding protein (RBP) is another value that can be used for assessing visceral protein status, but is not typically used in the hospital setting. It is responsible for transporting the alcohol of vitamin A, otherwise known as retinol. It has a very short half-life of 12 hours, therefore it reflects changes in protein malnutrition even earlier than albumin or prealbumin. As with albumin and prealbumin, it is affected post-surgery, by acute catabolism, and in liver disease as well as in cases of Vitamin A deficiency. In cases of renal failure, a high level of RBP is expected due to glomerular filtration and kidney metabolism.[41]

TRANSFERRIN

Transferrin functions as a carrier protein for iron and can be more useful than serum albumin in some cases. It has a half-life of 8 to 10 days, and is also synthesized in the liver. Ranges for transferrin are:

- Mild Depletion   150 to 200 mg/dL
- Moderate Depletion 100 to 150 mg/dL
- Severe Depletion   <100 mg/dL

Elevated levels are seen with pregnancy, iron-deficiency anemia, chronic blood loss, hepatitis, and dehydration. A low transferrin is seen in uremia, nephrotic syndrome, chronic infection, fluid overload, acute catabolic stress, and protein malnutrition.[42,43] Transferrin levels are often derived from total iron-binding capacity (TIBC) using a variety of equations. Derived transferrin values are most accurate for patients with normal iron levels.[44] Each institution should have an established formula that it uses to assure consistency. Some calculations for derived transferrin are listed here.

- Blackburn—transferrin (mg/dL) = 0.8 TIBC (mg/dL) − 43
- Heymsfield—transferrin (mg/dL) = 0.9 TIBC (mg/dL) − 4.5
- Grant—transferrin (mg/dL) = 0.87 TIBC (mg/dL) + 10

FIBRONECTIN

Fibronectin is a glycoprotein that functions as an opsonic factor. It has a half-life of 12 to 24 hours and thus is clinically sensitive to attempts at repletion. The significance of change is less relevant after 1 week of repletion. Critically ill patients are unable to synthesize adequate fibronectin; therefore, it is rarely used as a reliable parameter in the critical care setting.[45–47] However, it has been shown to correlate with morbidity and mortality.[48]

SOMATOMEDIN C

Somatomedin C (SM-C), also known as insulin-like growth factor, is a growth hormone–dependent peptide with a proinsulin-like structure and anabolic properties.[49] SM-C is synthesized in the liver and has a half-life of 2 to 4 hours. Unlike others, this value is not influenced by acute stress, inflammatory response, or physical exercise; however, it may not be accurate in those patients with kidney or liver failure or with autoimmune diseases. A normal value for SM-C is 0.10 to 0.40 mg/L.[46,50,51]

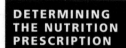

DETERMINING THE NUTRITION PRESCRIPTION

ASSESSING CALORIE REQUIREMENTS

Several methods can be used to determine calorie requirements. The most commonly used methods are predictive equations; however, nomograms and body surface area equations are also addressed in this section. These methods usually represent an estimation of metabolic rate or predicted energy expenditure as a means to determine estimated requirements. Three terms used often when describing caloric requirements are *basal metabolic rate* (BMR), *resting metabolic rate* (RMR), and *total energy expenditure* (TEE). The BMR is the amount of energy needed when a person is at complete rest or after a 12-hour fast. It is the energy we need for breathing, sending nerve and hormonal messages, and to keep our heart beating among the other involuntary activities that we perform each day. This figure varies with age, gender, and body composition. Fever, environmental temperature, fasting or starvation, malnutrition, thyroid function, and the stress from certain diseases and drugs also affect it. RMR is defined as the amount of energy expended 2 hours post-absorption of a meal under conditions of rest and thermal neutrality. RMR is approximately 10% higher than BMR. TEE shows the total amount of energy expended in a day. TEE takes into account several factors as well: basal requirements, activity, fever, effects of starvation, disease-related thermal loss, and the thermic effect of food.[15]

Indirect Calorimetry

Indirect calorimetry refers to the measurement of inspired and expired gas volumes and concentrations to arrive at energy expenditure within 4% accuracy. Indirect calorimeters are used in both clinical and research settings. These calorimeters measure oxygen consumption and carbon dioxide production, which is associated with the synthesis of adenosine triphosphate (ATP). This gas exchange that occurs via the lung is employed in a calculation that follows to assess cellular metabolism (VO2 and VCO2 are expressed in liters per day and urea nitrogen in grams per day).[52]

$$\text{Energy Expenditure (kcals per day)} = \text{VO2 (3.94)} + \text{VCO2 (1.11)}$$
$$- \text{Urea nitrogen excretion (2.17)}$$

Indirect calorimetry is a unique and highly accurate way to determine a patient's energy expenditure, but it can be too costly to use on a routine basis.

The most commonly used calorimeter in the clinical setting is a portable device. With a typical open-circuit unit (see Figure 1–11), the patient breathes room air or is assisted via mechanical ventilation and expired air is collected via facemask canopy or the ventilator. The calorimeter must be recalibrated before each use. Patients must have a stable breathing pattern and minute ventilation during the test. Air leaks present a problem, especially in the critically ill population where they are likely to be common. Examples of air leaks are from chest tubes, endotracheal or trachostomy cuffs, tubing connectors in the ventilator, or even the face mask or canopy of the calorimeter.[53]

Direct Calorimetry

Direct calorimetry was once used to measure energy expenditure. This method requires the subject to be placed in a special chamber or wear a specially designed suit that is water-cooled. Energy expenditure is measured through the loss of heat.[52] This method is impractical for the clinical setting and is reserved only for research settings.

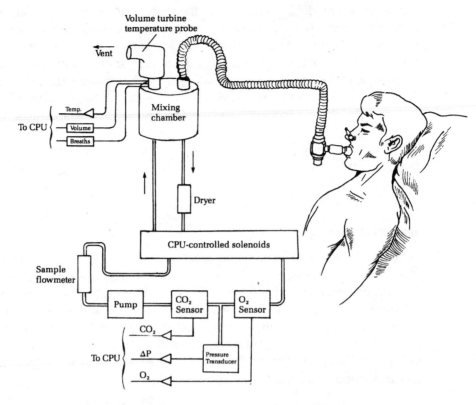

Figure 1–11 Open circuit indirect calorimeter

Cardiovascular Fick Equation

For those patients who require a pulmonary artery catheter (e.g., Swan Ganz catheter) for aggressive hemodynamic monitoring, the Fick equation can be calculated to measure energy expenditure. In this equation, the gas exchange of oxygen and carbon dioxide are derived from cardiac output, the mixed venous blood from the pulmonary artery, and arterial blood flow.[54,55]

Fick Equation:

Resting Energy Expenditure = CO $\times$ Hgb (Sao2 $-$ Svo2) $\times$ 95.18

In this equation, CO is cardiac output; Hgb is hemoglobin in gms per deciliter; and Sao2 and Svo2 are percent saturation of oxygen in arterial and mixed venous blood in fractions.[15]

Harris-Benedict Formula

A popular method to arrive at energy requirements is the Harris-Benedict equation, which represents basal energy expenditure (BEE). Harris and Benedict used a closed-circuit indirect calorimeter in their original studies, which were published in 1919.[56]

The Harris-Benedict equation is often criticized for overestimating energy requirements in severely metabolically stressed individuals by as much as 5% to 10%, and therefore good clinical judgment should always be exercised to interpret these numbers.[57] For most clinical settings and in situations where indirect calorimetry is not available, the Harris-Benedict equation offers a good method for determining energy expenditure.[15]

Male: BEE = 66.473 + 13.75(Wt in kg) + 5.0(Ht in cm) − 6.76(age in years)

Female: BEE = 655.1 + 9.56(Wt in kg) + 1.85(Ht in cm) − 4.68(age in years)

The sum of the BEE is then multiplied by activity and injury factors such as the ones listed in Table 1–5.

Calories per Kilogram Method

A simpler method for estimating calories or kilocalories (kcals) can be obtained by applying the following mathematical approach to actual body weight:[15]

- No stress, minimal activity—28 kcal/kg/day
- Mild stress—30 kcal/kg/day
- Moderate stress—35 kcal/kg/day
- Severe stress—40 kcal/kg/day

Most hospitalized patients fall into the mild to moderate categories when using this method. The exceptions are the elderly, children, and in cases of refeeding chronically starved patients. Providing more than 40 calories per kilogram is not often done and could cause serious complications for critically ill patients. Calculations and formulas should never replace clinical judgment. If the numbers seem inaccurate, a metabolic chart, if accessible, should be used to determine calorie needs.

Ireton-Jones Calculation

The Ireton-Jones equation is predictive of energy expenditure in critically ill or hospitalized patients.[58] The equation shown here has been revised from the

Table 1–5 Activity and Injury Factors

Activity Factor	Percentage	Injury Factor	Percentage
Confined to bed	1.2	Minor surgery	1.2
Out of bed	1.3	Skeletal trauma	1.3
Very active (athlete)	1.4	Major sepsis	1.6
		Severe burn	2.1
		Fever	1.1 for each degree above normal temperature (37 degrees C)

original reference.[59] Energy expenditure (EEE) is calculated and factors such as breathing dependency, trauma, burns, sex, and body composition are factored into the equation.

$$EEE (v) = 1784 - 11 (A) + 5 (W) + 244 (S) + 239 (T) + 804 (B)$$

$$EEE (s) = 629 - 11 (A) + 25 (W) - 609 (O)$$

Where:

EEE = kcal per day

v = ventilator dependent   T = trauma [present = 1, absent = 0]

s = spontaneous breather   B = burn [present = 1, absent = 0]

W = weight in kg   O = obesity [present = 1, absent = 0]

A = age in years   S = sex [male = 1, female = 0]

Nomograms

Figure 1–12 shows a nomogram to assess resting energy expenditure. Nomograms are fast, inexpensive tools. However, clinicians tend to be variable in their use of actual versus desirable weights. Nomograms are noted as having much room for error.[15]

A Final Word on Calculating Caloric Requirements

No matter which tool is used, the goal should be provision of calories to meet maintenance requirements or promote anabolism without overfeeding.

ESTIMATING PROTEIN REQUIREMENTS

As with estimating calorie needs, there are several methods for calculating protein requirements. As time allows, it can be useful to use more than one method for determining a protein requirement in order to verify accuracy.

- Grams of Protein per kg of Ideal Weight
- Healthy adult—0.8 g/kg
- Mild Stress—0.8 to 1.0 g/kg
- Moderate Stress—1.0 to 1.5 g/kg
- Severe Stress—1.5 to 2.0 g/kg

Inherent with this method is that the determination of ideal weight can vary greatly between clinicians and may be difficult to determine without accurate height, or issues such as obesity and stressed and disease states. Nonetheless, it is frequently used in the clinical setting.

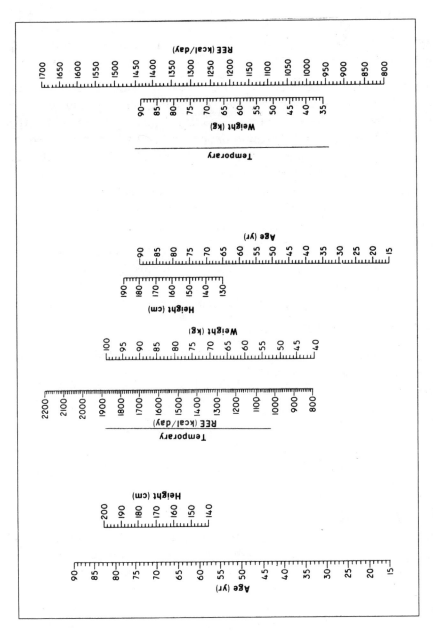

Figure 1–12 Resting energy expenditure for males and females.

NITROGEN BALANCE

Nitrogen is an end product of protein metabolism. If the body is being adequately nourished and healthy, it is usually in "nitrogen balance." This means that *nitrogen in* equals *nitrogen out*. In hospitalized patients suffering recent trauma, surgery, burns, or other catabolic conditions, nitrogen balance is often *negative* because the body is being forced to use protein reserves for energy.[60] A goal in this situation is to attain and maintain a *positive* nitrogen balance.

Nitrogen (N) balance is derived by an equation using urinary urea nitrogen (UUN) obtained in a 24-hour urine. N output equals UUN plus obligatory N losses. Obligatory losses are from feces, skin, urine, and respiration. Approximately 2 to 4 grams per day are estimated to be lost. The inconsistencies that occur with N balance studies are seen with the use of anabolic and catabolic hormones, fecal and skin losses, renal impairment, thermal injury, incontinence, draining wounds and fistulas, immobility, and in the nutrient composition of feedings. A precise collection of the 24-hour urine is critical to the outcome of this measurement. A goal for positive N balance is between 2 and 4 grams per day.[61,62]

Using the TUN is considered more accurate when calculating N balance; however, it is often not available in hospital laboratories. UUN is often substituted, but it only represents 80% to 90% of TUN in healthy, non-stressed individuals, which can equate to a significant 12 gram protein difference per day.[63]

The equation for N balance is:

N balance = N intake − N output whereas

$$\frac{\text{24-hour protein intake (gm)}}{6.25} - (\text{24-hour UUN (gm)} + 4 \text{ gm})$$

$$\frac{\text{24-hour protein intake (gm)}}{6.25} - (\text{24-hour TUN (gm)} + 2 \text{ gm})$$

UUN = Urinary Urea Nitrogen; TUN = Total Urinary Nitrogen

ASSESSING FLUID REQUIREMENTS

The provision of daily fluids is an important part of nutritional care. Fluids are provided in intravenous medications and nutrients, in oral medications and diet, enteral formula, water flushes, etc. The RD and physician often work closely together to calculate fluid requirements, while the pharmacist and/or nurse may implement a plan to deliver those fluids in the most efficient manner. Assuming the patient has no renal impairment where a fluid restriction is imposed, the following methods can be used to determine fluid needs.[64] As with calorie or protein requirements, using two or three methods before arriving at a final fluid requirement may prove more clinically relevant.

- **By Age**

18 to 64 years	30 to 35 mL/kg
55 to 65 years	30 mL/kg
> 65 years	25 mL/kg

- **By Weight**

  1500 mL for the first 20 kg

  Add 20 mL/kg over 20 kg
- **By Calories - RDA**

  1 mL/kcal (~3.5 mL/kg UBW)
- **By Calories and Protein**

  1 mL/kcal

  Add 100 mL/gm of nitrogen
- **By Height**

  1500 mL/m2 (squared)

CONCLUSION

In summary, it is important to treat each patient as an individual. Nutrition assessment takes a considerable amount of time. An accurate assessment guides the decision making for many other treatments—e.g., medication dosing, IV therapy, duration of therapy—and possibly even impacts a patient's length of hospital stay. Therefore, a well-trained clinician or clinicians should be in charge of gathering and documenting the appropriate data to yield the best possible therapeutic outcome.

REFERENCES

1. Butterworth C. The skeleton in the hospital closet. *Nutr Today* 1974;9:4–8.
2. Weinsier RL, Hunker EM, Krumdieck CL, Butterworth CE. Hospital malnutrition: a prospective evaluation of general medical patients during the course of hospitalization. *Am J Clin Nutr* 1979;32:418–426.
3. Coats KG, Morgan SL, Bartolucci AA, Weinsier RL. Hospital-associated malnutrition: a reevaluation 12 years later. *J Am Diet Assoc* 1993;93:27–33.
4. McClave S, Mitoraj T, Thielmeier K, Greenburg R. Differentiating subtypes of protein calorie malnutrition: incidence and clinical significance in a university hospital setting. *J Parenter Enteral Nutr* 1992;16:337–342.
5. Whitehead RG, Coward WA, Lunn PG. Serum albumin concentration and the onset of kwashiorkor. *Lancet* 1973;1:63–66.
6. Coward WA, Lunn PG. The biochemistry and physiology of kwashiorkor and marasmus. *Br Med Bull* 1981;37:19–24.
7. Klidjian AM, Archer TJ, Foster KJ, Karran SJ. Detection of dangerous malnutrition. *J Parenter Enteral Nutr* 1982;6:119–121.
8. Bistrian BR, Blackburn GL, Hallowell E, Heddle R. Prevalence of malnutrition in general surgical patients. *JAMA* 1974;230:858–860.

9. Reinhardt GF, Myscofski JW, Wilkens DB, et al. Incidence and mortality of hypoalbuminemic patients in hospitalized veterans. *J Parenter Enteral Nutr* 1980;4:357–359.

10. Karkeck J. Improving the use of dietary survey methodology. *J Am Diet Assoc* 1987;87: 869–871.

11. Kovacevich DS, Boney AR, Braunschweig CL, Perez A. Nutrition risk classification: a reproducible and valid tool for nurses. *Nutr Clin Pract* 1997;12:20–25.

12. Rindal J. Metabolic Nurse Clinician, Department of Surgery, University of Minnesota, Minneapolis, MN. 1996.

13. Baker JP, Detsky AS, Wesson DE, et al. Nutritional assessment: a comparison of clinical judgment and objective measurements. *N Engl J Med* 1982;306:969–972.

14. Detsky AS, McLaughlin JR, Baker JP, et al. What is subjective global assessment of nutritional status? *J Parenter Enteral Nutr* 1987;11:8–13.

15. Hopkins B. Assessment of nutritional status. In: Gottschlich MM, Matarese LE, Schronts EP, eds. *Nutrition Support Dietetics Core Curriculum*. 2nd ed. Silver Spring, MD: American Society for Parenteral and Enteral Nutrition; 1993.

16. Whitney EN, Cataldo CB, DeBruyne LK, Rolfes SR. Nutrition assessment: anthropometric and biochemical data. In: *Nutrition for Health and Health Care*. Minneapolis/St. Paul, MN: West Publishing Company; 1996.

17. Pirie P, Jacobs D, Jeffery R, Hannan P. Distortion in self-reported height and weight data. *J Am Diet Assoc* 1981;78:601–606.

18. Zeman FJ. *Clinical Nutrition and Dietetics*. New York, NY: MacMillan; 1991.

19. Guenter PA, Smithgall JM, Williamson West I, Rombeau JL. Nutrition assessment. In: Rombeau JL, Caldwell MD, Forlaw L, Guenter PA, eds. *Atlas of Nutritional Support Techniques*. Boston, MA: Little, Brown and Company; 1989.

20. Gray DS, Crider JB, Kelley C, et al. Accuracy of recumbent height measurement. *JPEN* 1985;9:712.

21. Grant JP. *Handbook of Total Parenteral Nutrition*. Philadelphia, PA: WB Saunders Company; 1980:15.

22. Abraham S. Height-weight tables: their sources and development. *Clin Consult Nutr Supp* 1983;3:5–8.

23. Frisancho AR. New standards of weight and body composition by frame size and height for assessment of nutritional status of adults and the elderly. *Am J Clin Nutr* 1984;40: 808–819.

24. Metropolitan Life Insurance Company. Statistical Bulletin. January–June, 1983.

25. Blackburn GL, Bistrian BR, Maini BS, et al. Nutritional and metabolic assessment of the hospitalized patient. *J Parenter Enteral Nutr* 1977;1:11–22.

26. Gray GE, Gray LK. Anthropometric measurements and their interpretation: principles, practices and problems. *J Am Diet Assoc* 1980;77:534–538.

27. Blackburn GL, et al. *J Parenter Enteral Nutr* 1977;1:1–12.

28. The Body Test—Silhouettes and Body Mass Index. Canadian Dietetic Association.

29. Bray GA. Pathophysiology of obesity. *Am J Clin Nutr* 1992;55:488S-494S.

30. Chicago Dietetic Association Manual.

31. Grant A, DeHoog S. *Nutritional Assessment and Support*. Seattle, WA: Grant and DeHoog Publishers; 1985:11.

32. Heymsfield S, McManus C, Seitz S, et al. Anthropometric assessment of adult protein-energy malnutrition. In: Wright R, Heymsfield S, eds. *Nutritional Assessment of the Adult Hospitalized Patient*. Boston, MA: Blackwell Scientific Publications; 1984:27–82.

33. Vansant G, Van Gaal L, Deleeuw I. Assessment of body composition by skinfold anthropometry and bioelectrical impedance technique: a comparative study. *J Parenter Enteral Nutr* 1994;18:427–429.

34. Schroeder SA, Krupp MA, Tierney LM, et al. *Current Medical Diagnosis and Treatment.* Norwalk, CT: Appleton and Lange; 1991.
35. Bioelectrical impedance analysis in body composition measurement. Paper presented at Technology Assessment Conference; National Institutes of Health; 1994; Bethesda, MD.
36. Spiekerman AM. Proteins used in nutritional assessment. *Clin Lab Med* 1993;13:353–369.
37. Boosalis MG, Ott L, Levine AS, et al. Relationship of visceral proteins to nutritional status in chronic and acute stress. *Crit Care Med* 1989;17:741–747.
38. Winkler MF, Gerrior SA, Pomp A, Albina JE. Use of retinol-binding protein and prealbumin as indicators of the response to nutrition therapy. *J Amer Diet Assoc* 1989;89: 684–687.
39. Ingenbleek Y, Young V. Transthyretin (prealbumin) in health and disease: nutritional implications. *Ann Rev Nutr* 1994;14:495–533.
40. Tuten MB, Wogt S, Dasse F, Leider Z. Utilization of prealbumin as a nutritional parameter. *J Parenter Enteral Nutr* 1985;9:709–711.
41. Smith FR, Suskind R, Thanangkul O, et al. Plasma vitamin A, retinol-binding protein and prealbumin concentrations in protein-calorie malnutrition, III: response to varying dietary treatments. *Am J Clin Nutr* 1975;28:732–738.
42. Roza AM, Tuitt D, Shizgal HM. Transferrin—a poor measure of nutritional status. *J Parenter Enteral Nutr* 1984;8:523–528.
43. Fletcher JP, Little JM, Gust PK. A comparison of serum transferrin and serum prealbumin as nutritional parameters. *J Parenter Enteral Nutr* 1987;11:144–147.
44. Miller SF, Morath MA, Finley RR. Comparison of derived and actual transferrin: a potential source of error in clinical nutrition assessment. *J Trauma* 1981;21:548–550.
45. McKone TK, Davis AT, Dean RE. Fibronectin: a new nutritional parameter. *Am Surg* 1985;51:336–339.
46. Bounpane EA, Brown RO, Boucher BA, et al. Use of fibronectin and somatomedin-C as nutritional markers in the enteral nutrition support of traumatized patients. *Crit Care Med* 1989;17:126–132.
47. Saba TM, Kiener JL, Holman JM Jr. Fibronectin and the critically ill patient: current status. *Intensive Care Med* 1986;12:350–358.
48. Harvey KB, Moldawer LL, Bistrian BR, Blackburn GL. Biologic measures for the formulation of a hospital prognostic index. *Am J Clin Nutr* 1981;34:2013–2022.
49. Russell MK, McAdams MP. Laboratory monitoring of nutritional status. In: Matarese LE, Gottschlich MM, eds. *Contemporary Nutrition Support Practice: A Clinical Guide.* Philadelphia, PA: WB Saunders Company; 1998.
50. Minuto F, Barreca A, Adami GF, et al. Insulin-like growth factor-1 in human malnutrition: Relationship with some body composition and nutritional parameters. *J Parenter Enteral Nutr* 1989;13:392–396.
51. Clemmons DR, Underwood LE, Dickerson RN, et al. Use of plasma somatomedin-C/insulin-like growth factor 1 measurements to monitor the response to nutritional repletion in malnourished patients. *Am J Clin Nutr* 1985;41:191–198.
52. Frankenfield D. Energy dynamics. In: Matarese LE, Gottschlich MM, eds. *Contemporary Nutrition Support Practice: A Clinical Guide.* Philadelphia, PA: WB Saunders Company; 1998.
53. Benedict FG. An apparatus for studying the respiratory exchange. *Am J Physiol* 1909; 24:345–374.
54. Liggett S, St. John R, Lefrak S. Determination of resting energy expenditure utilizing thermodilution pulmonary artery catheter. *Chest* 1987;91:562–566.
55. Cobean RA, Gentilello LM, Parker A, et al. Nutritional assessment using a pulmonary artery catheter. *J Trauma* 1992;33:452–456.

56. Harris JA, Benedict FG. *A Biometric Study of Basal Metabolism in Man.* Washington, DC: Carnegie Institute; 1919. Publication No. 279.

57. Mifflin MD, St. Jeor ST, Hill LA, et al. A new predictive equation for resting energy expenditure in healthy individuals. *Am J Clin Nutr* 1990;51:241–247.

58. Ireton-Jones C. Evaluation of energy expenditure in obese patients. *Nutr Clin Prac* 1989; 4:127–129.

59. Ireton-Jones CS. Indirect calorimetry. In: Skipper A, ed. *Dietitian's Handbook of Enteral and Parenteral Nutrition.* 2nd ed. Gaithersburg, MD: Aspen Publishers, Inc; 1998:161.

60. Russell M. Serum proteins and nitrogen balance: evaluating response to nutrition support. *Support Line* 1995;XVII:3–8.

61. Loder PB, Kee AJ, Horsburgh R, et al. Validity of urinary urea nitrogen as a measure of total urinary nitrogen in adult patients requiring parenteral nutrition. *Crit Care Med* 1989;17:309–312.

62. Konstantinides FN, Konstantinides NN, Li JC, et al. Urinary urea nitrogen: too insensitive for calculating nitrogen balance studies in surgical clinical nutrition. *J Parenter Enteral Nutr* 1991;15:189–193.

63. Hedberg AM, Garcia N. Macronutrient requirements. In: Skipper A, ed. *Dietitian's Handbook of Parenteral and Enteral Nutrition.* 1st ed. Rockville, MD: Aspen Publishers, Inc; 1989.

64. Food and Nutrition Board. *National Research Council: Recommended Dietary Allowances.* 10th ed. Washington, DC: National Academy of Sciences; 1989.

SUGGESTED READINGS

American Society for Parenteral and Enteral Nutrition: Definition of terms used in A.S.P.E.N. guidelines and standards. *J Parenter Enteral Nutr* 1995;10:1–3.

American Society for Parenteral and Enteral Nutrition: Standards of practice: nutrition support nurse. *Nutr Clin Pract* 1996;11(3):127–134.

American Society for Parenteral and Enteral Nutrition: Standards of practice for nutrition support: hospitalized patients. *Nutr Clin Pract* 1995;10(6):206–207.

American Society for Parenteral and Enteral Nutrition: Guidelines for the use of parenteral and enteral nutrition in adult and pediatric patients. *J Parenter Enteral Nutr* 1993;17(4 Suppl):1SA–52SA.

Arrowsmith H. A critical evaluation of the use of nutrition screening tools by nurses. *Br J Nurs* 1999;8:1483–1490.

Ayello EA, Thomas DR, Litchford MA. Nutritional aspects of wound healing. *Home Healthc Nurse* 1999; 17:719–729.

Bickford GR, Brugler LJ, Dolsen S, et al. Nutrition assessment outcomes: A strategy to improve health care. *Clin Lab Manage Rev* 1999;13:357–364.

Corish CA, Kennedy NP. Protein-energy undernutrition in hospital in-patients. *Br J Nutr* 2000;83:575–591.

Dudek SG. Malnutrition in hospitals. Who's assessing what patients eat? *Am J Nurs* 2000;100:36–43.

Gottschlich MM, Fuhrman P, Hammond K, Holcombe B, Seidner D (eds) *The Science and Practice of Nutrition Support: A Case Based Core Curriculum.* Dubuque, IA: Kendall/Hunt Publishing Company, 2001.

Jeejeebhoy KN. Nutrition assessment. *Nutrition* 2000;16:585–590.

Kubena KS. Accuracy in dietary assessment: On the road to good science. *J Am Diet Assoc* 2000;100:775–776.

Mahan LK, Arkin MT. Nutritional care in anemia. In: *Krause's Food, Nutrition, and Diet Therapy.* 8th ed. Philadelphia, PA: WB Saunders Company; 1992:557–568.

McMahon K, Brown JK. Nutritional screening and assessment. *Semin Oncol Nurs* 2000;26:106–112.

Nataloni S, Gentili P, Marini B, et al. Nutritional assessment in head injured patients through the study of rapid turnover visceral proteins. *Clin Nutr* 1999;18:247–251.

Smith Z. Failure to thrive: Early intervention to address dietary issues is vital. *Community Nurse* 1999;5:S3–S6.

Zulkowski K. Examining the nutritional status of independently living elderly. *Ostomy Wound Manage* 2000;46:56–60.

RESOURCES

American Dietetic Association (A.D.A.)
216 West Jackson Avenue
Chicago, IL 60606
(800) 877–1600
Consumer Nutrition Hotline—(800) 366–1655
www.eatright.org

American Society for Parenteral and Enteral Nutrition (A.S.P.E.N.)
8630 Fenton Street
Suite 412
Silver Spring, MD 20910–3805
(301) 587–6315
www.nutritioncare.org

American Society of Health-System Pharmacists
7272 Wisconsin Avenue
Bethesda, MD 20814
(301) 657–4383
www.ashp.com

2

Enteral Nutrition Basics

PEGGI GUENTER

Nursing care is key to positive outcomes in patients requiring specialized nutritional therapy. Enteral nutrition can be defined as nutrition provided via the gastrointestinal tract. Tube feeding is specifically enteral nutrition provided through a tube, catheter, or stoma that delivers nutrients distal to the oral cavity.[1] These terms are often used interchangeably and any reference to enteral nutrition in this book will be referring to tube feeding. This chapter will outline enteral nutrition basics including indications for feeding, general definitions of the process, formulation ingredients and selection, and organizational resources for professionals and consumers.

Enteral nutrition is indicated when a patient will not, should not, or cannot eat but has a functional GI tract. It should be used in appropriate patients who are or who will become malnourished and in whom oral feedings are inadequate to maintain nutritional status.[2] For example, some patients with dysphagia should not take nutrients orally due to the risk of aspiration pneumonia but would be able to tolerate tube feeding. Advantages of enteral nutrition over the use of parenteral (intravenous) nutrition include: (1) enteral nutrition is less expensive than parenteral, (2) enteral nutrition is considered safer than parenteral nutrition, although it is still associated with clinical complications, (3) enteral nutrition is considered more "physiologic" in that it is digested and absorbed via the GI tract, as opposed to being infused directly into the veins, which may better maintain gut structure and function, and (4) enteral nutrition is associated with better clinical outcomes in some instances as compared to parenteral nutrition.[3–5]

INDICATIONS FOR ENTERAL NUTRITION

Major considerations involved in selecting the patients' form of nutritional support are illustrated in the clinical decision algorithm presented in Figure 2–1.[6]

These special considerations include gastrointestinal function, expected duration of therapy, potential risk for aspiration, and level of organ function. Gastrointestinal function can be assessed by abdominal examination, presence of bowel sounds, stool output, and nasogastric output. Specific indications and contraindications for enteral feedings can be found in Exhibit 2–1. Contraindications are not absolute and must be evaluated on a case-by-case basis.

GENERAL STEPS IN FEEDING PROCESS

In order to prevent or treat malnutrition, tube feeding should be started as early as possible. Once the patient and physician decide that tube feeding will be the mode of nutritional support, several general steps need to be taken. These steps include nutritional assessment and determination of nutrient needs as outlined in Chapter 1, placement of an enteral access device (tube), formula selection,

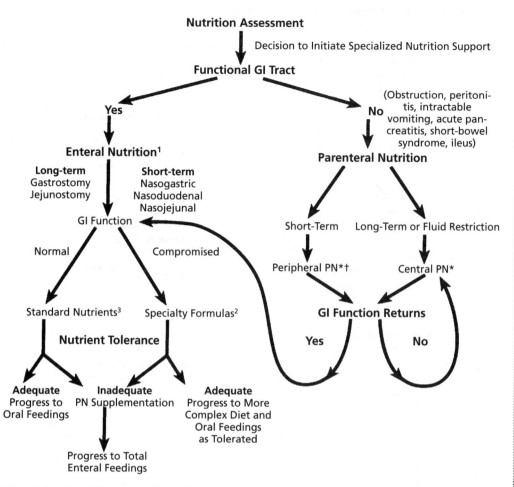

GI, gastrointestinal; PN, parenteral nutrition.

*Formulation of enteral and parenteral solutions should be made considering organ function (e.g., cardiac, renal, respiratory, hepatic).

†In selected patients, peripheral parenteral nutrition may be considered to provide partial or total nutrition support for up to 2 weeks in patients who cannot ingest or absorb oral or enteral tube-delivered nutrients, or when central vein parenteral nutrition is not feasible.

[1]Feedings may be more appropriate distal to the ligament of Treitz if the patient is at increased aspiration risk.

[2]Elemental low/high fat content, lactose-free, fiber-rich, and modular formulas should be provided according to patient's GI tolerance.

[3]Polymeric, complete formulas are appropriate.

Adapted with permission from A.S.P.E.N. Board of Directors: Guidelines for the use of parenteral and enteral nutrition in adult and pediatric patients. JPEN 17(Suppl 4):7SA, 1993. NOTE: This figure supercedes the algorithm published in the Guidelines.

Figure 2–1 Clinical nutrition support decision-making algorithm

feeding start-up and advancement to goal, monitoring, complication prevention, and transition to oral intake if possible. Feeding formula is defined as a ready-to-administer mixture of nutrient. Enteral access devices are defined as tubes placed directly into the gastrointestinal tract for the delivery of nutrients and/or drugs.[1]

Exhibit 2–1 Indications and contraindications for enteral nutrition

Indications *

- Neurologic and Psychiatric
  - Cerebrovascular accidents
  - Neoplasms
  - Trauma
  - Inflammation
  - Demyelinating diseases
  - Severe depression
  - Anorexia nervosa
  - Failure to thrive
- Oropharyngeal and Esophageal
  - Neoplasms
  - Inflammation
  - Trauma
- Gastrointestinal
  - Mild pancreatitis
  - Mild inflammatory disease

  - Short bowel syndrome (later stages)
  - Mild malabsorption
  - Preoperative bowel preparation
  - Bowel fistulas (non-midgut)
- Miscellaneous
  - Sepsis
  - Respiratory failure (ventilator dependence)
  - Burns
  - AIDS
  - Organ dysfunction (hepatic, cardiac, renal)
  - Chemotherapy, radiation therapy
  - Organ transplantation

Contraindications **

Early short bowel syndrome
Small intestinal obstruction beyond the duodenum
Intractable vomiting and diarrhea
Intestinal ischemia

Severe small intestine inflammatory bowel disease
General hypoperfusion/shock
High output midgut fistulas
Severe acute pancreatitis

* These indications may impair one's ability to take in oral nutrition but not universally so
** Are not absolute, must be evaluated on individual basis

FORMULA SELECTION

There is a huge variety of tube feeding formulas available to patients to meet their nutritional needs. In the past, the physician and registered dietitian were more involved in formula selection; in the current era of cross-training, this may now not be the case. The nurse needs to be aware of the reasons for formula selection, particularly in terms of cost-effectiveness and complication prevention. Most but not all tube feeding formulas are commercially prepared. Some patients do receive homemade tube-feeding formulas, which are made using the family meals and blenderized to a thin liquid for administration. This section will provide information for the nurse on formula composition (ingredients) and classifications of these formulas. Due to space limitations and the ever-changing market, all of the formulas will not be specified, but examples of the various types will be given for clarification. For a full list of products, contact the major formula manufacturers using the information found at the end of this chapter. Most of the manufacturers provide educational materials for nurses, generally at low or no cost.

Manufacturers produce some products that are similar to one another, thus substitution of products with another brand often happens as patients transition from one health care agency to another. This is due to the fact that many agencies purchase tube feeding formulas from buying groups and may have a restrictive contract with a particular manufacturer in order to reduce costs.[7] This limits choice and not all formulas are always available. Check with the prescribing physician and/or a registered dietitian before any substitutions are made in order to prevent formula intolerances.

FORMULA COMPOSITION

Tube-feeding formulas, like regular food, are made up of carbohydrates, fat, protein, micronutrients, and water. Formula ingredients vary in the complexity of the nutrients; some contain the complex form of the nutrient while others contain the nutrient as a simpler, more chemically broken down, smaller particle.

Carbohydrates

The carbohydrates used include maltodextrin, modified cornstarch, and corn syrup, all of which are derived from cornstarch and differ only in the carbohydrate polymer. Maltodextrin is the most complex carbohydrate source and corn syrup is a simpler source, thus adding to the osmolality of the formula.[8] Osmolality represents the number of dissolved particles in the volume of solution. An isotonic solution is 300 milliosmoles per liter and is close to that of body fluids. A majority of tube-feeding formulas are isotonic but concentrated formulas—that is, those with more particles per volume are hypertonic. Lactose, or milk sugar, is generally not included as an ingredient, as many ethnic groups are lactose intolerant. Lactose intolerance may also occur during illness due to decreased lactase production. Carbohydrate content in the range of formula varies from 30% to 90% of calories, but standard formulas contain about 55% of calories as carbohydrate.[9]

Fat

The fat source in formulas may include vegetable oils such as corn, canola, soybean, and safflower. These contain long-chain triglycerides (LCT), which keep the osmolality of the formula down and contribute essential fatty acids. Some formulas contain medium-chain triglycerides (MCT), which are easier to digest and absorb but do not contain essential fatty acids.

Other specialized formulas may contain fish oils (omega-3 fatty acids), and the use of these will be explained later in this section.[8] Fat content ranges from 1% to 55% in formulas, but the standard formula contains fat content of about 30% of total calories.[9]

Protein

The protein sources in formulas include casein or whey, which are intact proteins separated from milk,[10] and soy protein isolates. These are all larger protein polymers and keep osmolality down. Smaller protein particles (peptides) are created by enzymatic hydrolysis of casein or whey. These are easier to digest and absorb but increase the osmolality of formulas. The last source is free amino acids. In some specialized formulas, the amino acids glutamine and/or arginine are added to the mixture to promote specific physiologic actions.[8] The protein content of formulas ranges from 4% to 32% of calories; however, the standard formula contains about 15% of total calories as protein.[9]

Micronutrients

Micronutrients are the vitamins and minerals contained in a formula. Most nutritionally complete formulas contain 100% of the RDA in micronutrients in an adequate volume or daily dose ranging from 1.5 to 2 liters. Patients who do not receive this adequate volume may need daily micronutrient supplementation. Some specialized formulas contain enhanced vitamin and mineral doses to promote a physiologic action such as wound healing.[8]

Fiber

Fiber sources contained in formulas come in a variety of types. Soy polysaccharide, which is mostly insoluble fiber, is the most prevalent fiber source in formulas and helps decrease constipation and diarrhea. Another source is soluble fiber such as gum arabic, guar gum, or pectin, which may improve glucose tolerance, maintain ileal and colonic mucosa, and lower cholesterol.[8,11] Another fiber source that recently has been added to tube feeding formulas is fructooligosaccharides (FOS). These are not digested in the GI tract but are fermented by colonic bacteria. They improve intestinal flora, reduce constipation, and improve blood lipid levels.[8] Most formulas contain a range of 5 to 14 grams of fiber per liter.

Water

Water content of formulas ranges from 70% to 85% per volume. Caloric density is determined by amount of water contained in the formula. Formulas that provide 1 calorie per ml are approximately 85% water and those that provide 2 calories per ml contain 70% water. These calorically dense concentrated formulas are often for patients who are fluid restricted.

FORMULA CLASSIFICATIONS

Formulas are classified into types according to their product description and intended use.[12] These classifications and their characteristics are listed below.

Figure 2–2 is an algorithm for deciding on the type of formula needed for patients with a variety of conditions.

1. General purpose or standard formulas are also called polymeric (containing complex nutrient polymers); these are useful for most patients except those with condition-specific needs. Most of these formulas are isotonic, have a caloric density of 1.0 to 1.4 calories per ml, and have a protein content of 35 to 45 grams per 1000 calories. They may or may not contain fiber. Examples of these formulas include Jevity (Ross), Isocal (Mead Johnson), or Nutren 1.0 (Nestlé).

2. Calorically dense formulas are for patients requiring fluid restriction, such as those with congestive heart failure, or elevated caloric needs, such as those with multiple trauma. The caloric density of these formulas ranges from 1.5 to 2.0 calories per ml and they are somewhat hypertonic (400 to 700 Osm/L). Examples of this type of formula include Isosource 1.5 (Novartis), Nutren 1.5 (Nestlé), Deliver 2.0 (Mead Johnson), and Two-Cal HN (Ross).

3. High-protein or high-nitrogen formulas contain increased amounts of protein for patients with high protein losses, such as in burns and large wounds, and for those with increased protein needs, such as trauma or septic patients. These can have 1.0 to 2.0 calories per ml and be either isotonic or hypertonic but have protein amounts of 50 to 80 grams per liter. Examples of this type include Replete (Nestlé), Promote (Ross), Isosource VHN (Novartis), and Traumacal (Mead Johnson).

4. Chemically defined formulas are those also called elemental, semi-elemental, peptide-based, hydrolyzed, or oligomeric. These formulas contain simple nutrients. Proteins in particular are broken down into smaller-sized polymers or peptides. These smaller particles are more easily digested and absorbed and often better tolerated. Patients who might benefit from this type of formula are those with small-intestinal malabsorption or pancreatic or biliary deficiencies, or those with critical illness, especially after trauma, shock, or sepsis.[8] These formulas tend to be hypertonic and have little if any fiber. They usually contain only 1 calorie per ml in density. Examples of these formulas include Criticare HN (Mead Johnson), Perative (Ross), Peptamen (Nestlé), and Vivonex (Novartis).

5. Disease-specific products were developed to meet the needs of patients with specific organ dysfunction or disease. Examples include formulas for pulmonary, hepatic, renal, or diabetic disease or critically ill states. In general, these formulas have altered levels of nutrients or additional ingredients that correct or compensate for physiologic alterations secondary to the disease. These formulas are generally more expensive; not all are proven to be cost-effective over standard formulas, and they should be used judiciously.[13]

   a. Renal formulas are usually calorically dense (2.0 calories/ml), have restricted amounts of potassium, phosphorus, and magnesium and variable levels of protein—from low to moderate amounts depending whether the patient is dialyzed. Some of the formulas may not be complete, in that they may be vitamin- or mineral-free and thus

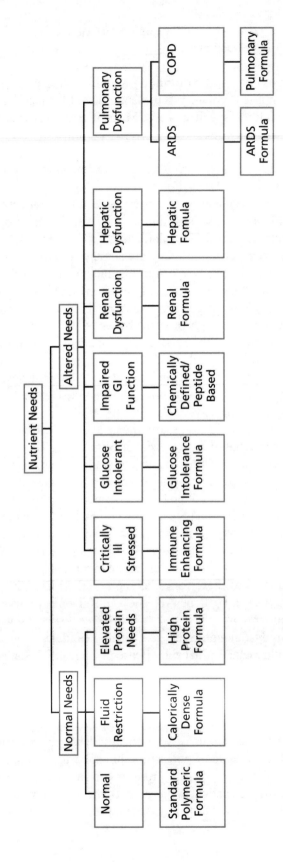

Figure 2–2 Guidelines for formula selection

require additional nutrient supplementation. Examples of these formulas are Nepro (Ross), Magnacal Renal (Mead Johnson), Renalcal (Nestle), and Novasource Renal (Novartis).

b. Hepatic dysfunction formulas are hypertonic and calorically dense (1.2–1.5 calories/ml). They are lower in protein but have high-branched chain and lower aromatic amino acids to decrease ammonia production and minimize hepatic encephalopathy. They are also lower in fat and contain MCT, which are easier to digest and absorb in the face of decreased bile synthesis and fat malabsorption.[8,9,12] Examples of these formulas include NutriHep (Nestlé) and Hepatic-Aid II (B. Braun, Irvine, CA).

c. Pulmonary formulas were designed for patients with respiratory conditions such as COPD or ventilator dependence. These products provide more calories from fat (40%–55% of calories) and less from carbohydrates as compared to standard formulas. In theory, these products are calorically dense (1.5 calories/ml), are somewhat hypertonic, and have an increased protein level. Some researchers have demonstrated a reduction in ventilator days but others have found no difference as compared to standard formulas.[14–16] Examples of these formulas include Pulmocare (Ross), NutriVent (Nestlé), Respalor (Mead Johnson), and NovaSource Pulmonary (Novartis). Another different type of respiratory formula is specifically targeted for patients at risk for or with Adult Respiratory Distress Syndrome (ARDS). This formula uses specific fat sources (eicosapentaenoic acid [EPA] from sardine oil and gamma-linolenic acid [GLA] from borage oil) and antioxidants (vitamin E, vitamin C, and beta-carotene) to decrease pulmonary inflammation and facilitate pulmonary vasodilation, thus increasing oxygenation and curbing this syndrome.[17] This formula is Oxepa (Ross) and should be used specifically in acute care settings due to its high cost and extreme specialty.

d. Glucose intolerance formulas were designed for diabetic patients and those who may have hyperglycemia due to their current medical condition or treatments such as sepsis or steroid use. These products contain high fiber, low carbohydrate, and high fat levels, therefore they are only indicated with brittle or very difficult to manage patients with diabetes. These formulas are also just slightly hypertonic, have a caloric density of 1.0 calorie per ml, and have a standard amount of protein. Carbohydrate sources are mostly complex. These formulas should be used in conjunction with serum glucose monitoring and standard glucose control therapies.[8,9,12] Examples of these products include DiabetiSource (Novartis), Glytrol (Nestlé), Choice dm (Mead Johnson), and Glucerna (Ross).

e. Immune enhancing formulas are used for patients in a state of immunosuppression. These include many critically ill patients, particularly those with trauma, burns, sepsis, surgical stress, cancer, AIDS, and those who are hypermetabolic and hypercatabolic. Use of these formulas as compared to standard formulas has demonstrated fewer days on mechanical ventilation, decreased length of hospitalization, and less antibiotic use, thus decreasing overall health costs.[8,9,17–20] These formulas contain several key ingredients, sometimes in different combinations, that have physiologic impact and cause immune enhancement. Arginine enhances wound healing and increases lymphocyte production, and glutamine is the primary energy source for lymphocytes and enterocytes, reduces infection, and helps maintain nitrogen balance. Omega-3 fatty acids cause less inflammation and immunosuppression, and nucleotides, which are the structural components of RNA, DNA, and ATP, help in energy transfer and have immunomodulating properties.[18,19] Examples of these formulas include Impact (Novartis), Crucial (Nestlé), Optimental (Ross), and Immun-Aid (B. Braun).

f. Wound-healing formulas were designed to provide extra protein and micronutrients (vitamin C, vitamin A, and zinc) to patients with surgical wounds, pressure ulcers, or burns. These are generally isotonic but provide about 60 grams of protein per liter. Examples of these formulas include Protain XL (Mead Johnson), Isosource VHN (Novartis), Replete (Nestlé), and Promote (Ross).

Modular supplements are another type of product used in modifying tube feeding formulas. These are also used to increase the concentration of certain nutrients in the formula. Examples of these are protein powders, fats or oils, and carbohydrate polymers. The protein modules contain either casein, whey, soy, or hydrolyzed protein. Some of these modulars are ProMod (Ross), Casec (Mead Johnson), Nutrisource Protein (Novartis), and Promix (CORPAK Medsystems, Wheeling, IL). Carbohydrate modular supplements are made of glucose polymers and generally used to add calories to existing formulas. They come in either powder or liquid form. Examples of these include Polycose (Ross), Nutrisource Carbohydrate (Novartis), and Moducal (Mead Johnson). Fat can be added to formulas either as MCT for easier digestion and absorption or as standard oils containing LCT. LCT add calories and the MCT add a different type of fat as a supplement. Examples include Microlipid (Mead Johnson), Nutrisource Lipid LCT (Novartis), and MCT Oil (Mead Johnson).

CONCLUSION

In summary, tube feeding formulas are varied and should be selected with the patient's specific medical conditions in mind. Use of specialty formulas should be frequently evaluated for ongoing appropriateness.

REFERENCES

1. A.S.P.E.N. Board of Directors. Definitions of terms used in A.S.P.E.N. guidelines and standards. *J Parenter Enteral Nutr* 1995;19:1–2.

2. A.S.P.E.N. Board of Directors. Guidelines for the use of parenteral and enteral nutrition in adults and pediatric patients. *J Parenter Enteral Nutr* 1993;17(4 Suppl):1SA–52SA.

3. Kudsk KA, Croce MA, Fabian TC, et al. Enteral versus parenteral feeding: effects on septic morbidity after blunt and penetrating abdominal trauma. *Ann Surg* 1992;215:503–513.

4. Moore FA, Feliciano DV, Andrassy RJ, et al. Early enteral feeding, compared with parenteral, reduces postoperative septic complications: the results of a meta-analysis. *Ann Surg* 1992;216:172–183.

5. Lipman TO. Grains or veins: is enteral nutrition really better than parenteral nutrition? A look at the evidence. *J Parenter Enteral Nutr* 1998;22:167–182.

6. Merritt RM. Introduction. In: Merritt RM, ed. *The A.S.P.E.N. Nutrition Support Manual.* Silver Spring, MD: American Society for Parenteral and Enteral Nutrition; 1998:i-1–i-7.

7. Durfee DA, Skinner-Domet VM. Cost effectiveness of an enteral products formulary. *Am J Hosp Pharm.* 1984;41:2352–2354.

8. Olree K, Vitello J, Sullivan J, Kohn-Keeth C. Enteral formulations. In: Merritt R, ed. *The A.S.P.E.N. Nutrition Support Manual.* Silver Spring, MD: American Society for Parenteral and Enteral Nutrition; 1998:4-1–4-9.

9. Lord LM, Lipp J, Stull S. Adult tube feeding formulas. *MEDSURG Nursing* 1996; 5:407–421, 432.

10. Gottschlich MM, Shronts EP, Hutchins AM. Defined formula diets. In: Rombeau JL, Rolandelli RH, eds. *Enteral and Tube Feeding.* 3rd ed. Philadelphia, PA: WB Saunders Company; 1997.

11. Palacio JC, Rombeau JL. Dietary fiber: a brief review and potential application to enteral nutrition. *Nutr Clin Pract* 1990;5:99–106.

12. Morita-Chan L. Choosing the right enteral formula. *Infusion* April 1998;4:21–29.

13. Matarese LE. Rationale and efficacy of specialized enteral nutrition. *Nutr Clin Pract* 1994;9:58–64.

14. Al-Saady N, Blackmore C, Bennet ED. High fat, low carbohydrate enteral feeding reduces PaCO2 and the period of ventilation in ventilated patients. *Intens Care Med* 1989;15:290–295.

15. Frankfurt JD, Fischer DE, Stansburg DW, et al. Effects of high- and low-carbohydrate meals on maximum exercise performance in chronic airflow obstruction. *Chest* 1991; 100:792–795.

16. Malone AM. Is a pulmonary enteral formula warranted for patients with pulmonary dysfunction? *Nutr Clin Pract* 1997;12:168–171.

17. Gadek JE, DeMichele SJ, Karlstad MD, et al. Effect of enteral feeding with eicosapentaenoic acid, gamma-linolenic acid and antioxidants in patients with acute respiratory distress syndrome. *Crit Care Med* 1999;27:1409–1420.

18. Barton RG. Immune-enhancing enteral formulas: Are they beneficial in critically ill patients? *Nutr Clin Pract* 1997;12:51–62.

19. Bliss DZ. Tube feeding: immune-boosting formulas. *RN* August 1999;62:26–28.

20. Heys SD, Walker LG, Smith I, et al. Enteral nutritional supplementation with key nutrients in patients with critical illness and cancer: a meta-analysis of randomized, control clinical trials. *Ann Surg* 1999;229:467–477.

SUGGESTED READINGS

Baxter J. A recipe for tackling malnutrition. *Community Nurse* 1999; 5:29–30.

Cheever KH. Early enteral feeding of patients with multiple trauma. *Critical Care Nurse* December 1999;19:40–53.

Dabrowski GP, Rombeau JL. Practical nutritional management in the trauma intensive care unit. *Surg Clin North Am* 2000;80:921–932.

Gottschlich MM, Fuhrman P, Hammond K, Holcombe B, Seidner D (eds) *The Science and Practice of Nutrition Support: A Case Based Core Curriculum.* Dubuque, IA: Kendall/Hunt Publishing Company, 2001.

Hall JC. Choosing nutrition support: How and when to initiate. *Nurs Case Manag* 1999; 4:212–223.

Ideno KT. Enteral nutrition formulas: An overview. *MEDSURG Nursing* 1996;5:264–268.

Mitchell SL, Berkowitz RE, Lawson FM, et al. A cross-national survey of tube-feeding decisions in cognitively impaired older persons. *J Am Geriatr Soc* 2000;48:391–397

Moss K. The Oley Foundation. *Infusion* February 1995;1:15–19.

Romand JA, Suter PM. Enteral nutrition: the right stuff at the right time in the right place. *Crit Care Med* 2000;28:2671–2672.

Senkal M, Zumtobel V, Bauer KH, et al. Outcome and cost-effectiveness of perioperative enteral immunonutrition in patients undergoing elective upper gastrointestinal tract surgery: a prospective randomized study. *Arch Surg* 1999;134:1309–1316.

Silk DB. Formulation of enteral diets. *Nutrition* 1999;15:626–632.

Weinstein DS, Furman J. Enteral formulas. *Nurs Clin North Am* 1997;32:669–683.

RESOURCES

Professional Organizations

American Dietetic Association (ADA)
www.eatright.org

American Society for Parenteral and Enteral Nutrition (A.S.P.E.N.)
1–800–727–4567
www.nutritioncare.org

Health Care Financing Administration (HCFA)
http://www.hcfa.gov

Intravenous Nurses Society (INS)
www.ins1.org

Joint Commission on Accreditation of Healthcare Organizations (JCAHO)
www.jcaho.org

Oncology Nursing Society (ONS)
www.ons.org

Patient Advocate Organization

Oley Foundation: Provides information and psychosocial support to consumers dependent upon home parenteral and enteral nutrition. 1–800–776–OLEY or 518/262–5079
www.oley.org

Major Formula Manufacturers

B. Braun, Inc.
2525 McGaw Ave.
Irvine, CA 92713
1–800–854–6851
www.bbraunusa.com

Mead Johnson Nutritionals
A Bristol-Myers Squibb Company
400 West Lloyd Expressway
Evansville, IN 47721
1–800–457–3550
www.meadjohnson.com

Nestlé Clinical Nutrition
Three Parkway North, Suite 500
PO Box 760
Deerfield, IL 60015–0760
1–800–422–2752

Novartis Nutrition
5100 Gamble Drive
St. Louis Park, MN 55416
1–800–999–9978
www.novartis.com/nutrition

Ross Products
Division of Abbott Laboratories
625 Cleveland Avenue
Columbus, OH 43215
1–800–544–7495
www.ross.com

3

Enteral Feeding Access Devices

PEGGI GUENTER

An enteral feeding access device is defined as the tube or device placed directly into the gastrointestinal tract for the delivery of nutrients and/or drugs.[1] These tubes are placed by a variety of techniques into the GI tract and have many important characteristics. This chapter will provide information on these enteral devices, including why, where, and how they are placed along with their characteristics and placement complications.

DEVICE SELECTION

Feeding access device selection is based on several patient-related factors. These include patient diagnoses, functional status, and anticipated length of time that tube feedings will be needed. The feeding formula itself can be administered into the stomach (called gastric or prepyloric feedings) or into the small intestine (also called postpyloric, duodenal, or jejunal feedings). It is essential that the nurse be aware of the type of tube the patient has and exactly where the end or tip of the tube is located at the time of feedings (stomach or small intestine). Gastric feedings are preferred over small intestinal feedings because it is more physiologic for digestion and absorption and it is often easier to gain access to the stomach as compared to the duodenum or jejunum. There are, however, conditions when small intestinal feeding is preferred, such as with delayed gastric emptying, gastric outlet obstruction, or high aspiration risk.

Anticipated length of time that tube feeding will be needed also dictates selection of the type of enteral access device. If the patient requires tube feeding for less than 3 or 4 weeks, a short-term, less invasive nasoenteric tube can be placed. If, however, it is anticipated that the patient will need tube feeding for longer than 3 or 4 weeks, a long-term feeding access device should be placed, such as a gastrostomy or jejunostomy tube.[2,3] Figure 3–1 illustrates a decision algorithm that helps in selection of the enteral access device.[4]

NASOENTERIC FEEDING TUBES

Nasoenteric short-term feeding tubes are the most common type of tube used, the easiest to place, and the least expensive.[5] These tubes are placed by nurses, physicians, dietitians, caregivers, or the patients themselves. They can be placed via the orogastric route if nasal insertion is undesirable, such as with nasotracheal intubation or nasal trauma. Once short-term feeding is decided upon, various characteristics of available tubes need to be considered. These characteristics include (1) material, (2) presence of a weight on the end of the tube, (3) length, (4) lumen size, (5) shape and size of tip, (6) stylets, (7) lubricant coating, and (8) adapters. All tubes should be radiopaque for easy identification on x-ray and have outside markings to aid in placement and checking for migration. Table 3–1 lists these characteristics and nursing considerations for each[6] and Figure 3–2 illustrates a prototypical tube.

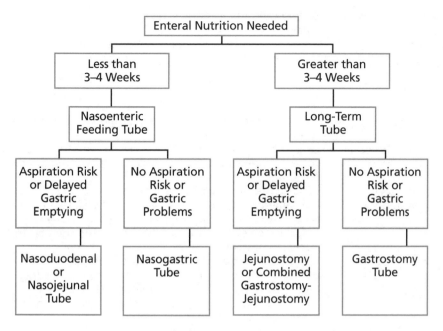

Figure 3–1 Selection of feeding access device

Nasoenteric tube placement should be done with the cooperation of the patient when possible. Exhibit 3–1 fully outlines this nursing procedure for placement of a nasoenteric feeding tube. For placement of the tip of the tube into the small intestine, a number of special techniques have been suggested. One nurse researcher[9] found that giving metoclopromide 10 mg IV, 10 minutes prior to insertion of a nonweighted tube and inserting most of the tube led to a 90% passage of the tip into the small intestine. Other successful techniques include bending the distal end of the stylet and rotating the tube during insertion,[11] air insufflation, and right lateral decubitus positioning.[12,13]

Fluoroscopic (radiologic) placement of the tube tip into the small intestine is the practice of choice in many institutions. This radiologic visualization of placement assures that the tip passes through the pylorus and can be manipulated into the jejunum.[14,15] Feeding tubes can also be placed through the pylorus with the aide of an endoscope, either over a wire or with a snare dragging the tube through the pylorus.[16] Both of these techniques are very successful but require physician time, particular equipment, and special scheduling and are more expensive than bedside insertion techniques.

Complications reported in the literature with small bore nasoenteric feeding tube placement include placement into the trachea, lung, brain, and through the esophagus or the gastrointestinal wall.[17–21] These nasoenteric feeding tubes must be placed cautiously by experienced professionals.

The nasoenteric tube tip position needs to be determined initially following tube placement and serially to monitor for tube migration. The ideal method

Table 3–1 Nasoenteric feeding tube characteristics

Characteristic	Nursing Considerations
Material	
Polyurethane	Adequate stiffness for insertion and checking residuals. Good patient comfort and durability. Most feeding tubes are made of this material.
Silicone	Too soft for insertion and checking residual. Excellent patient comfort but damages easily.
Polyvinylchloride or Rubber	Easy to insert and check residuals. Uncomfortable to patient and stiffens more with time. Standard nasogastric tubes for suction are made of these materials.[6]
Weighted vs. unweighted tubes	Weights are tungsten and range from 3–7 grams. The purpose of the weight is to prevent tube tip migration back into the stomach. Several studies have shown weights have no advantage in transpyloric passage of the tube tip.[7,8] Another study demonstrated an increased passage rate with unweighted tubes.[9]
Tube length	Lengths range from 22"–60". Generally it requires a 36" tube for gastric intubation and a 43"–55" tube for intestinal intubation.
Lumen size	Measured in French sizes, range from 8–16 French (8 smaller, 16 larger). Generally most formulas will flow through 8,10, or 12 Fr. lumens without clogging given proper care.
Shape and size of tip	Smooth tip easier to pass than bolus tip.
Stylet	Stylet stiffens tube for easier passage and then is removed once tube position confirmed. Stylet may perforate viscera during placement especially if force is used.
Activated lubricant coating	Easier removal of stylet after placement and more comfortable placement for patient. Activate with water.
Adapters	Should be incompatible with IV tubing to prevent parenteral administration of enteral formula.[10] Double and triple ports make for easier administration of medications and fluids without disconnecting tube from feeding bag.

for determining tube placement is x-ray verification. This assures that the tube tip is indeed in the GI tract as opposed to the lung. It also defines what portion of the upper GI tract (stomach vs. small intestine) the tube tip lies. The auscultation method of listening for insufflated air over the epigastrum has been used to document tube placement but is not always reliable. Bronchial sounds can be transmitted to the epigastric area and a pulmonary placed tube can sound like a gastrically placed tube.[22] A combination of this technique and checking the tube for gastric or intestinal contents is a fairly reliable predictor of placement.[2] Gastric contents can be further verified by using pH paper; gastric pH ranges between 1 and 4, but may be higher with the use of H_2 receptor antagonist or antacids. Duodenal or jejunal pH is generally greater or equal to 7.[23] If there is any question of tube migration or displacement, or if the nurse is unable to determine tube placement, an x-ray should be requested. The proper position of a nasointestinal feeding tube is shown in Figure 3–3.

PROXIMAL

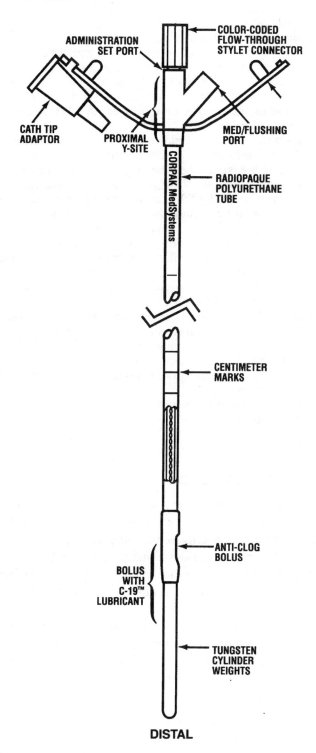

Figure 3–2 Characteristics of a nasoenteric feeding tube

Exhibit 3–1 Procedure for placing nasoenteric feeding tubes

1. Provide privacy.
2. Explain procedure and its purpose.
3. Place patient in sitting or right lateral decubitus position with neck flexed slightly and head of bed elevated to at least 45 degrees.
4. Estimate distance for placement into the stomach by measuring the length from the tip of the nose to the ear lobe and then from the ear lobe to the xiphoid process. Add 50 cm to this length. Observe markings on shaft of tube for guidance.
5. Inspect nares and determine optimal patency by having the patient breathe through one nostril while the other is occluded temporarily.
6. Lubricate the end of the tube or activate the self-lubricant with water and pass it posteriorly. If the patient is alert and cooperative, ask him or her to swallow water to facilitate passage of the tube. Coordinating each swallowing attempt with advancement of the tube is key.
7. Once the tube is beyond the nasopharynx, allow the patient to rest.
8. Have the patient flex his or her neck and swallow while the tube is advanced.
9. If patient is comatose or uncooperative, check the oropharynx for presence of the coiled tube.
10. If the patient begins to cough, withdraw the tube into the nasopharynx and then reattempt passage.
11. If the patient is unable to cough, listen for sounds of respiration through the tube. If audible, withdraw the tube and try again.
12. Confirm passage into stomach by aspiration of gastric contents first and then obtain x-ray.
13. Secure tube to bridge of nose or upper lip with nonallergenic tape or tube attachment device.
14. Once tube placement is confirmed, remove stylet. Do not try to reinsert stylet after removal.

LONG-TERM FEEDING ACCESS DEVICES

If it is anticipated that a patient will require more than 3 or 4 weeks of tube feedings, it is advisable to place a long-term feeding access device early in the tube feeding course. Long-term feeding tubes can be classified into two types, those placed with their feeding tips either in the stomach (gastrostomy tubes) or into the jejunum (jejunostomy tubes). They are placed using various methods including endoscopic, open surgical, laparoscopic, or radiologic techniques. Feeding tube names and abbreviations are often used interchangeably and sometimes incorrectly. Not every tube is a percutaneous endoscopic gastrostomy (PEG). The nurse should determine what type of tube has been placed in the patient, including the size, material, brand, and tip location, and should identify the inserting physician. This information is important to know in order to replace or repair the tube, and to properly administer enteral formula and medications.

Gastrostomy tubes are generally 12–28 French size, are made of polyurethane or silicone, and have a balloon, mushroom tip, or disc to secure them internally. The external portion has a disc or bumper at the skin level, an end adapter that links with the feeding bag tubing, and often a side port for medication administration.

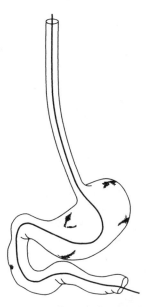

Figure 3–3 Proper position of nasointestinal feeding tube

The PEG tube is the preferred method of gastrostomy tube placement in patients not requiring abdominal surgery for some other reason.[24] It does not require general anesthesia, operating room time, or an abdominal incision, thus the procedure is generally faster, less invasive, less expensive, and easier to recover from.[25] The general method of insertion is described as follows: the patient first receives conscious sedation, and then undergoes a full esophagogastroduodenoscopy. The scope light is transluminated through the abdominal wall. A needle is inserted through the abdomen and a guidewire is passed through the esophagus and outside of the patient's mouth. A feeding tube is then tied to the guidewire and pulled down through the abdominal wall (see Figure 3–4).

The tube is secured externally with a disk while the endoscope is replaced in the stomach to visualize the internal bumper and surrounding gastric mucosa. The bumper should be snug against the mucosa but not too tight. See Figures 3–5 and 3–6 for proper placement of the PEG tube.

Gastrostomy tubes can be placed radiologically through the abdominal wall as well. These are often placed when an endoscope is unable to pass through the esophagus, such as with head and neck or esophageal cancer or when other oral, pharyngeal, or esophageal lesions are present. The procedure is somewhat similar to PEG placement except that once fluoroscopic identification of the stomach is obtained, a gastrostomy tube is pushed through the epigastrum, usually over a guidewire, and then secured internally with a balloon and externally with a skin disc.[26,27]

Surgically placed gastrostomy tubes are generally inserted in patients already undergoing a laparotomy for another reason or used with those patients who

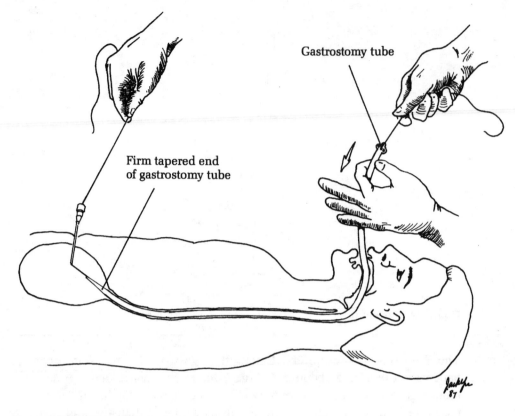

Figure 3-4 PEG insertion technique

cannot undergo endoscopic or radiologic placement, such as a patient with a completely obstructing esophageal tumor or with massive ascites. These procedures can be performed using an open laparotomy or with the less invasive laparoscopic techniques. The open procedure most often performed is a Stamm gastrostomy. This technique requires a small gastrotomy in the anterior wall of the stomach. A fairly large tube (24–30 Fr.) is inserted and secured with a purse string suture (see Figure 3–7).

The stomach is then approximated to the abdominal wall to minimize risk of leakage (see Figure 3–8).[27]

The minimally invasive laparoscopic techniques are improving, and these techniques entail less postoperative pain and quicker recovery.[27,28]

Jejunostomy tubes (J-tubes) are placed when it is desirable to bypass the stomach, as in those patients with upper GI obstruction or those at high risk for aspiration. The tube sizes are 8–14 French and are composed of polyurethane, silicone, or rubber. Adapters are often placed on the end of the tube to aid in feeding, flushing, and medication delivery. If the patient requires jejunostomy or postpyloric feedings long term, there are several techniques for placement. Like gastrostomy tubes, J-tubes can be placed endoscopically, radiologically, or surgically.

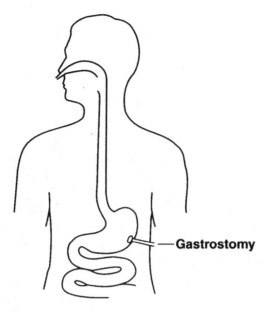

Figure 3–5 Proper position of PEG tube

Endoscopically placed J-tubes (PEJ) are usually inserted through a PEG tube and the J-tube tip is then endoscopically dragged through the pylorus and positioned in the jejunum (see Figure 3–9).[29–31]

Radiologically placed J-tubes are placed through existing PEG tubes or through radiologically placed gastrostomies.[32] Using fluoroscopy, the J-tube tip is guided into the jejunum. These techniques offer lower risk to patients who might otherwise require a surgically placed J-tube.

Like gastrostomies, surgically placed jejunostomy tubes can be inserted during an open laparotomy or using less invasive laparoscopic techniques. Open surgical

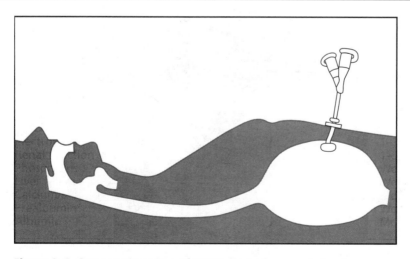

Figure 3–6 Cross-section view of PEG tube and support structures

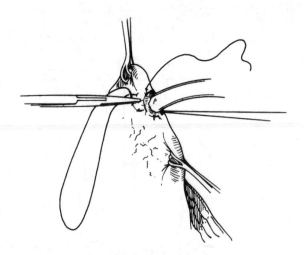

Figure 3–7 Insertion of surgical gastrostomy tube in stomach

J-tubes have been performed for more than 100 years and can be placed using a variety of techniques including the Witzel jejunostomy (most common), the Roux-en-Y jejunostomy, and the needle catheter jejunostomy.[2] The Witzel technique is one that uses a seromuscular tunnel to cover the jejunostomy in order to minimize bowel leakage and facilitate healing on tube removal (see Figure 3–10).

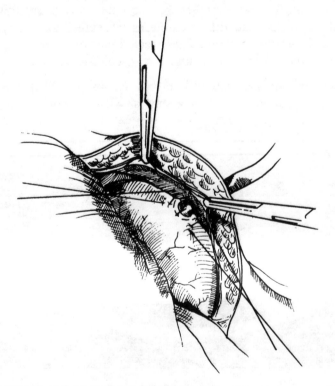

Figure 3–8 Suturing of stomach to abdominal wall

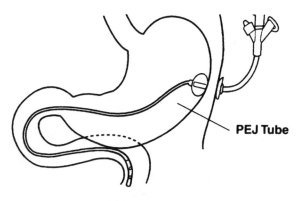

Figure 3–9 Correct position of PEJ tube

Larger bore tubes (10–14 Fr.) can be used to minimize tube clogging. A needle catheter jejunostomy tube is a much smaller lumen tube (5–8 Fr.), is placed through a needle into the jejunum during a laparotomy, and takes only a short time to insert. Disadvantages to these tubes are that they may be easily clogged with feeding formula or medications and can be difficult to replace if dislodged.[33,34] Laparoscopic jejunostomy tubes are placed using minimally invasive laparoscopic techniques and appear to have a faster postoperative recovery time when compared to standard open techniques.[35]

Occasionally patients require gastric decompression and simultaneous postpyloric enteral nutrition. This type of patient may be one with an increased risk for aspiration due to delayed gastric emptying or altered level of consciousness or have a need for decompression following gastroesophageal surgery.[36] Combined gastro-jejunal tubes will meet the needs of these patients. This double lumen tube has a gastric drainage port and a jejunal feeding port. This tube can be placed endoscopically, radiologically, or surgically.[37,38]

A low-profile feeding access device is also called a skin-level feeding device. Many manufacturers offer this type of device—for example, Button (Bard Interventional, Billerica, MA), Flexiflo Stomate with mushroom tip or Hide-a-Port with balloon (Ross Labs, Columbus, OH), Corflo cuBBy (CORPAK Medsystems, Wheeling, IL), MIC-KEY (Medical Innovations Corporation, Santa Clara, CA), or Passport (Wilson-Cook Med Inc., Winston-Salem, NC). These devices are selected for patients with body image concerns who may not want a traditional tube, or for confused patients or children in order to prevent accidental tube removal. See Figure 3–11 for an illustration of this type of device in place.

These devices are usually placed once a gastrostomy tract is well established, although they can be placed as the initial device.[39] The existing gastrostomy is removed and a measuring device is placed into the stomach to determine the device shaft length. The appropriate length device is then inserted into the gastrostomy tract using the device tip itself or with the aid of an obturator, depending on the brand of the device. The device is kept in place with the mushroom

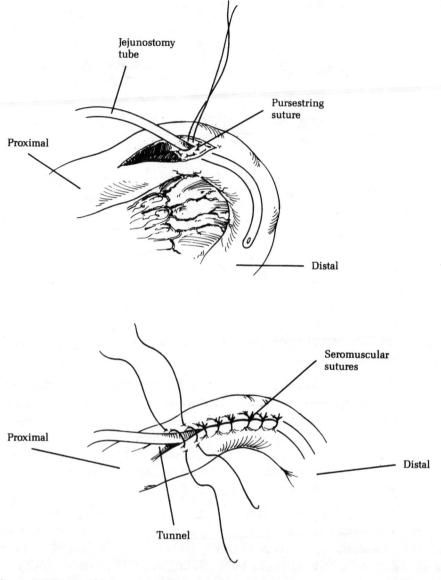

Figure 3–10 Witzel jejunostomy tube placement technique

tip or an inflatable balloon. These devices require an extension tubing to be attached during the feeding and removed once the feeding dose is completed. The device is then capped and a one-way valve inside the device prevents leakage of gastric contents.[5] In one adult study, these devices were surgically placed directly into the jejunum for postpyloric feedings and the investigators concluded that this appears to be an attractive alternative for selected patients requiring long-term jejunal feedings.[40]

Complications associated with initial placement of long-term feeding access devices can be seen in Table 3–2.[5,36] Other complications associated with the

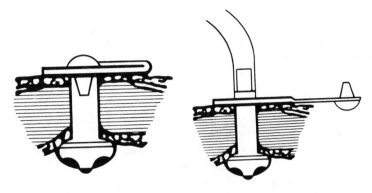

Figure 3–11 Low-profile feeding access device with cap on and with extension tube attached for feeding

use and maintenance of feeding tubes can be found in Chapter 7, Enteral Nutrition Complications.

CONCLUSION

An enteral feeding access device is selected based on patient related factors. These devices are placed in a variety of ways, and the nurse needs to understand the tube type and method of placement.

Table 3–2 Complications associated with initial placement of long-term feeding tubes

Technique	Tube Type	Complication
Endoscopic	Gastrostomy (PEG)	Puncture of colon, small intestine, or liver
	Jejunostomy (PEJ)	Peritube site infection
	Gastro-jejunal combination	Intraperitoneal leakage
Radiologic	Gastrostomy	Puncture of colon, small intestine, or liver
	Jejunostomy	Peritube site infection
	Gastro-jejunal combination	Inability to intubate small bowel
		Intraperitoneal leakage
Surgical	Open Gastrostomy	Bleeding
	Laparoscopic G-tube	General anesthesia
	Witzel Jejunostomy	Wound infection
	Laparoscopic J-tube	Bowel obstruction, volvulus
	Gastro-jejunal combination	Intraperitoneal leakage
		Pneumatosis intestinalis

REFERENCES

1. A.S.P.E.N. Board of Directors. Definitions of terms used in A.S.P.E.N. guidelines and standards. *J Parenter Enteral Nutr* 1995;19:1–2.
2. Kirby DF, Minard G, Kohn-Keeth C. Enteral access and infusion equipment. In: Merritt R, ed. *The A.S.P.E.N. Nutrition Support Manual*. Silver Spring, MD: American Society for Parenteral and Enteral Nutrition; 1998:3-1–3-12.
3. Rolandelli RH, Koruda MJ, Guenter P, et al. Techniques for administering enteral nutrition in the ICU. *J Crit Ill* October 1988;3:107–112.
4. Guenter P, Jones S, Sweed MR, et al. Delivery systems and administration of enteral nutrition. In: Rombeau JL, Rolandelli RH, eds. *Enteral and Tube Feeding*. 3rd ed. Philadelphia, PA: WB Saunders Company; 1997.
5. Lord LM. Enteral access devices. *Nurs Clin North Am* 1997;32:685–704.
6. Monturo CA. Enteral access device selection. *Nutr Clin Pract* 1990;5:207–213.
7. Levenson R, Turner WE, Dyson A, et al. Do weighted nasoenteric feeding tubes facilitate duodenal intubation? *J Parenter Enteral Nutr* 1988;12:135–137.
8. Rees RG, Payne-James JJ. Spontaneous transpyloric passage and performance of "fine bore" polyurethane feeding tubes: a controlled clinical trial. *J Parenter Enteral Nutr* 1988;12:469–472.
9. Lord LM, Weiser-Maimone A, Pulhamus M, et al. Comparison of weighted vs. unweighted enteral feeding tubes for efficacy of transpyloric intubation. *J Parenter Enteral Nutr* 1993;17:271–273.
10. Association for the Advancement of Medical Instrumentation. Enteral feeding set connectors and adapters. *Nutr Clin Pract* 1997;12(1):special insert.
11. Zaloga GP. Bedside method for placing small bowel feeding tubes in critically ill patients. *Chest* 1991;100:1643–1646.
12. Ugo PJ, Mohler PA, Wilson GL. Bedside postpyloric placement of weighted feeding tubes. *Nutr Clin Pract* 1992;7:284–287.
13. Thurlow PM. Bedside enteral feeding tube placement into duodenum and jejunum. *J Parenter Enteral Nutr* 1986;10:104–105.
14. Grant JP, Curtas MS, Kelvin FM. Fluoroscopic placement of nasojejunal feeding tubes with immediate feeding using a nonelemental diet. *J Parenter Enteral Nutr* 1983;7:299–303.
15. Ott DJ, Mattox HE, Gelfand DW, et al. Enteral feeding tubes: Placement by using fluoroscopy and endoscopy. *Am J Roentgenol* 1991;157:769–771.
16. Stark SP, Sharpe JN, Larson GM. Endoscopically placed naosenteral feeding tubes: Indications and techniques. *Am Surg* 1991;57:203–205.
17. Ghahremani GG, Gould RJ. Nasoenteric feeding tubes: radiographic detection of complications. *Dig Dis Sci* 1986;31:574–585.
18. Bouzarth WF, Intracranial nasogastric tube insertion. *J Trauma* 1978;18:818–819.
19. Valentine RJ, Turner WW. Pleural complications of nasoenteric feeding tubes. *J Parenter Enteral Nutr* 1985;9:605–607.
20. Olbrantz KR, Gelfand D, Choplin R, et al. Pneumothorax complication in enteral feeding tube placement. *J Parenter Enteral Nutr* 1985;9:210–211.
21. Bohnker BK, Artman LE, Hoskins WJ. Narrow bore nasogastric feeding tube complications. *Nutr Clin Pract* 1987;2:203–209.
22. Methany N, McSweeney M, Wehrle MA, et al. Effectiveness of the auscultatory method in predicting feeding tube location. *Nurs Res* 1990;39:262–267.
23. Methany N, Reed L, Wiersema L, et al. Effectiveness of pH measurements in predicting feeding tube placement: an update. *Nurs Res* 1993;42:324–331.
24. Gauderer MWL, Ponsky JL, Izant RJ. Gastrostomy with laparostomy: a percutaneous endoscopic technique. *J Pediatr Surg* 1980;15:872–875.

25. Stiegmann GV, Goff JS, Silas D, et al. Endoscopic versus operative gastrostomy: Final results of a prospective randomized trial. *Gastrointest Endosc* 1990;36:1–5.

26. Johnson MS. Radiologic placement of gastrostomy tubes. *Nutr Clin Pract* 1997;12: S20–S22.

27. Nance ML, Morris JB. Enteral nutritional support: techniques and common complications. *Hosp Physician* November 1992:24–29.

28. Georgeson KE. Laparoscopic versus open procedures for long-term enteral access. *Nutr Clin Pract* 1997;12:S7–S8.

29. Shike M, Schroy P, Ritchie MA, et al. Percutaneous endoscopic jejunostomy in cancer patients with previous gastric resection. *Gastrointest Endosc* 1987;33:372–374.

30. Ponsky JL, Gauderer MWL, Stellato TA, et al. Percutaneous approaches to enteral alimentation. *Am J Surg* 1985;149:102–105.

31. DeLegge MH, Duckworth PF, McHenry L, et al. Percutaneous endoscopic gastrojejunostomy: a dual center safety and efficacy trial. *J Parenter Enteral Nutr* 1995;19:239–243.

32. Ho C-S, Yee CAN, McPherson R. Complications of surgical and percutaneous nonendoscopic gastrostomy: review of 233 patients. *Gastroenterology* 1988;95:1206–1220.

33. Eddy VA, Snell JA, Morris JA. Analysis of complications and long-term outcome of trauma patients with needle catheter jejunostomy. *Am Surg* 1996;62:40–44.

34. Myers JG, Page CP, Stewart RM, et al. Complications of needle catheter jejunostomy in 2,002 consecutive applications. *Am J Surg* 1995;170:547–551.

35. Ota DM, Loftin RB. Research frontiers: Laparoscopic endoscopic techniques for enteral access. *J Crit Care Nutr* 1994;2(2):23–28.

36. Rombeau JL, Caldwell MD, Forlaw L, Guenter PA. *Atlas of Nutritional Support Techniques.* Boston: Little, Brown and Co.; 1989.

37. Shapiro T, Minard G, Kudsk KA. Transgastric jejunal feeding tubes in critically ill patients. *Nutr Clin Pract* 1997;12:164–167.

38. Baskin WN, Johanson JF. An improved approach to delivery of enteral nutrition in the intensive care unit. *Gastrointest Endosc* 1995;42:161–165.

39. Ferguson DR, Harig JM, Kozarek RA, et al. Placement of a feeding button ("one-step button") as the initial procedure. *Am J Gastroenterol* 1993;88:501–504.

40. Gorman RC, Morris JF, Metz CA, et al. The button jejunostomy for long-term jejunal feeding: Results of a prospective randomized trial. *J Parenter Enteral Nutr* 1993;17: 428–431.

SUGGESTED READINGS

Adams GF, Guest DP, Ciraulo DL, et al. Maximizing tolerance of enteral nutrition in severely injured trauma patients: A comparison of enteral feedings by means of percutaneous endoscopic gastrostomy versus percutaneous endoscopic gastrojejunostomy. *J Trauma* 2000;48:459–465.

Ahmed W, Levy H, Kudsk K, et al. The rates of spontaneous transpyloric passage of three enteral feeding tubes. *Nutr Clin Pract* 1999;14:107–110.

Bowers S. Tubes: A nurse's guide to enteral feeding devices. *MEDSURG Nursing* 1996; 5:313–326.

Burtch GD, Shatney CH. Feeding jejunostomy (versus gastrostomy) passes the test of time. *Am Surg* 1987;53:54–57.

Chen MYM, Ott DJ, Gelfand DW. Nonfluoroscopic, postpyloric feeding tube placement: Number and cost of plain films for determining position. *Nutr Clin Pract* 2000;15:40–44.

Clevenger FW, Rodriguez DJ. Decision-making for enteral feeding administration: the why behind where and how. *Nutr Clin Pract* 1995;10:104–113.

Gottschlich MM, Fuhrman P, Hammond K, Holcombe B, Seidner D (eds) *The Science and Practice of Nutrition Support: A Case Based Core Curriculum.* Dubuque, IA: Kendall/Hunt Publishing Company, 2001.

Huerta D, Puri VK. Nasoenteric feeding tubes in critically ill patients (fluoroscopy vs. blind). *Nutrition* 2000;16:264–267.

Kelley E, Gokhale CB. Replacing displaced PEG tubes with a Foley catheter. *Gastroenterol Nurs* 1998;21:254–255.

Maccabee D, Dominitz JA, Lee SW, et al. Acute presentation of transverse colon injury following percutaneous endoscopic gastrostomy tube placement: Case report and review of current management. *Surg Endosc* 2000;14:296.

Mathus-Vliegen LM, Koning H. Percutaneous endoscopic gastrostomy and gastrojejunostomy: a critical reappraisal of patient selection, tube function and the feasibility of nutritional support during extended follow-up. *Gastrointest Endosc* 1999; 50:746–754.

Metheny NA, Stewart BJ, Smith L, et al. pH and concentration of bilirubin in feeding tube aspirates as predictors of tube placement. *Nurs Res* 1999;48:189–197.

Nicholson FB, Korman MG, Richardson MA. Percutaneous endoscopic gastrostomy: A review of indications, complications and outcome. J *Gastroenterol Hepatol* 2000;15: 21–25.

Sarr MG. Appropriate use, complications and advantages demonstrated in 500 consecutive needle catheter jejunostomies. *Br J Surg* 1999;86:557–561.

Scolapio JS, Romano M, Meschia JF, et al. PEG feeding tube placement following stroke: When to place, when to wait. *Nutr Clin Pract* 2000;15:36–39.

Simon T, Fink AS. Recent experience with percutaneous endoscopic gastrostomy/jejunostomy (PEG/J) for enteral nutrition. *Surg Endosc* 2000;14:436–438.

Van Rosendaal BM, Verhoef MJ, Kinsella TD. How are decisions made about the use of percutaneous endoscopic gastrostomy for long-term nutritional support? *Am J Gastroenterol* 1999;94:3225–3228.

Weltz CR, Morris JB, Mullen JL. Surgical jejunostomy in aspiration risk patients. *Ann Surg* 1992;215:140–145.

RESOURCES

Selected Feeding Tube Manufacturers

Bard Interventional Products
C. R. Inc.
129 Concord Road
Billerica, MA 01821
1–800–225–1332
www.bardinterventional.com

CORPAK Medsystems, Inc.
100 Chaddick Drive
Wheeling, IL 60090
800–323–6305
www.corpakmedsystems.com

Kendall Healthcare Products Company
15 Hampshire St.
Mansfield, MA 02048
1–800–962–9888
www.kendallhq.com

Medical Innovations Corporation
1600 Wyatt Dr.
Santa Clara, CA 95654
www.aedi.com

Nestlé Clinical Nutrition
Three Parkway North, Suite 500
PO Box 760
Deerfield, IL 60015
800–422–2752

Novartis Nutrition
5100 Gamble Drive
St. Louis Park, MN 55416
800–999–9978
www.novartis.com/nutrition

Ross Laboratories
Division of Abbott Laboratories
625 Cleveland Avenue
Columbus, OH 43215
800–544–7495
www.ross.com

Wilson-Cook Medical, Inc.
4900 Bethania Station Road
Winston-Salem, NC 27105
1–336–744–0157
www.cookgroup.com

ZEVEX International, Inc.
4314 ZEVEX Park Lane
Salt Lake City, UT 84123
800–970–2337
www.zevex.com

4

Nursing Care of Patients with Enteral Feeding Devices

PEGGI GUENTER

INTRODUCTION

Optimal care is key to prevention of feeding-tube access complications. This chapter provides the reader with a variety of nursing procedures that aid in the delivery of optimal nursing care for the patient with an enteral access device. A thorough review of mechanical, gastrointestinal, metabolic, and infectious complications along with prevention measures and treatments can be found in Chapter 7, Enteral Nutrition Complications.

NASOENTERIC TUBES

Basic care of the patient with a short-term nasoenteric feeding tube includes frequent nose and mouth care, securing the device, and flushing the tube. Frequent mouth care is essential particularly for patients who are without any oral intake. At least daily the nurse should examine the mouth and oropharynx for any irritation, pressure necrosis, or lesions. Teeth should be brushed twice daily and if inflammation is present, an oral antiseptic rinse may be needed.[1] If the mouth is extremely dry, frequent rinsing or artificial saliva can be considered.

Securing the nasoenteric tube is done initially when the device is placed and then daily according to the procedure listed in Exhibit 4–1.

Other methods of securing the tube include placing the tape solely on the side of the cheek to keep the device in place. Unless the skin on the bridge of the nose is severely excoriated, this method should not be used, as it allows the tube to be displaced easily or accidentally removed out of the nose even while the tape on the cheek remains in place. It is acceptable, however, to secure the tube with tape both on the nose and on the cheek to get the tube end away from the front of the patient's view.

Patients who are very confused and prone to frequent tube removal may benefit from the use of sutures on the nares, mittens to cover the hands, or a nasal bridle to keep the tube secure.[2]

FLUSHING OR IRRIGATION OF THE FEEDING ACCESS DEVICE

To maintain patency of any feeding access device and provide the patient with additional fluid, the tube or device should be flushed with water at least every 4 to 6 hours. This should be done when the patient is receiving continuous feedings, when the tube is not in use, before and after medication administration, and after residual checks and intermittent feedings. This flushing schedule may be altered if an automatic flush enteral pump is being used. The tube flushing procedure is outlined in Exhibit 4–2. The flush solution can be sterile water or tap water depending on your institutional preference and local water supply. Sterile water may be preferable in immunocompromised patients or where the local water supply may contain harmful microbes.[3] Sterile water is, however, more expensive

Exhibit 4–1 Procedure for securing the nasoenteric feeding tube

1. Explain procedure to the patient.
2. Remove the existing tape.
3. Note the position of the tube at the level of the nares according to the incremental markings on the tube. If there are no markings, mark the tube with a permanent marker at that level.
4. Document the tube position information in the nursing record.
5. Inspect the nares and skin on the nose.
6. Clean the nares with warm water or use half-strength hydrogen peroxide to remove crusty debris.
7. Apply a small amount of petroleum to the nares to keep moist.
8. Apply adhesive tape as shown in (a). A 3–4″ piece of tape is torn halfway lengthwise and the intact portion of the tape is placed downward on the bridge of the nose. The two torn halves are alternately looped around the tube. Those torn ends should have their distal ends folded over about ¼″ prior to wrapping to allow for easier removal the following day. Some diaphoretic patients may need skin adhesive to allow for better tape adherence. Avoid having tape pull up on nares to prevent pressure necrosis.
9. In lieu of tape, a Feeding Tube Attachment Device (Hollister, Libertyville, IL) or some other commercially available device can be used to secure the tube. This device adheres to the nose and uses an adjustable clip to hold the tube in place. See (b) for an illustration of the placement of this device. Proceed through the above steps except do not remove the device daily but replace it every 5–7 days and as needed.

(a)

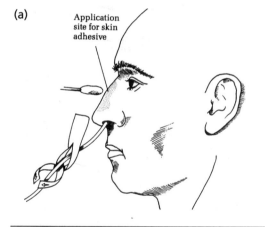

Application site for skin adhesive

(b)

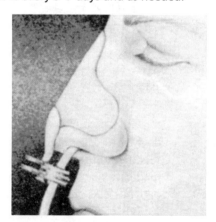

and each facility should make a decision on its water flush supply. Routine flushes should be made with water only. Use of routine flush solutions containing cranberry juice, carbonated beverages, or meat tenderizer solutions may actually precipitate protein in the feeding solution and cause tube clogging.[4]

ADAPTERS

Some feeding access devices, particularly longer term tubes, may not have a "nurse friendly" adapter on the end of the tube. This is often the case when urinary catheters are used for feeding gastrostomy tubes or when abdominal drainage devices or red rubber tubes are used for jejunal tubes. Often there is

Exhibit 4–2 Tube flushing procedure

1. Gather supplies—water and a 30–60 ml catheter tip or luer slip tip syringe depending on the feeding tube proximal end. Do not use a smaller sized syringe (less than 20 ml) due to increased pressure on the tube and potential for tube rupture.
2. Draw up 20–30 ml of room temperature water into the syringe.
3. Place the syringe tip into the feeding tube, either in the proximal end following disconnection from the formula source or through the side medication/flushing port. See (a) and (b).
4. Do not use excessive force to flush the feeding tube.
5. Record the time and amount of water used on the fluid intake record.

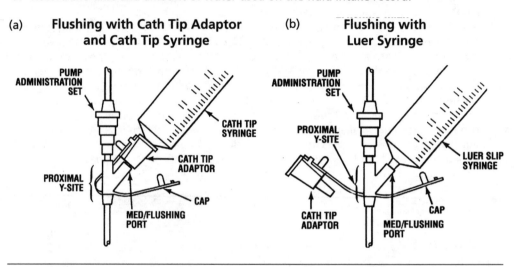

(a) **Flushing with Cath Tip Adaptor and Cath Tip Syringe**

(b) **Flushing with Luer Syringe**

no way to cap the tube when the feeding is completed. Additionally, when the feeding administration set needs to be disconnected to flush the tube or give medications, the end of the feeding administration set either is placed on the patient's bed or, worse, falls on the floor. How many times have metal surgical clamps been used to close off feeding tubes? The ideal type of adapter should have a side port for flushing/medication administration and should have a proximal end and side port that can be capped when the feedings are not being administered. These adapters do not turn a single lumen tube into a double lumen tube but simply provide a "Y" for flushing or medication delivery.

There are several adapter devices available on the market that can be used to transform these makeshift tubes into ones useful to the nurse and comfortable to the patient. See Figure 4–1 for an example. Several manufacturers market a variety of these adapters. See Table 4–1 for currently available devices.

These adapters are different from those needed to administer feeding through a skin-level gastrostomy device. Those devices need their own specific manufacturer's feeding adapter, which must be obtained from the device manufacturer. The patient must take care of those adaptive devices and bring them to hospital or physician's visits.

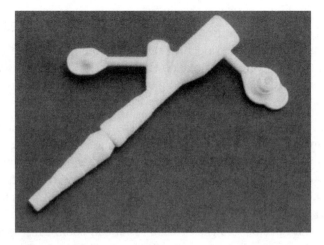

Figure 4–1 Example of a commercially available adapter to be added to a feeding tube

LONG-TERM FEEDING TUBES

The nursing care for patients who receive long-term feeding access devices such as gastrostomies or jejunostomies include post-procedure and maintenance site care, checking placement and tube fit, and tube stabilization. Following placement of a gastrostomy or jejunostomy, a sterile dressing is generally placed around the insertion site and left in place for about 24 hours. After that time, the dressing can be removed and the site inspected by the nurse and inserting physician. Normally there may be a small amount of serosanguineous drainage on the dressing. Clean under the external bumper or around the sutures with half-

Table 4–1 Commercially available feeding tube adapters

Brand Name	Manufacturer	City	Phone	Comments
Clintec Y-port Adapter	ZEVEX, Inc	Salt Lake City, UT	800-970-2237	Graduated tip
Dual-Port Feeding Adapter	Bard Interventional	Billerica, MA	800-826-2273	
Flexiflo Y-port Connector	Ross Products	Columbus, OH	800-544-7495	Use with PEGs 14-20Fr
Flexiflo Feeding Tube Irrigation Adapter	Ross Products	Columbus, OH	800-544-7495	Use with NG or G-tube
Replacement Plug-In Adapter	Novartis	Minneapolis, MN	800-999-9978	Small–large; Large fits urinary catheters
Replacement Side Port Adapter	Novartis	Minneapolis, MN	800-999-9978	

strength hydrogen peroxide to remove any crusty drainage and thereafter with mild soap and water, rinse and dry well.[5] A dressing is generally not needed and the site should be left open to air to promote healing and prevent moist dressings from causing skin breakdown. Occasionally patients with sutures around a jejunostomy site may want a light, dry dressing for comfort. Change dressings immediately if they become damp from drainage or perspiration.

The feeding access device should be checked for placement and fit daily. Inspect the tube for any inward or outward migration. Measure the tube length from the skin level out, document the measurement, and place a mark with waterproof marker on the tube at skin level. Some tubes have incremental markers and these can also be used to note tube position—for example, "Skin level is at the ___ cm mark." It is essential that the tubes stay in their original position. If inward migration occurs, the gastric tube distal end could cause pyloric obstruction. If outward migration occurs, the tube tip may slip out of the gastrointestinal tract and peritonitis can ensue. A percutaneous endoscopic gastrostomy (PEG) tube or low profile (skin level) device should move slightly and have a bit of space between the skin and external bumper. One expert[6] recommends 2 mm be left at the time of initial tube placement. This space can be confirmed by rotating the tube 360 degrees to make sure there is some tube independence (see Figure 4–2).

If the tension is great and the bumper too tight against the skin, skin breakdown or pressure necrosis may occur.[7] This space may decrease as the patient gains weight; thus it is recommended that the bumper be pulled back or outward about 1 cm once the tract has been well developed in order to allow for this "growing room."[8]

Tube stabilization is important to prevent tube migration, accidental tube removal, or enlargement of the tube site stoma, which could allow for leakage of GI fluids and formula. For most radiologically placed gastrostomies and jejunostomies, an external disk or bumper holds the tube externally and a mushroom tip or balloon

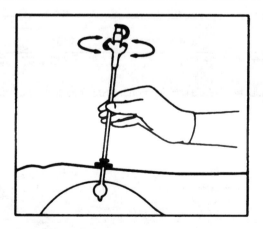

Figure 4–2 Rotate the PEG tube 360 degrees to check for adequate space between the external disk and the skin

holds the tube internally. If the device has an internal balloon, check the volume of the fluid in the balloon weekly and compare it to the previous week. Occasionally these balloons have a slow leak. Refill the balloon with the original volume and document these findings. If the tube balloon has ruptured, replace the tube.

Jejunal tubes and some surgically placed gastric tubes are often held in with sutures. This may not always prevent the tube from pulling on the stoma and causing stoma enlargement. These patients may need some additional type of stabilizing device. Often physicians will use tape and sterile dressings, but this may cause a buildup of moisture around the tube leading to skin breakdown, or it may not stabilize the tube adequately. Stabilizing devices are available commercially. One in particular, Vertical Tube Attachment Device (Hollister Inc., Libertyville, IL, 1–800–323–4060, www.hollister.com), provides a protective skin barrier surrounding a clip device that secures the tube in place. It eliminates the need for suturing, protects the skin, and minimizes tube movement. Experience has found these to be extremely helpful in many patients. The device can be changed weekly depending on wear and can accommodate a variety of tube diameters (see Figure 4–3). If these devices are used, the peritubular area needs to be cleaned daily to remove any drainage or debris.[1]

Some of the most frequent complications following feeding tube placement are exit site problems.[5] These problems can include exit site infection, pressure necrosis, skin breakdown secondary leakage, and hypergranulation tissue. The site or stoma should be inspected for purulent or gastrointestinal drainage, redness, swelling, tenderness, rashes, or warmth. Also look for skin breakdown, pressure necrosis, or hypergranulation tissue.[1] Exit site infections may present as redness, edema, warmth, or purulent drainage at the site. These often require systemic and local antimicrobial therapies but usually can be cleared up with-

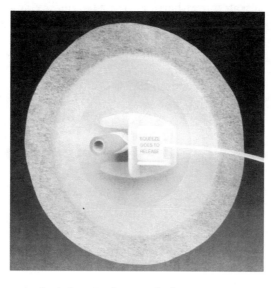

Figure 4–3 Placement of a tube attachment device

out removal of the feeding device. Meticulous nursing care of the site and adequate stabilization may help in infection prevention.

Skin breakdown can occur from external moisture or pressure or leakage around the tube. To prevent external moisture, keep the skin clean and dry and open to air. Occasionally the tube is placed in skin folds or under pendulous breasts, which may not be apparent when the patient is lying supine on a procedure table. This has led to site complications and can be easily prevented by using the enterostomal therapy nurse techniques of preplacement marking for gastrostomy or jejunostomy tube sites.[9] To relieve bumper pressure, have the bumper loosened. In cases where the bumper pressure is extreme, perhaps due to weight gain, the patient can develop pressure necrosis and "buried bumper," as shown in Figure 4–4. This can cause internal and external pressure ulcers that generally require aggressive wound care and/or tube removal.[7]

Other skin breakdown can be caused by leakage of formula and gastrointestinal fluids that well up through the stoma site. These leaks can be caused by the patient's position (keep patient up at least 30 degrees during and 1 hour after intermittent feeding), by the feeding being infused too rapidly or in too large volume (can switch to continuous lower volume feedings), or by increased size of the gastrostomy or jejunostomy tract. (In the last case, keep the tube well stabilized, increase balloon volume by 2 to 5 ml if balloon tube is present, and be sure internal bumper or balloon is pulled up snugly against abdominal wall. Do not expand balloon beyond volume capacity. Sometimes loosening the external bumper can correct the leak. One that is too tight can distort the external opening, permitting leaks.[5] Replacing the tube with a larger tube may just further increase the stoma size.) Often removing the gastrostomy tube for a few hours, allowing the tract to shrink before replacing the tube, can help with the leak as well.

Skin irritation and breakdown from moisture or leakage can be prevented by applying a waterproof barrier such as a zinc oxide ointment. Mildly broken-down skin can be treated with Stomadhesive powder or hydrocolloid and pectin

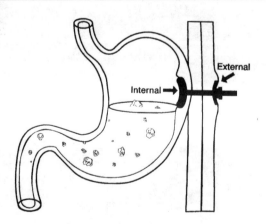

Figure 4–4 Buried bumper PEG

wafers such as Stomadhesive wafers (ConvaTec, Cranbury, NJ).[1] If this redness appears to be due to a yeast infection, an antifungal cream will help. Hyper-granulation tissue or "proud flesh" may form around the stoma site due to excessive movement, retained moisture, or rapid epithelialization. This can be eliminated by cautery with silver nitrate sticks as needed. Untreated, this tissue can bleed easily.[1,2,5] Patients can also have peritubular allergic reactions due to use of strong soaps, solutions, or ointments around the site or if a latex urinary catheter is used as a replacement gastrostomy.[10]

TUBE REPLACEMENT

Feeding tubes need to be replaced under three circumstances: (1) emergently, when a long-term feeding tube inadvertently falls out; (2) routinely, when a tube is worn or clogged; or (3) when a gastrostomy is replaced by a low-profile skin-level device. In some practice settings, either staff nurses or advance practice nurses replace these tubes. Nurses need to check with state nursing practice acts, institutional clinical privileges, and credentialing boards to determine whether or under what circumstances they are allowed to replace long-term feeding tubes.[1]

In general, gastrojejunostomies and jejunostomies, regardless of the insertion method, are replaced by physicians either endoscopically, radiologically, or manually with radiological confirmation.[11] In the case of accidental removal of any long-term feeding tube, the tube needs to be replaced as soon as possible, as the tube tract can close quickly due to rapid cell turnover in the GI tract. The physician should be notified immediately or a tube replacement protocol should be followed. For the patient at home, the home care agency should be notified. Patients can be taught to replace the tube themselves or can visit a local emergency department for tube replacement.[1] Often scheduled replacements may prevent emergency visits. Gastrostomy tubes should not be replaced routinely until the tract is matured and adhesions have formed between the stomach and the internal abdominal wall. This maturation generally takes about 3 weeks unless the patient is very malnourished, immunocompromised, or diabetic.[1] During this time, only a physician should replace a gastrostomy tube when necessary.

Those who replace gastrostomies must be aware of the tube characteristics and the initial tube insertion procedure. Some PEG tubes require endoscopy for removal. Many newer ones have been designed for manual removal without endoscopy.[12] There are many commercially available gastrostomy replacement tubes. These tubes are generally silicone with a balloon on the distal end. If a latex, Foley-type tube is selected, latex allergies may be an issue. Those tubes generally do not have an external bumper to stabilize the replacement tube and often lead to the exit site problems described above. Low-profile devices are often chosen as replacement feeding devices and have the same indications as previously described in Chapter 3, Enteral Feeding Access Devices. A step-by-step procedure for gastrostomy tube replacement can be found in Exhibit 4–3.

Exhibit 4–3 Gastrostomy tube replacement procedure

1. Explain procedure to the patient.
2. Gather equipment including same diameter tube as the one in place.
3. Remove the existing tube by deflating the balloon with a luer tip syringe, or by placing hand pressure on the abdomen and pulling on the tube until the invertable or collapsible tip emerges through the site. Note: Do not remove the tube unless you are sure of its internal fixation device. Some tubes need to be endoscopically removed.
4. Cleanse the area around the stoma with half-strength hydrogen peroxide or mild soap and water.
5. Inflate the replacement tube balloon with sterile water to assess for leaks and then deflate.
6. Lubricate the tube tip and stoma site with water-soluble lubricant.
7. Insert the tube tip gently into the stoma and through the tract into the stomach.
8. Inflate the balloon with 10–20 ml sterile water.
9. Gently pull tube up so that balloon is snug but not tight against stomach and internal abdominal wall.
10. Slide the external bumper or disk down onto abdominal skin to stabilize tube allowing for about 2 mm of space.
11. Check for placement by aspirating back gastric contents.
12. Irrigate tube well using flush procedure.
13. Document change procedure noting type and size of replacement of tube, skin condition, cm mark at skin level, amount of fluid in balloon, and patient tolerance to procedure. If performed as an outpatient be sure to provide written communication of these findings to patient or receiving institution.

CONCLUSION

Nursing procedures that attend to the patient's tube site, replacement, patency, and stabilization will do much to prevent painful and costly complications related to the feeding tube and will help assure that the optimal nutrition is delivered.

REFERENCES

1. Kirby DF, Minard G, Kohn-Keeth C. Enteral access and infusion equipment. In: Merritt R, ed. *The A.S.P.E.N. Nutrition Support Manual.* Silver Spring, MD: American Society for Parenteral and Enteral Nutrition; 1998.
2. Lord LM. Enteral access devices. *Nurs Clin North Am* December 1997;32:685–704.
3. Perez SK, Brandt K. Enteral feeding contamination: comparison of diluents and feeding bag usage. *J Parenter Enteral Nutr* 1989;13:306–308.
4. Frankel EH, Enow NB, Jackson KC, et al. Methods of restoring patency to occluded feeding tubes. *Nutr Clin Pract* 1998;13:129–131.
5. Ireton-Jones CS, Hennessy K, Orr M. Care of patients receiving home enteral nutrition. *Infusion* March 1996;2:30–43.
6. Foutch G. Complications of percutaneous endoscopic gastrostomy and jejunostomy. *Gastrointest Endosc Clin North Am* 1992;2:236–237.

7. Heximer B. Pressure necrosis: Implications and interventions for PEG tubes. *Nutr Clin Pract* 1997;12:256–258.
8. Shapiro G, Edmundowicz S. Complications of percutaneous endoscopic gastrostomy. *Gastrointest Endosc Clin North Am* 1996;2:412–414.
9. Hanlon MD. Preplacement marking for optimal gastrostomy and jejunostomy tube site locations to decrease complications and promote self-care. *Nutr Clin Pract* 1998;13:167–171.
10. Bey D, Browne B. Clinical management of latex allergy. *Nutr Clin Pract* 1997;12:68–71.
11. Stogdill BJ, Page CP, Pestana C. Nonoperative replacement of a jejunostomy feeding catheter. *Am J Surg* 1984;147:280–282.
12. Baskin WN, Johanson JF. An improved approach to delivery of enteral nutrition in the intensive care unit. *Gastrointest Endosc* 1995;42:161–165.

SUGGESTED READINGS

Bockus S. When your patient needs tube feedings: making the right decisions. *Nursing 93* July 1993:34–42.

Bowers S. Tubes: A nurse's guide to enteral feeding devices. *MEDSURG Nursing* 1996; 5:313–326.

Gottschlich MM, Fuhrman P, Hammond K, Holcombe B, Seidner D (eds) *The Science and Practice of Nutrition Support: A Case Based Core Curriculum.* Dubuque, IA: Kendall/Hunt Publishing Company, 2001.

Kirby DF, Delegge MH, Fleming CR. American Gastroenterological Association technical review on feeding for enteral nutrition. *Gastroenterology* 1995;108:1282–1301.

O'Brien B, Dabis S, Erwin-Toth P. G-tube site care: a practical guide. *RN* 1999; 62:52–56.

Smarszcz RM, Proicou GC, Dugle JE. Microbial contamination of low-profile balloon gastrostomy extension tubes and three cleaning methods. *Nutr Clin Pract* 2000; 15:138–142.

Wilson RE. Case study: a system for stabilizing percutaneous tubes. *Ostomy Wound Management* 1994;40:44–49.

RESOURCES

ConvaTac
Cranbury, NJ
www.convatec.com

Hollister, Inc.
Libertyville, IL
1–800–323–4060
www.hollister.com

Wound, Ostomy and Continence Nurses Society
www.wocn.org

5

Tube Feeding Administration

PEGGI GUENTER

There are a variety of tube feeding administration methods that can be utilized to give patients optimal nutritional support. Nurses are key to positive outcomes and complication prevention. Adequate knowledge and practice protocols assist nurses in providing the best care possible for patients requiring enteral nutrition. This chapter will outline the variety of administration methods, progression to goal protocols, monitoring steps, and equipment selection and care.

ADMINISTRATION METHODS

Methods of tube feeding delivery include those administered via gravity control and those that are infused using a pump. This section will outline the delivery method definitions, indications, and step-by-step protocols for practice. Gravity-controlled methods include bolus, intermittent, and continuous gravity drips, and are almost always used for gastric feedings. The bolus feeding method and the intermittent method terms are often used interchangeably but not always correctly. Intermittent/bolus feedings are given periodically throughout the 24-hour day, usually 4 to 8 times per day. A prescribed dose is administered (such as 250 ml) followed by a water flush. This type of method is generally used in ambulatory patients, allowing for disruption from a constant infusion and freedom from a pump. This will allow for participation in other activities such as physical rehabilitation.[1] See Figure 5–1 for a feeding method decision-making algorithm. These methods are suggestions only and should be adapted to the individual patient's tolerance and schedule.

The difference between bolus and intermittent methods is that bolus feedings are administered using a larger volume of formula ($\geq$250 ml) and a large syringe attached to the feeding tube. The formula is poured into the syringe and held up for 15 to 20 minutes until all of the prescribed formula has dripped in. It may also be pushed in with the syringe, which will speed up the infusion rate even further. This dose is given about 4 to 6 times per day and may be associated with some gastrointestinal discomfort due to the rapid infusion. It is very time-consuming for the nurses and it may not be cost-effective to have nursing staff stand with the patient to hold the syringe for that amount of time. This method is most often used when patients self-administer feedings and are on a stable regimen at home. These feedings may be best tolerated when given at less than 60 ml/ per minute.[2] An example of the nursing order for this type of feeding would read as follows: 240 ml of formula every 3 hours via bolus method over at least 10 minutes followed by 30 ml of water flush.

For better utilization of nursing time and better gastrointestinal tolerance, the intermittent method using a feeding bag may be employed. This allows the prescribed volume of formula to be infused over 30 to 60 minutes using a feeding

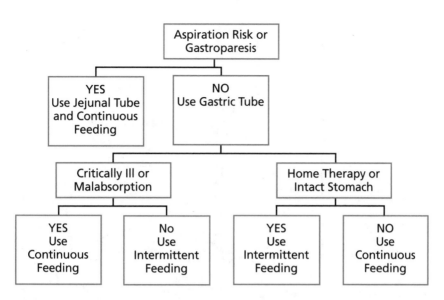

Figure 5–1 Algorithm for decision making for administration method

bag with a roller clamp on the tubing to control the drip rate. See Figure 5–2 for correct patient position and equipment for intermittent feeding method.

The nurse fills the bag, sets the drip rate, and can attend to other patient care activities while the formula is infusing. An example of the nursing order for this type of feeding would read as follows: 300 ml of formula every 4 hours over 60 minutes via intermittent method followed by 100 ml of water flush. See Exhibit 5–1 for a step-by-step nursing protocol for intermittent feeding administration. Intermittent feedings can be infused using a pump, although this may not always be available or reimbursed for in the home setting. However, it is often used with hospitalized, acutely ill patients.

Continuous feedings can be given using a feeding bag and roller clamp. However, most continuous feedings, particularly in acute care, are infused via an enteral pump. Small bowel feedings are administered using a pump in order to provide for strict control of the infusion. Continuous feedings are generally given over 24 hours at lower volumes per hour. The infusion enteral pumps are recommended to provide a more accurate volume of formula over a prescribed period of time and may prevent feeding intolerance.[1] Continuous feedings into the stomach have been shown to decrease incidence of gastric distention and aspiration when compared with intermittent feedings.[3] Pump-controlled continuous feedings are essential in jejunal or small bowel feedings as large volumes of bolus feedings may cause osmotic diarrhea. In the patient in intensive care, continuous feedings have been shown to produce fewer metabolic complica-

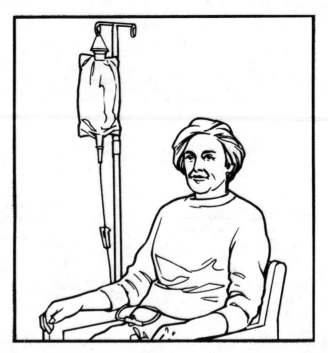

Figure 5–2 Correct patient position and equipment for intermittent feeding method

tions.[4,5] An example of the nursing order for this type of feeding would read as follows: Infuse 80 ml per hour of formula over 24 hours continuously via enteral pump. See Exhibit 5–2 for a step-by-step nursing protocol for continuous feeding administration.

Cyclic feeding is a continuous feeding regimen given over 10 to 16 hours. This is also called the nocturnal or transitional feeding method, as it is often given

Exhibit 5–1 Protocol for intermittent feeding administration

1. Gather necessary supplies at bedside, including tube feeding formula, enteral feeding bag, and syringe.
2. Wash hands and top of formula cans.
3. Close roller clamp on feeding bag before pouring formula into the bag.
4. Pour specified amount of formula into the bag.
5. Hang bag on an IV pole. Squeeze drip chamber 1/2 to 1/3 full of formula and manually prime tubing.
6. Confirm proper feeding tube placement and raise head of bed to 30 degrees.
7. Check gastric residuals.
8. Attach feeding tube to feeding bag, adjust roller clamp to infuse.
9. Allow feeding to run over 30–60 minutes as ordered.
10. When feeding completed, flush feeding tube with at least 30 ml of water and cap tube.
11. Record formula and flush separately on intake and output sheet.
12. Change feeding bag, syringe, and containers daily.

Exhibit 5–2 Protocol for continuous feeding administration

1. Gather necessary supplies at bedside, including tube feeding formula, enteral feeding bag, and syringe.
2. Wash hands and top of formula cans.
3. Close roller clamp on feeding bag before pouring formula into the bag.
4. Pour specified amount of formula into the bag.
5. Hang bag on pump pole. Squeeze drip chamber 1/2 to 1/3 full of formula and manually prime tubing or load enteral pump with feeding set.
6. Confirm proper feeding tube placement and raise head of bed to 30 degrees with gastric feedings.
7. Check gastric residuals for gastric feedings.
8. Attach feeding tube to feeding bag, start enteral pump.
9. Allow feeding to run over 30–60 minutes as ordered.
10. When feeding completed, flush feeding tube with at least 30 ml of water and cap tube.
11. Record formula and flush separately on intake and output sheet.
12. Change feeding bag, syringe, and containers daily.

---

during the night so that the patient can be free from the pump during the day. The patient may eat during the day without feeling full from the feedings. Cyclic feeding prescriptions often use higher calorie formulas at higher volumes if the plan is to try to give the patient all of their daily requirement during this cycled regimen. Particular attention should be given to monitoring fluid status, because fluids are not evenly dispensed throughout the day.[1] An example of a nursing order for this type of feeding would read as follows: Infuse 120 ml per hour of formula continuously from 7 PM to 7 AM followed by 50 ml water flush.

STARTER REGIMEN AND PROGRESSION TO GOAL

Starter regimens for enteral feeding are based on three main issues: (1) the location of the enteral access in the gastrointestinal tract, (2) the patient's clinical status, and (3) how long the patient has been NPO. Enteral regimens can be started either by continuous infusion or intermittent delivery. Reports recommend starting with a low rate of an isotonic formula fed into either the stomach or small bowel. Hypertonic formulas may cause abdominal distress and diarrhea when delivered into the small intestine.[4] Initial dilution of these concentrated formulas may assist in tolerance; however, it is unnecessary to heavily dilute concentrated formulas (quarter strength) when utilizing gastric administration, as they provide patients very little nutritional value.[5] Table 5–1 describes a starter regimen and progression that maximizes nutritional intake and tolerance. Formulas are then advanced as tolerated by 10 to 25 ml per hour every 8 to 12 hours until a goal rate is reached. Depending on the patient's tol-

Table 5–1 Starter regimen and progression based on delivery method

	Intermittent Method	Continuous Method
Initial Regimen	120 ml isotonic formula q 4 hours followed by 30 ml water flush	30–40 ml/hr isotonic formula
Rate and method of advancement	Check residuals prior to next feeding. Residuals acceptable up to half of previously administered volume.	Check residuals q 4 hours. Hold for ≥2 hours worth of rate up to maximum of 150 ml

erance to feedings and their long-term nutrition care plan, the feeding schedule may be changed to intermittent or cyclic feedings.[6]

Progression and tolerance to feeding should be assessed by the nurse measuring several parameters. Bowel function is evaluated by auscultating the abdomen and listening for bowel sounds in all four quadrants. Observing the patient for nausea, vomiting, or symptoms of aspiration should occur. Measuring abdominal girth and assessing for bloating and distention are essential.[7] Checking gastric residuals every 4 to 6 hours or before each intermittent feeding is vital to assessing for adequate gastric emptying. Studies have shown that staff nurses are successful only half of the time in checking residuals from small-bore nasogastric tubes.[8]

The physician should specify how much residual should be present in order to hold the feedings. Residuals should be checked with a large syringe; this best works on a tube that is at least 10 French. Sometimes insufflating 20 ml of air into the tube may move the tube away from the gastric wall and clear the tube of any residual water, formula, or medications.[1] Residual volume should be returned to the stomach, as it contains needed nutrition, fluid, and electrolytes. If the residual volume exceeds the limit, hold the feeding and recheck residuals in 1 hour. Flush the tube with 10 to 30 ml of water following these residual checks. The exact volume that is considered too high remains controversial, and limited research has been conducted in this area. One researcher found that residual volume had little correlation with physical examination, and concluded that low residual volume does not guarantee tolerance to tube feeding nor does one high residual volume indicate intolerance.[9] A recent comprehensive review on this topic was written by a nurse and dietitian who concluded that there is no good data to guide practice so clinicians must use sound judgment. Elevating the head of the bed, careful abdominal examination, use of promotility agents and formulas that promote gastric emptying are techniques that should be employed to prevent high gastric residuals.[10] A general rule is that maximum residuals are 2 times the hourly rate for continuous feedings and one-half of the volume of the intermittent feeding with an upper limit of 150 ml. The study by McClave[9] includes a more in-depth discussion on this topic of residual volumes.

Stool output should also be monitored as tube feedings are started and advanced. Stool frequency, consistency, and volume should be noted, as definitions of diarrhea vary greatly.[11]

There are often many reasons why a patient is unable to be advanced to their goal enteral formula dose. In a recent study in critically ill patients, investigators found that the patients received only 51.6% of nutritional goal.[12] Some of this low intake was due to underordering by physicians, slow progression to goal, and gastrointestinal intolerance. All nursing measures should be focused to advance the regimen to goal in order to optimize the nutrition support.

MODULAR ADMINISTRATION

As noted in Chapter 2, Enteral Nutrition Basics, patients often require additional nutrients such as protein powders or liquid fat modules. Although the literature is extremely limited in this area, some recommendations can be made. Most often the nutrient should be given at a certain time like a medication, not simply mixed into the formula bag. This assures the nurse that the patient is actually receiving all of the nutrient and that it doesn't get wasted. Also, some of these nutrients may not mix thoroughly with the formula, may clump at the bottom of the feeding bag, and may either interfere with the enteral pump mechanism or clog the feeding tube. Also some institutions use ready-to-hang formula bags that would preclude one from adding anything to the formula. It has been suggested that the protein powder, or a specific protein module such as glutamine powder, be mixed with water. A typical nursing order for this module would read as follows: Add 5 grams of powder to 30 ml of water, mix well and infuse via large syringe every 6 hours. Flush with an additional 20 ml water and continue tube feeding.[13]

ENTERAL DELIVERY EQUIPMENT

Feeding containers and sets vary between manufacturers and have evolved greatly since the first feeding bag back in ancient times was made from a pig's bladder.[5] Feeding bags, or containers, come with or without attached tubing. This administration tubing is often referred to as an administration set. The container's form can be rigid or collapsible. See Figure 5–3 for a variety of containers.

Since tube feeding formulas and lipid-containing intravenous nutrition may appear similar, it is important that tubing sets attached to feeding bags not be compatible with IV systems. The Association for the Advancement of Medical Instrumentation developed manufacturing guidelines to prevent such a complication.[14]

The containers range in size from 500 to 1500 ml and usually fill from the top. The ideal container should be easy to fill, close, and hang. It should also be leakproof, have easy-to-read calibrations, and directions for use. The container and set should be compatible with the institutional enteral pumps, and the distal tubing end should fit a variety of feeding tubes.[5] The containers and sets come as pump compatible or are designed for gravity drip delivery method. Many manu-

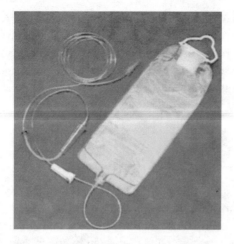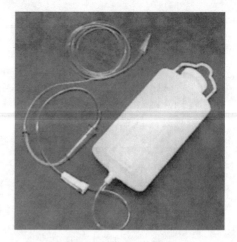

Figure 5–3 Variety of containers

facturers also provide prefilled containers, which generally come in 1-liter sizes and contain their commonly used full-strength formulas. Use of prefilled containers saves nursing time and decreases potential bacterial contamination by eliminating the need to open cans and transfer formulas from can to container.

Enteral formula is a good growth medium for microbial growth. When using formula from cans that is transferred to a container, use the following guidelines to decrease potential bacterial growth:

- Hang enough formula for just 8 hours of infusion
- Do not add new formula to formula already hanging
- Wash hands and tops of cans before opening
- Use clean technique when handling all administration items (including syringes and irrigation containers)
- Change the entire administration system along with syringe and irrigation containers daily

Rinsing administration sets was once the standard of care; however, a recent study refuted that rinsing decreases microbial contamination.[15]

OPEN SYSTEM VERSUS CLOSED SYSTEM

Enteral nutrition is delivered to patients either via an "open" or "closed" system. Open delivery systems employ an open-top container or syringe for tube feeding administration. Formulas for open systems may come in flip-top cans or as powdered mixtures that require reconstitution with water. Hang time, or amount of time that the enteral formula should remain at room temperature in the bag, is limited to 4 to 8 hours. If formulas are diluted or if modulars are added, 4 hours should be the limit. Closed delivery systems utilize a prefilled sterile container that is spiked with enteral tubing and connected to the enteral pump. Prefilled containers usually hold 1 liter of formula and can hang safely for 24 to 48 hours, according to manufacturer's recommendations.[16] This system works best with long-term stable patients who will not be changing formulas frequently. The "closed" system is seemingly more expensive to use but is cost-effective when weighed against benefits, such as decreased formula contamination and decreased nursing time.[17] Further detail on this issue can be found in Chapter 11, Improving the Quality of Enteral Nutrition Care, under "Quality Improvement Programs."

ENTERAL PUMPS

Enteral feeding infusion pumps are mechanical devices that control the delivery rate of feeding formula. They can be used with continuous or intermittent feeding regimens. Pump-controlled tube feedings have been found to be beneficial in delivering large volumes of formula with good reliability ($+/-$ 10%).[18] Pumps guarantee a constant flow rate, thus reducing the amount of gastric pooling associated with aspiration risk, although the differences were not statistically significant.[19] The use of an enteral pump has proven to decrease the incidence of osmotic diarrhea and lessen abdominal discomfort.[3,20] These results suggest improved tolerance and rapid advancement of enteral feedings to goal rate. Other advantages of enteral pumps include the ability to infuse a more viscous formula through a smaller diameter feeding tube. Nursing time is saved with such devices, thus making pumps more cost-effective.[21] Disadvantages to pump use include the cost and lack of reimbursement for such devices, the time it takes to instruct nurses in using such devices, and the need for an electricity source to operate the pump and/or charge the battery.

Important features included on most pumps are an alarm system that alerts the practitioner to an empty container, occlusion, or low battery; a battery feature to allow patient mobility; and flow rate up to 300 ml/ per hour. Many of the pumps also have memory that retains the rate and amount infused.[18] The ideal pump should be easy to use; have safety features such as prevention of free-flow, sets incompatible with IV pumps, and rate accuracy; and have an automatic priming feature, an easily readable visual display, and extended battery life.[5]

Three pump manufacturers provide a portable lightweight (less than 5 pounds) enteral pump, which can be utilized for ambulatory patients who require pump-controlled feedings. These pumps are housed in carrying cases that can be placed over the shoulder or as a backpack. A comprehensive list of enteral pumps and their manufacturers can be found updated annually in *Infusion*.[22] See Exhibit 5–3, which contains contact information for enteral pump manufacturers.

A recent development in pump technology is the automatic water flush system designed to decrease clogged feeding tubes and provide additional water.[23] Several clinical trials using the automatic flush pump have demonstrated decreased clogging of tubes as compared to manual flushing.[24–26] In addition to the feeding formula, the pumps provide up to hourly water flushes, which often assist in meeting a patient's daily fluid requirements. When the patient is fluid restricted, the automatic water flush feature can be turned off and a manual water flush (30 ml per shift) performed to maintain tube patency. The two automatic flush

Exhibit 5–3 Enteral pump manufacturers

CORPAK Medsystems, Inc.
100 Chaddick Drive
Wheeling, IL 60090
800-323-6305
www.corpakmedsystems.com

Kendall Healthcare Products
15 Hampshire Street
Mansfield, MA 02048
800-962-9888
www.kendallhq.com

Novartis Nutrition
5100 Gamble Drive
St. Louis Park, MN 55416
800-999-9978
www.novartis/nutrition

Nestlé Clinical Nutrition
Three Parkway North, Suite 500
PO Box 760
Deerfield, IL 60015
800-422-2752

Ross Laboratories
Division of Abbott Laboratories
625 Cleveland Avenue
Columbus, OH 43215
800-544-7495
www.ross.com

ZEVEX International, Inc.
4314 ZEVEX Park Lane
Salt Lake City, UT 84123
800-970-2337
www.zevex.com

pumps currently on the market are the Flexiflo Quantum Pump (Ross Laboratories, Columbus, OH) and the Kangaroo Entriflush Pump (Kendall Healthcare, Mansfield, MA). See Figure 5–4 for an example of a flush pump.

In an unpublished cost analysis conducted by this author, it was found to be highly cost-effective to use the more expensive flush bag sets and the automatic flush pump system as compared to the standard non-flush system. Clogging complications cost over $2,000 per month and included nursing and physician time to replace clogged tubes, new tubes, x-rays, and operating room costs to replace clogged permanent jejunostomies. These costs far outweighed the difference in the cost of the flush pump sets over the standard sets.

MONITORING

Nurses are responsible for initiating tube feeding and monitoring tolerance for the duration of therapy. To assess tolerance, a nurse measures several subjective and objective parameters. Patients who are alert and oriented should be asked to describe their symptoms of tolerance to enteral feeding. The nurse must examine the abdomen, auscultate for presence of bowel sounds, and evaluate stool patterns as described above in progression to goal. Urine output as well as weight changes should be monitored and documented for review. Tube-fed patients should be observed for any signs of aspiration such as coughing during feedings. Initial serum labs typically requested include electrolytes, liver and kidney function, prealbumin, albumin, glucose, calcium, magnesium, and phosphorus. Table 5–2 suggests general guidelines for ordering lab work in hospitalized patients receiving enteral nutrition.[27] Lab monitoring will vary,

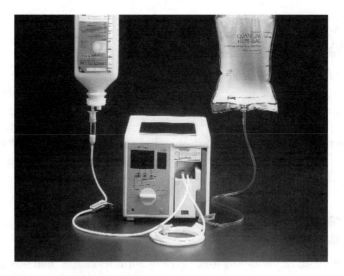

Figure 5–4 Automatic flush pump and pump set

increasing in frequency for a patient in the ICU and less frequent for a stable home patient. Monitoring is key to complication prevention and detection.

Complications that occur as a result of tube feeding will be more thoroughly discussed in Chapter 7, Enteral Nutrition Complications. Clinical pathways and care algorithms are often helpful in determining monitoring patterns. The American Society for Parenteral and Enteral Nutrition (www.nutritioncare.org) has a clinical pathway available that outlines monitoring guidelines for the adult patient receiving enteral nutrition.

Table 5–2 Monitoring measures for the tube-fed patients

Baseline Tests	Until on stable rate	When on goal**
Body weight	Twice weekly	Weekly
Fluid intake/input	Daily	Daily
Adequacy of nutrient intake	Daily	Weekly
Abdominal exam	2–3 times day	Daily
Glucose		
*Nondiabetic	Daily	2–3 times/week
*Diabetic	Daily	Daily
Electrolytes	Daily	1–3 times/week
Renal function	Daily	1–3 times/week
Phosphorus	2–3 times/week	Weekly
Liver function	1–2 times/week	Weekly
Calcium/Magnesium	2–3 times/week	Weekly
Prealbumin	2 times/week	Weekly
Albumin	Weekly	Monthly

**In the hospitalized patient (patients at home or at long-term care facilities may require less frequent monitoring)

ORDER SETS OR PROTOCOLS

Many institutions have established enteral nutrition order sets or protocols. These often are preprinted order sheets that include tube placement and verification orders, formula and flush administration rates and methods, monitoring procedures, and special treatment orders for complications such as clogged tubes or suspected aspiration. These types of protocols have been shown to improve delivery of enteral tube feeding.[28] An example of such an order set can be found in Exhibit 5–4.[5]

CONCLUSION

There are a variety of tube feeding administration methods that can be utilized to give patients optimal enteral nutrition. Practice protocols assist nurses in providing the best care possible.

Exhibit 5–4 Enteral nutrition standard order set

Feeding tube type and location of tip _____

Check items to be completed:

_____ 1. Obtain chest x-ray after tube placement to confirm position.

_____ 2. Prior to feeding, confirm placement of tube by aspirating for gastric contents.

_____ 3. Elevate head of bed 30 degrees when feeding into stomach.

_____ 4. Name of formula _____
      a. Intermittent: Give _____ ml over 30 minutes every _____ hours.
      b. Continuous: Give _____ ml per hour for _____ hours.

_____ 5. Check for residual every _____ hours with gastric feedings. Return residual to stomach. Hold feedings for 1 hour if residual is greater than _____ ml and recheck in 1 hour.

_____ 6. Routinely flush tube with _____ ml of water every _____ hours for hydration.

_____ 7. Weigh patient every Monday and Thursday and record on chart.

_____ 8. Record intake and output daily. Chart volume of formula separately from flush water or other oral intake for each shift.

_____ 9. Record number, volume, and consistency of bowel movements.

_____ 10. Change administration tubing, feeding bag, and irrigation syringe daily.

_____ 11. Obtain complete blood count, complete serum chemistry profile, and prealbumin weekly.

_____ 12. Obtain basic chemistry profile every Monday and Thursday.

_____ 13. Begin 24-hour urine collection for urea nitrogen and creatinine at 7:00 AM on _____.

_____ 14. Notify physician for nausea, vomiting, severe diarrhea, or shortness of breath.

_____ 15. Institute tube clogging protocol if unable to flush feeding tube.

REFERENCES

1. Guenter P, Jones S, Ericson M. Enteral nutrition therapy. *Nurs Clin North Am* December 1997;32:651–668.
2. Lord L, Trumbore L, Zaloga G. Enteral nutrition implementation and management. In: Merritt R, ed. *The A.S.P.E.N. Nutrition Support Manual*. Silver Spring, MD: American Society for Parenteral and Enteral Nutrition, 1998, 5-1–5-16.
3. Hiebert JM, Brown A, Anderson RG, et al. Comparison of continuous vs. intermittent tube feedings in adult burn patients. *J Parenter Enteral Nutr* 1981;5:73–75.
4. Clevenger FW, Rodriguez DJ. Decision-making for enteral feeding administration: the why behind where and how. *Nutr Clin Pract* 1995;10:104–113.
5. Guenter P, Jones S, Sweed M, et al. Delivery systems and administration of enteral nutrition. In: Rombeau JL, Rolandelli RH, eds. *Enteral and Tube Feeding*. 3rd ed. Philadelphia, PA: WB Saunders Company; 1997.
6. Forloines-Lynn S. How to smooth the way for cyclic tube feedings. *Nursing* 1996;26:57–60.
7. Bowers S. Tubes: a nurse's guide to enteral feeding devices. *MEDSURG Nursing* 1996; 5:313–326.
8. Methany N, Reed L, Worseck M, et al. How to aspirate from small-bore feeding tubes. *Am J Nurs* 1993;93:86–88.
9. McClave SA, Snider HL, Lowen CC, et al. Use of residual volume as a marker for enteral feeding intolerance: prospective blinded comparison with physical examination and radiographic findings. *J Parenter Enteral Nutr* 1992;16:99–105.
10. Murphy LM, Bickford V. Gastric residuals in tube feeding: how much is too much? *Nutr Clin Pract* 1999;14:304–306.
11. Bliss DZ, Guenter PA, Settle RG. Defining and reporting diarrhea in tube-fed patients: beginning to clean up the mess! *Am J Clin Nutr* 1992;55:753–759.
12. McClave SA, Sexton LK, Spain DA, et al. Enteral tube feeding in the intensive care unit: factors impeding adequate delivery. *Crit Care Med* 1999;27:1252–1256.
13. Savy GK. Enteral glutamine supplementation: clinical review and practice guidelines. *Nutr Clin Pract* 1997;12:259–262.
14. Association for the Advancement of Medical Instrumentation. Enteral feeding set connectors and adapters. *Nutr Clin Pract* February 1997;12:special insert.
15. Kohn-Keeth C, Shott S, Olree K. The effects of rinsing enteral delivery sets on formula contamination. *Nutr Clin Pract* 1996;11:269–273.
16. Wagner DR, Elmore MF, Knoll DM. Evaluation of "closed" vs. "open" system for the delivery of peptide-based enteral diets. *J Parenter Enteral Nutr* 1994;18:453–457.
17. Silkroski M, Allen F, Storm H. Tube feeding audit reveals hidden costs and risks of current practice. *Nutr Clin Pract* 1998;13:283–290.
18. Goff KL. The nuts and bolts of enteral infusion pumps. *MEDSURG Nursing* 1997;6:9–15.
19. Ciocon J, Galindo-Ciocon D, Thiessen C, et al. Comparison of intermittent versus continuous tube feeding among the elderly. *J Parenter Enteral Nutr* 1992;16:525–528.
20. Freeman JB, Fairhull-Smith RJ. Improved nitrogen equilibrium with constant infusion pumps in enteral feeding. *J Parenter Enteral Nutr* 1979;3:27–30.
21. Jones BJ, Payne S, Silk DB. Indications for pump assisted enteral feeding. *Lancet* 1980; 1:1057–1058.
22. Saladow J. History in the making: health care delivery and pump technology continue to evolve. *Infusion* June 1999;5:15–51.
23. Jones SA, Guenter P. Automatic flush feeding pumps: A move forward in enteral nutrition. *Nursing 97* 1997;27:56–58.

24. Brennan K, McCamish M, Ross J. The effect of automatic flushing on gastrostomy tube clogging rates (abstract). *FASEB J* 1993;7:A377.
25. Krupp K, McCamish M, Ross J. The effect of automatic flushing on nasogastric tube clogging rates (abstract). *J Am Coll Nutr* 1993;12:598.
26. Petnicki PJ. Cost savings and improved patient care with use of a flush enteral feeding pump. *Nutr Clin Pract* June 1998;13:S39–S41.
27. Ideno KT. Enteral nutrition. In: Gottschlich MM, Matarese LE, Shronts EP, eds. *Nutrition Support Dietetics Core Curriculum*. 2nd ed. Silver Spring MD: American Society for Parenteral and Enteral Nutrition; 1993.
28. Spain DA, McClave SA, Sexton LK, et al. Infusion protocol improves delivery of enteral tube feeding in the critical care unit. *J Parenter Enteral Nutr* 1999;23:288–292.

SUGGESTED READINGS

Bliss DZ, Lehmann S. Tube feeding: administration tips. *RN* August 1999;62:29–32.

Booker KJ, Niedringhaus L, Eden B, et al. Comparison of 2 methods of managing gastric residual volumes from feeding tubes. *Am J Crit Care* 2000;9:318–324.

Gottschlich MM, Fuhrman P, Hammond K, Holcombe B, Seidner D (eds) *The Science and Practice of Nutrition Support: A Case Based Core Curriculum*. Dubuque, IA: Kendall/Hunt Publishing Company, 2001.

Hebuterne X, Vaillon F, Perouz JL, et al. Correction of malnutrition following gastrectomy with cyclic enteral nutrition. *Dig Dis Sci* 1999;44:1875–1882.

Kirkland LL. Factors impeding enteral tube feedings. *Crit Care Med* 1999;27: 1383–1384.

Klodell CT, Carroll M, Carrillo EH, et al. Routine intragastric feeding following traumatic brain injury is safe and well tolerated. *Am J Surg* 2000;179:168–171.

Lord LM, Lipp J, Stull S. Adult tube feeding formulas. *MEDSURG Nursing* 1996; 5:407–432.

6

Medication
Administration

PEGGI GUENTER

The primary goal for medication administration in patients who are tube fed is to maximize the therapeutic response to the medication without adversely affecting enteral nutrition delivery and tolerance.[1] This is best accomplished using a multidisciplinary approach involving the nursing staff, pharmacist, dietitian, and physician. Knowledge of the medications, feeding tube characteristics and position, nutritional formulas and specific nursing procedures are needed, as is the medical history of the patient. Successful delivery of the medications and nutrients is key to prevention of complications such as tube occlusion and drug-nutrient interactions.

NURSING KNOWLEDGE

Two recent surveys of nursing practice demonstrated that nurses may need additional information on how to properly prepare and administer medications through feeding tubes. In a study by Seifert and colleagues,[2] 223 registered nurses (RNs) and licensed practical nurses (LPNs) who worked in a variety of health care settings reported that 50% of feeding tube obstructions were caused by medications. Even though 97% of the nurses perceived that medications given in a liquid form decreased clogging and 94% made an effort to seek liquid dose forms, only about 55% of the time did they use that dosage form; the rest of the time, crushed tablets were used. Assistance from the pharmacy department did influence administration practices. Nurses who received that assistance were significantly more likely than nurses who received no pharmacy assistance to administer liquid forms and were less likely to administer medications that needed to be crushed. Nurses who reported pharmacy assistance also reported significantly less feeding tube clogging due to medications. The survey also reported that 78% of nurses crushed and administered an enteric-coated dosage form and 50% of nurses crushed a sustained-release dosage form. Additionally, only 69% of those surveyed flushed the feeding tube with water prior to medication administration, only 59% diluted liquid medications, and 57% administered several medications together.[2] In a more general survey of nursing management of enteral tube feedings, Mateo found similar results: 47% flushed before medication delivery and only 38% flushed between medications.[3]

In order to best deliver medications through feeding tubes, the following questions need to be answered:

1. What are the properties of the medications to be administered?
2. Can this medication be crushed or does it come in liquid form?
3. Where is the tip of the feeding tube (gastric or intestinal)?
4. What is the enteral formula administration method (continuous vs. intermittent)?
5. Are there particular drug-nutrient interactions to be aware of?

The following information will aid the nurse in answering these questions so that the goal of maximizing medication therapeutic response without affecting nutrition delivery can be met.

MEDICATION CONCEPTS

The important concepts to understand for optimal medication delivery via a feeding tube include nutrient-drug incompatibilities, drug dosage forms that can or cannot be given through feeding tubes, and specific drug-nutrient interactions.

NUTRIENT-DRUG INCOMPATIBILITIES

All medications have the potential to cause incompatibilities when administered to the tube-fed patient. The types of incompatibilities are physical, pharmaceutical, physiologic, pharmacologic, and pharmacokinetic. Physical incompatibilities result in an actual physical change when substances are combined. The end result is usually a precipitate (curdling) or a change in viscosity (thickening or separation). Physical incompatibilities often cause feeding tubes to occlude. Examples of medications that cause this interaction with tube feeding formula include iron elixir, pseudoephedrine syrup, paragoric, and clarithromycin suspension.[4,5] The tube size, inner diameter of the tube lumen, and exit hole size will affect the medication flow. Pharmaceutical incompatibilities occur when there is a change in the dosage form itself that interferes with drug efficacy, potency, or tolerance. Medications in certain dosage forms, such as enteric coated or sustained release, should be evaluated by the pharmacist to determine whether the form of medication may be changed prior to delivery into a feeding tube. Physiologic incompatibilities are due to a nonpharmacologic action brought on by the medication itself or by the medium in which it is suspended. This incompatibility often occurs when liquid medications have a high osmolality or have a high sorbitol content. Patients can experience diarrhea from these medications if given undiluted. Pharmacologic incompatibilities refer to medications that alter tolerance to the tube feeding regimen because of the action of the medication itself, such as diarrhea related to generous use of prokinetic agents. Pharmacokinetic incompatibilities refer to changes that can occur with bioavailability, absorption, distribution, metabolism, and/or excretion of the medication. Impaired absorption of phenytoin due to tube feeding represents a pharmacokinetic incompatibility.[1,6]

DRUG DOSAGE FORMS THAT MAY BE ADMINISTERED VIA FEEDING TUBE

Medications that can be administered via enteral tubes include immediate-release oral tablets, soft gelatin capsules, and liquid medications. Immediate-release oral medications are the basic compressed tablets, including film or sugar-coated, and hard gelatin capsules filled with fine powder that can be opened and given via a feeding tube. Soft gelatin capsules filled with liquid can be given by poking a pinhole in the capsule and squeezing out the contents. Liquid medications are often the best alternative for administration via a feeding tube because of decreased risk of tube clogging and better absorption of the medication. However, liquid medications may cause physiologic incompatibilities such as gastrointestinal distress. Often patients are labeled as tube feeding intolerant when that distress is likely medication related.[7] The intolerance is attributed to either a high osmolality of the liquid medication or to large amounts of sorbitol required for medication formulation. This happens more often with a jejunal tube as compared with a gastric tube. The small bowel is more sensitive to higher osmotic loads. The stomach can better dilute hyperosmolar medications and/or enteral formulas. Examples of liquid medications that are often cited to be problematic include acetaminophen elixir, theophylline solution, and potassium chloride liquid. Liquid medications can be up to 6000 mOsm whereas the GI tract secretions are 300 mOsm. Some clinicians prescribe the intravenous form of a medication to be delivered via a feeding tube, as this may be the only liquid form of a medication. See Table 6–1 for some examples of hyperosmolar medications.

Sorbitol is a common additive to liquid medications. It is considered an inert ingredient and thus manufacturers are not required to list it as an ingredient, nor are they required to list the amount of sorbitol in each dose. This carbohydrate, often prescribed for its laxative effects, can cause diarrhea, bloating, or cramping, and these side effects are dose-related. See Table 6–2 for examples of medications that contain high levels of sorbitol. Lists of liquid medications with their osmolality level and sorbitol content can be found in a variety of references.[1,6,8–10]

Table 6–1 Osmolality of selected commonly used liquid medications

Medication	Average Osmolality (mOsm/kg)
Acetaminophen elixir	5400
Aminophylline liquid	450
Cimetidine solution	5550
Digoxin elixir	1350
Ferrous sulfate liquid	4700
Furosemide solution	2050
Metoclopramide syrup	8350
Multivitamin liquid	5700
Phenytoin sodium suspension	1500–2000
Potassium chloride liquid	3000–4350
Theophylline elixir	6550

Table 6–2 Sorbitol content of commonly used liquid medications

Medication	Percent Sorbitol (w/v)
Acetaminophen elixir	35.0
Cimetidine	46.1
Diazepam	21.0
Digoxin	21.0
Furosemide	49.0
Lithium	54.0
Metoclopramide	35.0
Theophylline	45.5

Medication suspensions have few compatibility problems but may be hypertonic and need dilution. Antibiotics are often in this form and may be associated with diarrhea, but it is often the antibiotic and not the dosage form that contributes to this problem. Unless these medications are diluted, the GI tract will pull water into the lumen to dilute this high osmotic load and cause osmotic diarrhea. This is especially true when the medication is delivered directly into the small intestine via a jejunostomy tube. These complications can be avoided by diluting the liquid medications with an appropriate amount of water. The following formula can be used to calculate the exact amount of water needed to bring the osmolality down to isotonic levels:

$$\text{Final volume} = \text{Volume of liquid med} \times \frac{\text{mOsm of liquid med}}{\text{desired mOsm (300–500)}}$$

then subtract the volume of liquid medication from the final volume to get the final water volume to use for dilution.[11] For example, a dilution with 30 cc of water can reduce a 10 cc amount of medication with an osmolality of 2000 mOsm/kg to 500 mOsm/kg. It is recommended that all liquid medications be diluted with at least 30 cc of water when fluid status allows.

It is important to consider the patient's clinical status when calculating additional free water needs, as some patients may be unable to tolerate the large volumes of water needed for multiple medications. Many tube-fed patients do not receive adequate amounts of water in the tube feeding formula. They may need additional flushes and tolerate liberal amounts of fluid used to dilute their medications. A general rule for water requirements is to give 35 ml per kg of body weight per day.[12]

If a liquid form of a medication is not available and the medication can be crushed, it must be pulverized to a fine powder to prevent tube clogging. A helpful device that saves nursing time in crushing and administering medications is the HandiCrush Irrigation Syringe (Nestlé Clinical Nutrition, Deerfield,

IL). This single syringe device crushes, dissolves, and administers crushable tablets and water without having to transfer the medication to another container, thus decreasing risk of contamination and loss of dose. See Figure 6–1 for an illustration of this device.

DRUG DOSAGE FORMS NOT RECOMMENDED TO BE ADMINISTERED VIA FEEDING TUBE

Crushing of enteric-coated medications can induce pharmaceutical incompatibilities; therefore, other therapeutic equivalents or administration routes should be considered. Enteric coating provides protection to the lining of the stomach, as in the case of enteric-coated aspirin. This coating also often protects the integrity of the medication from destruction in the acidic environment of the stomach. Once the medication moves into the alkaline environment of the small bowel, the enteric coating dissolves and the medication can be absorbed. An example of this type is pancrealipase (pancreatic enzymes).[13] Other medications that should not be administered via a feeding tube include sublingual or buccal medications, sustained-release tablets or capsules, and syrups. Acidic syrups hold a high risk of physical incompatibility when mixed with enteral formulas and often lead to tube clogging. A classic example of this type is iron elixir. A comprehensive list of medications that cannot be crushed can be found in a widely referenced article by Mitchell.[13] These include common slow-release medications such as Cardiazem (Hoechst Marion Roussel, Kansas City, MO), MS Contin (Purdue Frederick, Norwalk, CT), and Quinidex Extentabs (A.H. Robins, Richmond, VA) and enteric-coated medications such as Ecotrin (SmithKline Beecham, Pittsburgh, PA).

Some medications should not be given into duodenal or jejunal tubes. That is, they need to be delivered into the stomach for direct action or proper absorption. These include sucralfate and antacids. If administered into a jejunostomy tube, proton pump inhibitors such as omeprazole may need to be administered in a bicarbonate slurry in order to be best absorbed.

DRUG-NUTRIENT INTERACTIONS

There are a few medications that have been studied that are clearly influenced by enteral formulas. Drug-nutrient interactions apply to any situation in which the incompatibility involves changes in drug bioavailability, absorption, distribution, metabolism, and excretion.

Phenytoin: Impaired absorption of phenytoin is a pharmacokinetic incompatibility and is well documented in the literature.[14,15] There appears to be an impairment in absorption but the exact mechanism is yet to be defined. Possible reasons for this interaction include the protein source in the enteral formula (calcium caseinate) binding the drug, binding of the drug to the feeding tube, or poor solubility of the phenytoin itself and thus poor absorption. Phenytoin doses may need to be increased in tube-fed patients in order to maintain therapeutic blood levels. There are several medication administration strategies that can be

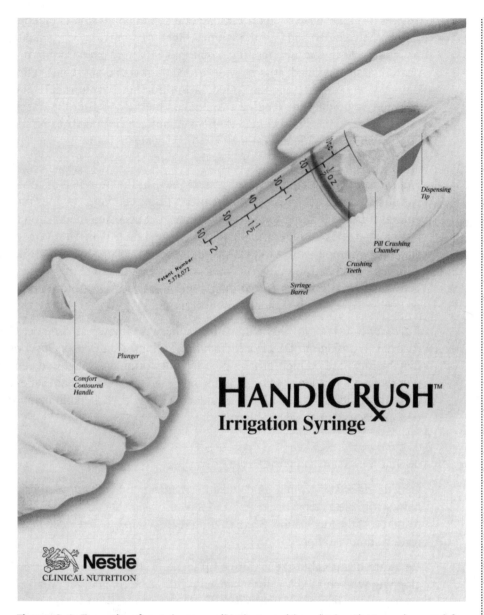

Figure 6–1 Example of a syringe medication-crushing device that can be used for medication delivery as well

used to promote optimal therapeutic levels. These include (1) holding the feeding 2 hours before and after the phenytoin dose and adjusting the tube feeding schedule to meet nutritional requirements, (2) diluting the phenytoin with 30 ml of water to enhance solubility and improve absorption, and (3) monitoring blood phenytoin levels carefully, especially if the patient is changing tube feeding regimens or moving from the parenteral to enteral dosage form.[14,15]

Warfarin: Resistance to warfarin has been documented in case reports and is believed to be related to the vitamin K content of formulas.[16] Subsequently, enteral formulas have been reformulated to contain only small amounts of vitamin K (between 10 and 75 micrograms/ liter).[17] Even with these small amounts of vitamin K in the tube feeding, some patients may have trouble being adequately anticoagulated. It is helpful to maintain stable and consistent formula delivery to facilitate accurate medication dosing. Formula delivery can be adjusted by holding the feeding 1 to 2 hours before and after the warfarin dose in order to increase absorption. Anticoagulant activity needs to be monitored closely while the patient is on tube feedings; evaluate warfarin dose, anticoagulant goals, and parameters closely as the patient transitions to an oral diet.[18]

Ciprofloxacin: The ciprofloxacin is decreased in the presence of tube feeding formula. This is secondary to the cations (e.g., calcium, magnesium) in the enteral formula binding to the medication.[19,20] Suggested medication administration strategies include dissolving the crushed drug with 50 ml of water and flushing the tube well with 120 ml of water to ensure maximum delivery.[1] Alternate medication delivery times with intermittent feeding doses; do not give together. Strategies for holding continuous feedings before and after the drug dose have not been thoroughly researched.

Carbidopa-levodopa: This medication, otherwise known as Sinemet (Dupont Pharma, Wilmington, DE) is a therapy for Parkinson's disease. Onset of action may be impaired by high-protein tube feeding formulas. Suggested administration therapies include holding tube feeding 1 hour before and after the Sinemet dose or providing tube feeding continuously at night, thus maximizing medication efficacy during waking hours.[21]

MEDICATION ADMINISTRATION PROCEDURE

General rules and written guidelines for medication administration can provide nurses with clear steps to take to avoid tube occlusion and to optimize therapeutic response of the medication. See Exhibit 6–1 for a step-by-step procedure for medication administration.

Be aware of the tube size and tube tip location. It is important to prevent tube clogging with small diameter tubes, and if the tube tip is in the small bowel, be aware of the osmotic sensitivity of this area and dilute liquid medications accordingly. General rules for delivering medications via enteral feeding tubes include the following: Use the oral route if at all possible. If the tube must be used, use liquid medications. Flush before and after medication administration with 30 ml of water. Dilute liquid medications with at least 30 ml of water to decrease osmolality. Avoid mixing any medications with the feeding formula. If liquid medications are not available, check to see that the tablet medication can be crushed. Administer each medication separately to avoid drug-drug interactions and flush well between with 15–30 ml of water. Consider the timing of the medication; check whether it should be given on an empty or a full stomach. Provide exact tube location information to the dispensing pharmacist in order to best provide the correct dosage form. Use only water to flush tubes, as cranberry juice or cola may actually promote tube occlusion.

Exhibit 6–1 Step-by-step medication administration procedure

1. Verify tube placement.
2. Check tube for patency and flush with 30 ml of water. Use a syringe no smaller than 30 ml to avoid excessive pressure and potential tube rupture.
3. Prepare medication by diluting liquid medication with 30 ml of water or by crushing tablet with a mortar and pestle to a fine powder and mix with water. A tablet-crushing syringe is now available that allows for crushing meds, drawing up water, and administering medication all with one device (HandiCrush, Clintec Nutrition, Deerfield, IL).
4. Connect syringe to medication port on tube or to end of tube if medication port not available and gently push in medication.
5. Flush tube with 30 ml water and administer next medication.
6. Flush tube well following all medications to assure patency and reconnect feeding bag unless otherwise contraindicated (such as with phenytoin).

CONCLUSION

By maximizing the therapeutic response to medication and preventing occlusion of the drug delivery access, the patient receiving enteral nutrition will have optimal feeding outcomes.

REFERENCES

1. Johnson DR, Nyffeler MS. Drug-nutrient considerations for enteral nutrition. In: Merritt R, ed. *The A.S.P.E.N. Nutrition Support Practice Manual.* Silver Spring, MD: American Society for Parenteral and Enteral Nutrition; 1998: 6-1–6-20.
2. Seifert CF, Frye JL, Belknap DC, Anderson DC. A nursing survey to determine the characteristics of medication administration through enteral feeding catheters. *Clin Nurs Res* August 1995;4:290–305.
3. Mateo MA. Management of enteral tubes. Nursing management of enteral tube feedings. *Heart Lung* 1996;25:318–323.
4. Cutie AJ, Altman E, Lenkel L. Compatibility of enteral products with commonly employed drug additives. *J Parenter Enteral Nutr* 1983;7:186–191.
5. Burns PE, McCall L, Wirsching R. Physical compatibility of enteral formulas with various common medications. *J Am Diet Assoc* 1998;88:1094–1096.
6. Thomson CA, Rollins CJ. Nutrient-drug interactions. In: Rombeau JL, Rolandelli RH, eds. *Enteral and Tube Feeding.* 3rd ed. Philadelphia, PA: WB Saunders Company; 1997: 523–539.
7. Edes TE, Walk BE, Austin JL. Diarrhea in tube-fed patients: feeding formula not necessarily the cause. *Am J Med* 1990;88:91–93.
8. Guenter P, Jones S, Ericson M. Enteral nutrition therapy. *Nurs Clinics North Am* December 1997;32:651–668.
9. Dickerson RN, Melnik G. Osmolality of oral drug solutions and suspensions. *Am J Hosp Pharm* 1988;45:832–834.
10. Lutomski DM, Gore ML, Wright SM, et al. Sorbitol content of selected oral liquids. *Ann Pharmacotherapy* 1993;27:269–274.

11. Estoup M. Approaches and limitations of medication delivery in patients with enteral feeding tubes. *Crit Care Nurse* 1994;14:68–81.

12. Ireton-Jones CS, Hennessy K, Orr M. Care of patients receiving home enteral nutrition. *Infusion* March 1996;2:30–43.

13. Mitchell JF. Oral dosage forms that should not be crushed:1998 update. *Hospital Pharmacy* 1998;33:399–415.

14. Bauer LA. Interference of oral phenytoin absorption by continuous nasogastric feeding. *Neurology* 1982;32:570–572.

15. Gilbert S, Hatton J. How to minimize interaction between phenytoin and enteral feedings: two approaches. *Nutr Clin Pract* 1996;11:28–31.

16. Martin JE, Lutomski DM. Warfarin resistance and enteral feedings. *J Parenter Enteral Nutr* 1989;13:206–208.

17. Melnick G. Pharmacologic aspects of enteral nutrition. In: Rombeau JL, Caldwell MD, eds. *Enteral and Tube Feeding*. 2nd ed. Philadelphia, PA: WB Saunders Company; 1990.

18. Speerhas RA. Administering medications with enteral feedings. *Support Line* 1994;16:1–4.

19. Wright DH, Pietz SL, Konstantinides FN, Rotschafer JC. Decreased in vitro fluoro-quinolone concentrations after admixture with an enteral feeding formulation. *J Parenter Enteral Nutr* 2000;24:42–48.

20. Nyffler MS. Ciprofloxacin use in the enterally fed patient. *Nutr Clin Pract* 1999;14:73–77.

21. Hurka B. Pharmacotherapy for Parkinson's disease. *Advance for Nurses* February 28, 2000;2:8–11.

SUGGESTED READINGS

Beckwirth MC, Barton RG, Graves C. A guide to drug therapy in patients with enteral feeding tubes: dosage form selection and administration methods. *Hosp Pharm* 1997;32:57–64.

Brown RO, Dickerson RN. Drug-nutrient interactions. *Am J Manag Care* 1999;5:345–355.

Cerulli J, Malone M. Assessment of drug-related problems in clinical nutrition patients. *J Parenter Enteral Nutr* 1999;23:218–221.

Chan LN. Redefining drug-nutrient interactions. *Nutr Clin Pract* 2000;15:249–252.

Engle KK, Hannawa TE. Techniques for administering oral medications to critical care patients receiving continuous enteral nutrition. *Am J Health Syst Pharm* 1999;56:1441–1444.

Gottschlich MM, Fuhrman P, Hammond K, Holcombe B, Seidner D (eds) *The Science and Practice of Nutrition Support: A Case Based Core Curriculum*. Dubuque, IA: Kendall/Hunt Publishing Company, 2001.

Klang M. Medicating tube-fed patients. *Nursing 96* 1996;26:18.

Miyagawa C. Drug-nutrient interactions in critically ill patients. *Crit Care Nurse* October 1993;69–90.

RESOURCES

Pronsky ZW. *Food Medication Interactions*. Pottstown, PA: Food-Medication
Interactions; 1995.
To Order:
PO Box 659
Pottstown, PA 19464
1–800–746–2324
www.foodmedinteractions.com
Medscape (Need to register but at no charge; you can access site and under Drugs sec-
tion can get full medication profile with food-drug interactions)
www.medscape.com

7

Enteral Nutrition Complications

PEGGI GUENTER

Tube feeding, although a relatively safe method of nutritional support, has been associated with major and minor complications, many of which can be prevented or treated. Complications associated with enteral nutrition are generally classified into three main types: mechanical, gastrointestinal, and metabolic. This chapter will review tube feeding–related complications including detection, prevention, and treatment measures. A comprehensive list of common complications, possible causes, and treatment measures can be found in Table 7–1.[1] Most complications can be prevented with close monitoring and timely and accurate assessment of patients' tolerance to feedings. The nurse plays a vital role in making these observations and can easily assist in complication prevention and treatment. Clinical pathways are useful tools allowing clinicians to track patient outcomes related to enteral therapy and to document variances as they occur.[2]

MECHANICAL COMPLICATIONS

Mechanical complications can most often be prevented with vigilant nursing care. These complications can be categorized into 5 types: tube displacement, tube injury, tube clogging, injury due to presence of the tube, and pulmonary aspiration. Each of these complications will be defined, causes identified, prevention measures noted, and interventions suggested. Details on tube insertion complications can be found in Chapter 3, Enteral Feeding Access Devices, and exit site complications in Chapter 4, Nursing Care of Patients with Enteral Feeding Devices.

TUBE DISPLACEMENT

Displacement can occur by the tube either sliding into or being pulled out of the GI tract. If a gastrostomy tube slides down into the lower stomach, the distal end can block the gastric outlet, causing nausea and vomiting. An unsecured jejunal tube can be pulled by peristalsis further into the small bowel, causing obstruction, or can be pulled out. If the internal gastric balloon becomes deflated or if the external tube suture, bumper, or disk is inadvertently removed, the tube may slide out and the tube tract will quickly close. This loss of enteral access will often precipitate a return to the operating, endoscopy, or radiology suite for tube replacement. Having the tube tip out of position may also deliver the formula into the wrong anatomical area such as into the esophagus or peritoneal cavity, potentially causing aspiration or peritonitis.[3]

Causes of displacement include intense coughing, nasotracheal suctioning or vomiting, accidental pulling on the tube by patients or staff, or loss of a secur-

Table 7–1 Common complications associated with enteral feeding

Complications	Possible Causes	Prevention
Mechanical		
Tube occlusion	Inadequate flushing	Routine flush
	Administration of crushed meds	Use liquid meds
Site breakdown	Exit site tube movement	Stabilize tube, skin care protocol
Tube displacement	Improper securing of tube	Secure tube
Aspiration	Improper tube placement	Verify placement
	Improper patient position	Keep head of bed up
	Neurologic impairment	Recommend post-pyloric feeding
Gastrointestinal		
Nausea or vomiting	Delayed gastric emptying	Monitor residuals
	Medications	Review meds
	Tube displacement	Verify placement
	Improper patient position	Keep head of bed up
	Rapid infusion rate	Decrease rate
Diarrhea	Rapid infusion rate	Decrease rate
	Hyperosmolar feedings or meds	Dilute formula and meds
	Lactose intolerance	Use lactose-free formulas
	Antibiotic therapy	D/C antibiotics
	Hypoalbuminemia	Improve nutritional status
	Formula contamination	Infection control measures
	Low residue formula	Use fiber formula
Constipation	Low-residue formula	Use fiber formula
	Dehydration	Give adequate fluid
	Inactivity	Exercise program
	Medications	D/C constipating meds
Metabolic		
Dehydration	Fever or infection	Treat infection
	Inadequate fluid intake	Give adequate fluid
	Excessive fluid losses	Prevent and replace losses
Elevated serum electrolytes	Excessive electrolytes in formula	Change formula
	Inadequate fluid intake	Give adequate fluid
	Excessive fluid losses	Prevent losses
Depressed serum electrolytes	Excessive water administration	Hold water flush
		Use calorically dense formula
	Inadequate electrolyte intake	Change formula
Hyperglycemia	Metabolic stress	Reduce stress
	History of diabetes	Administer insulin
	Excessive glucose intake	Change formula to lower CHO

CHO = Carbohydrate

ing device such as tape, suture, gastrostomy disk, or balloon.[4] The incidence of accidental tube removal varies from less than 1% in one large series of surgically placed jejunostomies[5] up to 68% with small-bore nasoenteric feeding tubes, the most commonly displaced.[3]

Prevention of tube displacement can be accomplished using a combination of measures. Using the external marks on the tube, assess the length of the tube outside of the body. If no marks exist on the tube, place a mark at the level of the exit site and document this length in the nursing record. The external length needs to be verified by the nurse on each subsequent shift. The nurse should check that the disk, suture, or attachment device holding the tube externally is secure and the attached tubing set is not being pulled on by the patient or staff. Assess the residual tube fluid for presence of GI secretions (gastric juice or bile) to determine that the tube is within the GI tract. Sometimes flushing the tube with 5 to 10 ml of air will allow for residual volume to be pulled out. If you are unable to pull any fluid from the tube and suspect the tube has migrated, a confirmatory x-ray may be required prior to restarting feedings. A number of tube-anchoring devices are available on the market to help secure the tubes (see Chapter 4 for further details). Signs of displacement include difficulty in infusing formula or flushing, leakage of fluid around the exit site, change in length of external portion of the tube,[4] and, of course, absence of the tube from the nose or stoma site.

If the feeding tube is suspected to have been dislodged, the formula should obviously be discontinued. It is essential that the tube be replaced or repositioned within a few hours to ensure adequate caloric intake and/or prevent closure of the tract. Depending on practice area, practice act or privileges, and the type of tube, the nurse may be able to replace or reposition the feeding tube. Otherwise, the physician should be notified immediately and arrangements made for replacement. Patient and/or staff must be reeducated on methods to prevent further tube displacement.

TUBE INJURY

Tube injury includes tube rupture, detachment of the weighted end,[6] tube deterioration, or balloon breakage. Causes of tube injury include perforation of the tube with the inserting guidewire, injecting more than the allowable volume into the securing balloon, flushing with a syringe smaller than 30 ml (this increases pressure per square inch, causing tube rupture), and deterioration of the tube material due to prolonged exposure to acidic gastric fluids.[7] Feeding tubes are not routinely replaced, and the life of a tube can be extended with preventive measures. Follow a regular flushing schedule, using a syringe larger than 30 ml in size. Inspect the tube for cracking, wall aneurysm areas, and deteriorating anchoring devices. Never reinsert a guidewire into a nasoenteric feeding tube while it is in place. Check the internal balloon for proper inflation every 7 to 10 days by withdrawing the balloon fluid, noting the volume, and comparing that to the amount initially injected into the balloon. If it is significantly less, refill the balloon with the correct volume and check again in 1 hour. If the balloon has lost more fluid, it is leaking and the tube needs to be replaced. Document the date and time that the balloon was checked and the amount of fluid instilled into the balloon. If a tube injury occurs at the connection to the feeding bag, it can sometimes be repaired using an available tube adapter. Request that a damaged or worn tube be replaced as soon as possible.[8]

TUBE OCCLUSION

Tube occlusion or clogging is one of the most frequent complications of enteral nutrition. Occlusions in general can be caused by inappropriate administration of medications, poor flushing techniques, thick formulas, formulation contamination that leads to coagulation, or even reflux of gastric or intestinal contents up into the tube. This change in pH from digestive enzymes mixing with the formula's intact protein in the tube tip causes protein denaturation (similar to curdling) and thus a clog in the tube.[9] In one study, tube clogging occurred significantly more often in continuous rather than intermittent[10] feedings. This led to the conclusion that nurses need to flush the tubes with water even though the patient is on a continuous infusion of formula.

Many nurses use a variety of flush fluids to prevent clogging or restore patency for occluded tubes. Cranberry juice and carbonated cola beverages have been used and noted in the literature. These beverages are acidic and may actually contribute to tube clogging from protein denaturation. Water has been shown thus far to be the best flush solution.[11] Flushing with 20 to 30 ml of water before and after checking for residuals, administering medications, or intermittent feedings—and every 4 to 6 hours during continuous feedings—is ideal for preventing tube occlusion. Other clogging-prevention measures include choosing the appropriate size tube to maximize formula flow (usually 8 French or greater), selecting a less calorically dense formula, and using a feeding pump with an automatic water flush feature.[12] General rules and written guidelines for medication administration can provide nursing staff with clear steps to take to avoid tube occlusion and optimize therapeutic response of the medication. See Chapter 6, Medication Administration, for further details.

If an occlusion does occur, immediate attention to the clog is important. The first step would be to check whether the feeding tube is kinked. Once you have determined that the tube is straight, place your flushing syringe into the tube end and gently pull back on the plunger to dislodge the clog. If the blockage remains, instill warm water into the tube. Gentle pressure alternating with syringe suction will relieve most obstructions. The tube can also be milked with the fingers from the insertion site out. A successful technique of declogging includes instillation of a pancreatic enzyme and sodium bicarbonate solution as described by Mancuard.[13] See Exhibit 7–1 for detailed instructions for this unclogging procedure.

Another product, which combines a thin hollow catheter and chemical declogging powder to be put into solution and instilled into the clog via the catheter, has met with success as well (Clog-Zapper, CORPAK Medsystems, Wheeling, IL).[9] See Figures 7–1 and 7–2 for an illustration of this product.

A few noteworthy mechanical instruments to unclog tubes are now available. These instruments include a plastic declogger device with a corkscrew tip and a cytology brush. These devices are inserted into the feeding tube and mechanically break up the clog by using a twisting motion.[14] These devices must be premeasured so that they do not exceed the tube length and cause mucosal damage. They include the Declogger (Bionix, Toledo, OH) and the PEG Cleaning Brush

Exhibit 7–1 Procedure for unclogging feeding tube

1. With a 30–60 ml irrigation syringe, aspirate as much liquid as possible from the feeding tube and discard the fluid.

2. Instill 5–10 ml of warm water with that same syringe under manual pressure for 1 minute and use a back-and-forth motion to help dislodge the clot.

3. Clamp the tube for 5–15 minutes.

4. Try to aspirate and flush with warm water.

5. If tube remains clogged, repeat the above procedure with the following solution: 1 crushed sodium bicarbonate tablet (325 mg) and 1 crushed Viokase tablet dissolved in 5 ml of water.

(Bard Interventional Products, Billerica, MA). Prior to using any of these devices or products, be sure that your nursing practice act or clinical privileges allow for such procedures. These mechanical devices should generally be used only by practitioners experienced in using such devices due to the risk of tube rupture.

FEEDING TUBE INJURY TO SURROUNDING TISSUES

Injuries can occur to surrounding tissues due to the presence of a feeding tube. These include nasal pressure necrosis due to improper taping of a nasoenteric tube, nasopharyngeal erosion, and stomach or duodenal ulceration. These complications occur more often with larger, stiffer tubes that are in place for gastric decompression. To prevent these problems, tape the tube to the nose properly and use smaller, softer tubes specifically designed for tube feeding and for use when the patient no longer needs decompression.

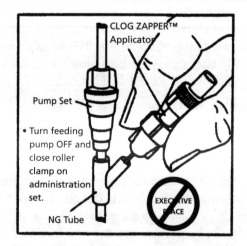

Figure 7–1 Commercially available feeding tube declogging system—insertion of applicator

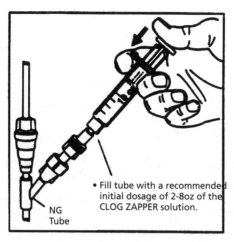

Figure 7–2 Commercially available feeding tube declogging system—infusion of clog zapper solution

ASPIRATION

Aspiration is defined as entry of material from the oropharynx into the larynx below the true vocal folds. Patients can aspirate oral secretions (most commonly), or refluxed stomach contents containing tube feeding formula.[15] Although aspiration of tube feeding formula into the lungs is a less frequently reported complication of enteral nutrition, it represents a significant hazard because it may cause pneumonia, asphyxiation, and/or death. Aspiration pneumonia is especially serious in the debilitated, frail elderly patient whose ability to fight infection is diminished. Much of what the nurse does in administering tube feedings is directed at preventing this event. The literature varies on how often aspiration pneumonia actually occurs in tube-fed patients, and the associated risk factors are not clearly defined. Conflicting reports exist about the frequency with which pulmonary aspiration occurs, ranging from less than 1% to 40%.[16] This may be due to the lack of consensus on a set definition of aspiration and the lack of a clinically practical method of measuring aspiration.

Associated risk factors most frequently mentioned in the literature include: a reduced level of consciousness that is often associated with diminished cough or gag reflex,[17] ileus or gastroparesis,[18] use of a large bore nasoenteric feeding tube,[19] dislodgement of tubes,[20] failure to elevate head of bed during feedings,[21] older age,[22] mechanical ventilation,[23] and those with previous history of pneumonia.[24] Signs and symptoms of aspiration include restlessness, decreased level of consciousness, or dyspnea that may indicate hypoxia. The patient may also have a new onset productive cough, wheezing, rales, rhonchi, or fever.[25]

Many patients aspirate without overt symptoms and thus detection is key to both prevention and treatment. First it is vital to determine whether the patient is aspirating oral secretions or tube feeding. This can be accomplished by adding blue dye to the tube feedings and noting the color of expectorated or suctioned respiratory secretions. Recovery of blue-tinged tracheal secretions is considered evidence of aspiration.[15] For years nurses have added either blue food coloring or methylene blue to tube feedings. There are several disadvantages and controversies associated with this practice. Food coloring can become contaminated and cause bacterial infections.[26] Methylene blue is not indicated for internal use, does not mix well with enteral formula, can be absorbed into the tissue, and should not be used. There are now commercially available sterile, single-use blue dyes that can be added to the tube feeding. There are also pre-colored, prefilled formula bags available. See Table 7–2 for some of those products and manufacturers.[27]

The other questions about use of blue dye to detect aspiration is when to use it, for how long, and how specific it is. Speaking simply from experience and anecdotal data, it should probably not be used routinely in all patients on enteral nutrition. It should be used in high-risk patients on an individual basis when aspiration is suspected, and then only for a few days until aspiration is ruled in or out. The specificity and sensitivities on this test remain questionable—that is, it does not definitely always determine presence or absence of aspiration.

Another detection method discussed in the literature is the use of glucose oxidase reagent strips to check the presence of glucose in tracheal secretions. This methodology is based on the assumption that tracheal secretions do not contain measurable amounts of glucose whereas enteral nutrition formulas do contain significant glucose.[15] There are questions about this method as well, in that investigators have found glucose in tracheal secretions without a patient receiving enteral nutrition.[28.] Some clinicians have abandoned this method[15] while others continue to support it.[29,30]

Nursing methods to decrease the potential for pulmonary aspiration in patients receiving tube feeding should be utilized. These include elevating the head of the bed 30 to 45 degrees, checking gastric residuals every 4 to 6 hours and holding if greater than 100 to 150 ml, using small-bore feeding tubes, using continuous feedings, using percutaneous endoscopic gastrostomy (PEG) tubes instead of nasogastric tubes, and feeding beyond the stomach into the small bowel when possible. Although none of these suggestions has been thoroughly proven to decrease risk, they are the best practice guidelines to follow until further research is completed.[31]

Table 7–2 Commercially available blue dyes to add to tube feeding

Product	Manufacturer
Steriblue single-use 5 ml ampule	Nestlé Clinical Nutrition Deerfield, IL
Blue Dye single-use 4 ml ampule	Novartis Minneapolis, MN
Flexiflo Colormark Pump Set: Solid tablet of dye in drip chamber	Ross Products Division Columbus, OH

Gastrointestinal complications associated with enteral nutrition include nausea, vomiting, diarrhea, and constipation. These are often the most frustrating and limiting complications for both the nurse and the patient. A very important role of the nurse is to quantify and document these conditions, as this information will help in diagnosis and treatment of these complications.

Nausea, vomiting, or gastroparesis can be caused by medications, critical illness, rapid formula infusion rate, diabetes, neurological dysfunction, or improper tube placement.[1] A large recent study in critically ill patients found that 39% of patients had high gastric residuals and 12% had vomiting.[32] Treatment for these problems includes assessing the medication list for drugs that contribute to these symptoms and eliminating or changing them when possible. The clinician needs to evaluate the patient's current clinical status and its effect on GI function. Checking and documenting residual volumes is essential. Occasionally patients receiving jejunal feedings need gastric decompression via an NG tube to alleviate these problems. On occasion, changing the formula, reducing the infusion rate, or adding a prokinetic agent can help with the intolerance.

Diarrhea is a commonly described problem in patients receiving tube feeding with the incidence ranging from 2.3% to 63%[33,34] depending on which study is cited and how the problem is defined. Diarrhea is generally defined in the clinical setting as the passage of more than 200 grams of stool per day, but it is more frequently defined as 3 or more liquid stools per day.[35] Stool may be more soft or pasty than usual with tube feedings. Common causes for this problem include medications (either hyperosmolar medications or antibiotics), as discussed in Chapter 6; GI infection; rapid or bolus infusion; formula contamination, as discussed in Chapter 5, Tube Feeding Administration; GI dysfunction (hypermotility, malabsorption, or fecal impaction); or hyperosmolar or low-fiber formula. The cause of diarrhea is often multifactorial, particularly in critically ill patients.[36] The clinician must consider each one of these factors to identify the cause and adjust the plan of care. Simply turning off the tube feeding usually does not correct the problem and will result in underfeeding. See Table 7–3 for a list of common causes and prevention and treatment measures for tube feeding–related diarrhea.

It is essential that the nurse quantify the stool output in a fashion that can be serially tracked over time in order to assess treatment effectiveness. Nurses often state that patients have "diarrhea" whether they have 3 loose stools or 12 watery stools per day. Exhibits 7–2 and 7–3 illustrate a valid and reliable stool assessment tool for nurses. The patient receives a daily stool output score that quantifies the condition.[37]

In general, while the exact cause of the diarrhea is being determined, symptom management can begin. The patient's stool must be collected and checked for infection, particularly *Clostridium difficile*, before antimotility agents can be used. Nursing measures include:[38]

Table 7–3 Common causes and management of tube feeding–associated diarrhea

Potential Cause	Management Option
Infectious Process	Reduce potential formula contamination
	Narrow or discontinue antibiotic course
	Treat identified pathogen
Formula Related	Use lactose-free and fiber-containing formulas
	Avoid hyperosmolar formulas
	Change to peptide-based formula
	Slow rate or return to previously tolerated regimen
Medications	Dilute hyperosmolar medications
	Avoid medications with high sorbitol content
	Avoid magnesium containing antacids or laxatives

- Provide adequate fluid and electrolyte replacement
- Monitor and document associations between administration of enteral nutrition or medications and change in stool output
- Administer antidiarrheal agents
- Maintain perianal skin integrity
- Provide psychosocial support

Perineal pouching using the Drainable Fecal Incontinence Collector (Hollister, Libertyville, IL) during fecal incontinence prevents skin breakdown and adds to patient comfort.[39]

Antidiarrheal medications include antimotility agents such as loperamide, diphenoxylate with atropine paragoric, or tincture of opium, all of which slow GI motility to decrease diarrhea, and adsorbents such as kaolin-pectin, which adsorb bacteria and toxins and reduce water loss.[14] Nurses should work closely with the physician and pharmacist to develop the best antidiarrheal medication regimen tailored to each individual patient. Antidiarrheal agents not considered standard medications include fiber sources and probiotics. Fiber sources made of soluble fiber such as pectin are from citrus or banana sources. One product that has met with good success and found to have a significant impact on a group of enterally fed patients with diarrhea[40] is Kanana Banana Flakes (CORPAK MedSystems, Wheeling, IL). Two tablespoons of the flakes can be mixed with 50 ml of warm water three times per day administered like a medication; then flush well with water and restart feedings. This can be added to begin symptom management of the diarrhea even before the *Clostridium difficile* test results come back. Some clinicians also use probiotics such as active acidophilus yogurt cultures or lactobacillus (Lactinex, Becton Dickinson Microbial, Franklin Lakes, NJ) powder or tablets to recolonize the colon following broad spectrum antibiotic–induced diarrhea.

Constipation is another gastrointestinal complication associated with enteral nutrition and can be caused by lack of adequate hydration, long term fiber-free feedings, bedrest, impaction, obstruction, and narcotics. Prevention and treatment include assuring adequate hydration, including fiber in the formula, restricting narcotic and antimotility agents, promoting activity and exercise, and

Exhibit 7–2 Stool output assessment tool

DATE: _____

	CONSISTENCY		
VOLUME	**SOLID FORMED**	**SOFT PASTY**	**LIQUID WATERY**
SMALL	1	2	3
LARGE	3	6	9

Rate each stool from the stool output assessment tool (Appendix A) and then add individual stool scores for 24-hour period to derive total stool output score _____

utilizing stool softeners and laxatives as needed.[14] Obtaining a history of what laxatives the patient has used in the past can be helpful. A thorough discussion on managing constipation can be found in a review by Hall and colleagues.[41]

METABOLIC COMPLICATIONS

Metabolic complications include alterations in hydration, hyperglycemia, and elevated or depressed electrolyte and mineral levels. Dehydration can occur due to inadequate fluid intake or excessive fluid losses through diarrhea, diuresis, ostomies, fistulae, wounds, or fever. Determining the patient's baseline fluid requirements coupled with accurate intake and output measurements will help maintain optimal fluid balance. Usually the fluid requirements can be met with water flushes for patency and medication administration. Additional water can be scheduled throughout the day as needed. Patients with automatic flush pumps can receive additional water via those pumps each day to meet these fluid requirements.[12] Overhydration during enteral feeding is possible when organ function (cardiac, renal, or hepatic) is impaired.

Hyperglycemia can occur with enteral nutrition but not as often as with parenteral nutrition. It is most common in patients with diabetes, metabolic stress,

Exhibit 7–3 Daily scoring form for the Stool Output Assessment Tool

TIME	VOLUME		CONSISTENCY		
	SMALL (<1/2 CUP)	LARGE (>1/2 CUP)	SOLID FORMED	SOFT PASTY	LIQUID WATERY
6 AM					
7 AM					
8 AM					
9 AM					
10 AM					
11 AM					
12 NOON					
1 PM					
2 PM					
3 PM					
4 PM					
5 PM					
6 PM					
7 PM					
8 PM					
9 PM					
10 PM					
11 PM					
12 MN					
1 AM					
2 AM					
3 AM					
4 AM					
5 AM					

or sepsis in which cellular glucose utilization is impaired or there is use of steroids or excessive glucose administration. Management of this complication includes reducing the glucose load, eliminating the source of stress and sepsis, administering insulin, or reducing steroids if possible. Sometimes a formula higher in fat and lower in carbohydrate can be helpful.[12]

Electrolyte and mineral abnormalities like hyperkalemia can occur with enteral nutrition but are uncommon. Refeeding syndrome—a state of hypokalemia, hypophosphatemia, and hypomagnesemia—can occur when enteral nutrition therapy is administered to a severely malnourished individual.[42] Formula components and the patient's disease and medical condition can contribute to those abnormalities in electrolyte and mineral levels and should be monitored frequently, especially in the early feeding stages. It is important to know the amounts of electrolytes and minerals in each of the formulas to know if a patient with potential for elevated or depressed levels will run into problems.

CONCLUSION

Complications related to enteral nutrition can often be prevented or detected early with optimal nursing care. Complication prevention will allow the patient to receive an adequate level of the nutrition required during illness recovery.

REFERENCES

1. Guenter P, Jones S, Sweed MR, et al. Delivery systems and administration of enteral nutrition. In: Rombeau JL, Rolandelli RH, eds. *Enteral and Tube Feeding*. 3rd ed. Philadelphia, PA: WB Saunders Company; 1997.
2. Board of Directors, American Society for Parenteral and Enteral Nutrition. *Clinical Pathways and Algorithms for Delivery of Parenteral and Enteral Nutrition Support in Adults*. Silver Spring, MD: American Society for Parenteral and Enteral Nutrition; 1997.
3. Hamaoui E, Kodsi R. Complications of enteral feeding and their prevention. In: Rombeau JL, Rolandelli RH, eds. *Enteral and Tube Feeding*. 3rd ed. Philadelphia, PA: WB Saunders Company; 1997:554–574.
4. Ireton-Jones CS, Hennessy K, Orr M. Care of patients receiving home enteral nutrition. *Infusion* March 1996;2:30–43.
5. Myers JG, Page CP, Stewart RM, et al. Complications of needle catheter jejunostomy in 2,022 consecutive applications. *Am J Surg* 1995;170:547–551.
6. Sood AK, Pardubsky PD, Gacuson M, et al. Nasoenteric tube complication: a case report of tip detachment. *Nutr Clin Pract* 1998;13:40–42.
7. Gowen GF. The management of complications of Foley feeding gastrostomies. *Am Surg* 1988;54:582–585.
8. Bowers S. Tubes: A nurses' guide to enteral feeding devices. *MEDSURG Nursing* 1996; 5:313–324.
9. Frankel EH, Enow NB, Jackson KC, et al. Methods of restoring patency to occluded feeding tubes. *Nutr Clin Pract* 1998;13:129–131.
10. Ciocon J, Galindo-Ciocon D, Thiessen C, et al. Comparison of intermittent versus continuous tube feeding among the elderly. *J Parenter Enteral Nutr* 1992;16:525–528.
11. Methany N, Eisenberg P, McSweeney M. Effect of feeding tube properties and three irrigants on clogging rates. *Nurs Res* 1988;37:165–169.
12. Jones SA, Guenter P. Automatic flush feeding pumps: a move forward in enteral nutrition. *Nursing 97* 1997;27:56–58.
13. Mancuard SP, Stegall KL, Trogdon S. Clearing obstructed feeding tubes. *J Parenter Enteral Nutr* 1989;13:81–83.
14. Lord L, Trumbore L, Zaloga G. Enteral nutrition implementation and management. In: Merritt R, ed. *The A.S.P.E.N. Nutrition Support Practice Manual*. Silver Spring, MD: American Society for Parenteral and Enteral Nutrition; 1998:5-1–5-16.

15. Elpern EH. Pulmonary aspiration in hospitalized adults. *Nutr Clin Pract* 1997;12:5–13.
16. Methany NA, Eisenberg P, Spies M. Aspiration pneumonia in patients fed through nasoenteral tubes. *Heart Lung* 1986;15:256–261.
17. Cameron J, Zuidema G. Aspiration pneumonia: magnitude and frequency of the problem. *JAMA* 1972;19:1194–1196.
18. Bartlett J, Gorbach S. The triple threat of aspiration pneumonia. *Chest* 1975;68:550–556.
19. Del Rio D, Williams K, Miller B. *Handbook of Enteral Nutrition.* El Segundo, CA: Medical Specifics Publishing; 1982.
20. Murphy L, Hostetler C. Tube feeding reconsidered. *Natl Intravenous Ther Assoc* 1981; 4:409–412.
21. Taylor T. A comparison of two methods of nasogastric tube feedings. *J Neurosurg Nurs* 1982;14:49–52.
22. Winterbauer RH, Durning RB, Barron E, McFadden MC. Aspirated nasogastric feeding solution detected by glucose strips. *Ann Int Med*;95:67–68.
23. Elpern EH, Scott MD, Petro L, et al. Pulmonary aspiration in mechanically ventilated patients with tracheostomies. *Chest* 1994;105:563–566.
24. Cogen R, Weinryb J. Aspiration pneumonia in nursing home patients fed via gastrostomy tubes. *Am J Gastro* 1989;84:1509–1512.
25. Davis AE, Arrington K, Fields-Ryan S, et al. Preventing feeding-associated aspiration. *MEDSURG Nurs* 1995;4:111–119.
26. File TM, Tan JS, Thomson RB, et al. An outbreak of Pseudomonas aeruginosa ventilator-associated respiratory infections due to contaminated food coloring dye—further evidence of the significance of gastric colonization preceding nosocomial pneumonia. *Infect Control Hosp Epidemiol* 1995;16:417–418.
27. Frankel EH. To add or not to add blue dye to tube feeding, that is the question. *A.S.P.E.N. 24th Clinical Congress Proceedings.* Memphis, TN, January 25, 2000. Silver Spring, MD: American Society for Parenteral and Enteral Nutrition; 288–289.
28. Kinsey GC, Murray MJ, Swensen SJ, et al. Glucose content of tracheal aspirates: implications for detection of tube feeding aspiration. *Crit Care Med* 1994;22:1557–1562.
29. Methany NA, Clouse RE. Bedside methods for detecting aspiration in tube-fed patients. *Chest* 1997;111:724–725.
30. Methany NA, Aud MA, Wunderlich RJ. A survey of bedside methods used to detect pulmonary aspiration of enteral formula in intubated tube-fed patients. *Am J Crit Care* 1999;8:160–164.
31. Hamaoui E, Kodsi R. Complications of enteral feeding and their prevention. In: Rombeau JL, Rolandelli RH, eds. *Enteral and Tube Feeding.* 3rd ed. Philadelphia, PA: WB Saunders Company; 1997.
32. Montejo JC. Enteral nutrition-related gastrointestinal complications in critically ill patients: a multicenter study. *Crit Care Med* 1999;27:1447–1453.
33. Cataldi-Betcher EL, Seltzer MH, Slocum BA, et al. Complications occurring during enteral nutrition support. *J Parenter Enteral Nutr* 1983;7:546–552.
34. Smith C, Marien L, Brodgen C, et al. Diarrhea following tube feeding in ventilated critically ill patients. *Nurs Res* 1990;39:148–152.
35. Bliss DZ, Guenter PA, Settle RG. Defining and reporting diarrhea in tube-fed patients: beginning to clean up the mess! *Am J Clin Nutr* 1992;55:753–759.
36. Guenter PA, Settle RG, Perlmutter S, et al. Tube feeding related diarrhea in acutely ill patients. *J Parenter Enteral Nutr* 1991;15:277–280.
37. Guenter P, Sweed M. A valid and reliable tool to quantify stool output in tube fed patients. *J Parenter Enteral Nutr* 1998;22:147–151.

38. Smith CE, Faust-Wilson P, Lohr G. A measure of distress reaction to diarrhea in ventilated tube fed patients. *Nurs Res* 1992;41:312–313.
39. Fruto LV. Current concepts: management of diarrhea in acute care. *J WOCN* 1994;21: 199–205.
40. Emery EA, Ahmad S, Koethe JD, et al. Banana flakes control diarrhea in enterally fed patients. *Nutr Clin Pract* 1997;12:72–75.
41. Hall GR, Karstens M, Rakel B, et al. Managing constipation using a research-based protocol. *MEDSURG Nurs* 1995:4:11–20.
42. Solomon M, Kirby DF: The refeeding syndrome: a review. *J Parenter Enteral Nutr* 1990: 14:90–97.

SUGGESTED READINGS

Bliss DZ, Johnson S, Savik K, et al. Fecal incontinence in hospitalized patients who are acutely ill. *Nurs Res* 2000;49:101–108.

Burns PE, Jairath N. Diarrhea and the patient receiving enteral feedings: A multifactorial problem. *J WOCN* 1994;21:257–263.

Chapman MJ, Fraser RJ, Kluger MT, et al. Erythromycin improves gastric emptying in critically ill patients intolerant of nasogastric feeding. *Crit Care Med* 2000;28: 2334–2337.

Goff K. Metabolic monitoring in nutrition support. *Nurs Clin North Am* December 1997;32:741–753.

Gottschlich MM, Fuhrman P, Hammond K, Holcombe B, Seidner D (eds) *The Science and Practice of Nutrition Support: A Case Based Core Curriculum.* Dubuque, IA: Kendall/Hunt Publishing Company, 2001.

Guenter P. Mechanical complications in long-term feeding tubes. *Nurs Spectr* 1999; 9:12–14.

Guenter P, Jones S, Ericson M. Enteral nutrition therapy. *Nurs Clin North Am* December 1997;32:651–668.

Hammond K. Preventing refeeding syndrome. *Home Healthc Nurse* 1999; 17:526–527.

Lord LM. Enteral access devices. *Nurs Clin North Am* December 1997;32:685–704.

MacLaren R, Kuhl DA, Gervasio JM, et al. Sequential single doses of cisapride, erythromycin, and metoclopramide in critically ill patients intolerant to enteral nutrition: a randomized, placebo-controlled, crossover study. *Crit Care Med* 2000;28:438–444.

Mathus-Vliegen LM, Binnekade JM, de Haan RJ. Bacterial contamination of ready-to-use 1-L feeding bottles and administration sets in severely compromised intensive care patients. *Crit Care Med* 2000;28:67–73.

Reese JL, Means ME, Hanrahan K, et al. Diarrhea associated with nasogastric feedings. *ONF* 1996;23:59–68.

Storm HM, Skipper A. Closed-systems enteral feedings: Point-counterpoint. *Nutr Clin Pract* 2000;15:193–200.

Vanek VW. Closed vs. open enteral delivery systems: A quality improvement study. *Nutr Clin Pract* 2000;15:234–243.

Transitional Feeding

MARCIA SILKROSKI

Zibrida and Carlson define transitional feeding as a directed change in the feeding modality that bridges the gap between one feeding and another.[1] Transitioning feeding modalities is perhaps the most important aspect of nutritional care. Progressing to an oral diet is the goal if the patient is physically able to ingest and digest one. Certain diagnoses may limit a patient's tolerance to oral feeds and may require a patient to utilize enteral (tube feeds) or total parenteral nutrition (TPN). However, most patients with a normal or semi-normal digestive tract will be able to tolerate an oral diet, even if modifications are made in texture or nutrient content. For many patients, transition to oral feeds occurs in the acute care setting. The exact circumstances in which advancement of a patient's diet is undertaken is not always clear. Each institution should develop its own protocol, and the patient should be treated individually in order to achieve the best outcome.

Looking beyond the patient's clinical picture for a moment, consider the basic cost difference between specialized nutrition support and the oral diet. It is far more expensive to maintain an individual on TPN or tube feedings than it is to feed the patient by mouth.[2] Most third-party payers will not pay for more specialized nutrition if the digestive tract can be utilized safely and in any capacity.[3] It is judicious for providers of health care to monitor patients carefully and transition their diet as soon as they appear ready in order to avoid an economic burden. This chapter will outline how to assess when a patient is ready to begin transition feedings. This chapter also refers to the use of TPN in more detail than the others; therefore, a brief description follows.

Developed in the 1960s, TPN is a liquid nutrient formula containing nutrients (protein, carbohydrate, fat, vitamins, minerals, and water) and delivered directly into the veins for patients unable to assimilate nutrients via the gastrointestinal (GI) tract. It is indicated for patients with a non-functioning GI tract (due to short bowel syndrome, intractable diarrhea or vomiting, severe malabsorption, for example); for bowel rest following severe pancreatitis; for hemodynamic instability, or in extreme cases of malnutrition. It is normally provided for greater than 5 days and requires adequate venous access.[4] Central venous access is used over peripheral access due to the hypertonicity of TPN. Examples of long-term central venous access devices include Hickman, Broviac, Groshong, ports, and peripherally inserted central catheters or "PICC" lines.[5]

Peripheral parenteral nutrition (PPN) is a less concentrated form of TPN. The major difference is that the PPN solution is provided through a peripheral vein, which has a limited capacity of 900 mOsm per liter. Glucose concentration is significantly reduced with PPN and, therefore, this limits the amount of calories one is able to provide. While PPN is associated with fewer central access complications, it is difficult to maintain peripheral access for more than 3 or 4 days. Maintaining viable access combined with the limited provision of calories may make PPN ineffective from a cost perspective.[4,5]

Determining readiness for the next step in nutritional care is the professional judgment of the clinician, and should be a multidisciplinary decision. If a patient has been tolerating the nutritional regimen well and is healing from an injury or illness, it may be time to progress to the next step. Using a tool similar to the algorithm shown in Figure 8–1 can help to assess a patient's physiological readiness for transitional feeding.

Emotionally, a patient may be afraid or unwilling to change when first trying to advance the diet. Utilize various people on the health care team to assist the patient in making this change. Social workers or behavior therapists can address this fear, which often rises from lack of knowledge. Informing the patient of plans may help to alleviate fear. Patient education helps to diminish fear. Unwillingness to change is often associated with fear or can stem from

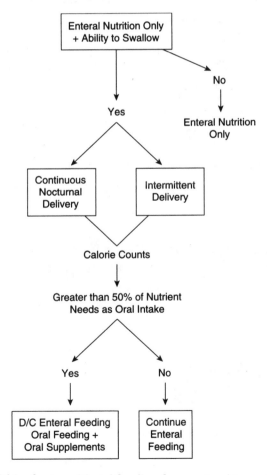

Figure 8–1 Algorithim for transitional feeding from enteral to oral nutrition

dependency. Change is not an easy action for some, but a necessary one nonetheless. Again, getting assistance from members of the health care team and family members may help.

Depending on patient goals, nutritional status may play a role in when to transition a feeding. Improvement in the clinical picture is the goal of making any change. Failure to upgrade a feeding modality may cause stagnation in appetite. Once feedings have been advanced, and oral intake resumes, nutritional status may improve. If nutritional status significantly declines with the change, it may be necessary to revert to the previous method. However, a slight decline followed by improvement would be considered normal in the adjustment process and the upgraded nutritional therapy continued.

Before a patient is transitioned, it is wise to update nutritional requirements. Energy and protein requirements change as patient status progresses. What was needed on admission may be quite different in a more stable patient. Reassessment observing biochemical markers, clinical findings, anthropometric measurements, and nutritional intake should all be factors considered. See Chapter 1, Nutrition Screening and Assessment, for more on assessment. It may be beneficial to involve the patient to motivate him or her in an upward trend. For the patient with dementia or another condition where brain function is limited, and for patients with psychological issues such as anorexia nervosa, it is more effective to reinforce the goals with the family and health care team.

As with any change, the goal is long-term success. If at any time in the progression toward oral intake a patient is unable to maintain adequate consumption, then other measures should be considered. It is possible and oftentimes necessary to provide nutrients in several combination therapies until a patient is able to tolerate oral nutrition exclusively.[1] The issue of insurance reimbursement may again become a problem. For example, a patient may *tolerate* oral nutrition, but is not capable of getting adequate amounts during the day. A tube feeding can be delivered to the patient on a cyclic basis overnight to compensate for the losses the patient would otherwise experience.[6] Feeding the patient at night also allows food to be taken during the day at normal meal times. This method of feeding often takes place in alternate sites such as long-term care facilities or even at home. This option allows patients to enjoy oral feedings and social interaction with their peers, maintain the sense of mastication (chewing), yet avoid the risks of malnutrition.[7]

CONCERNS WITH TRANSITIONING

OVERFEEDING AND REFEEDING SYNDROME

One of the biggest risks with the transition of nutrition support is that of overfeeding. Overfeeding may seem a minor problem, but it can have serious consequences for a critically ill patient. With sicker patients being discharged earlier, practitioners may feel impelled to push the patient to a "normal" intake faster than an acceptable time frame given their circumstances. In a malnourished patient starting on tube feedings, it is likely that the GI tract will not tolerate the rapid influx of nutrients, and the tube feeding may need to be stopped or slowed to accommodate the problem. GI complaints such as abdominal cramping, bloating, distension, diarrhea, and reflux are common when patients have been rapidly advanced. Overfeeding can lead to hyperglycemia and weight gain—accumulation of fat stores, especially in patients who are bedfast. Refer to Chapter 7, Enteral Nutrition Complications, for additional information on gastrointestinal complications of feeding. Once tube feedings have started, overfeeding can be prevented by slowly progressing the tube feeding to provide adequate calories. Use of indirect calorimetry and other assessment tools for accurately predicting energy expenditure may be beneficial in critical cases to provide adequate substrates for metabolism without being too overzealous.

Refeeding syndrome is significantly different from overfeeding. *Refeeding syndrome* is defined as the metabolic consequences and possibly even death resulting from rapid replacement of nutrients after a period of starvation.[8,9] At highest risk are those with severe malnutrition, often caused by anorexia nervosa, alcoholism, malabsorption, diabetes mellitus, cancer, and limited food availability. Intracellular shifts in phosphorus, magnesium, and potassium may be seen once nutritional therapy is started.

There are several reasons for refeeding syndrome. High carbohydrate loads cause the intracellular shift of these minerals and the resultant hyperglycemia. High blood sugars trigger the need for more potassium in order to synthesize glycogen. Magnesium and phosphorus are needed for the synthesis of adenosine triphosphate (ATP).[10] Figure 8–2 represents the Krebs cycle, where the synthesis of ATP happens.[11]

This demand causes a rapid depletion of phosphorus, magnesium, and potassium.[12,13] Signs and symptoms of a deficiency in these important nutrients are listed in Table 8–1.

Additionally, excess sodium provided to an already overhydrated patient causes fluid retention. If the heart muscle is weak, pumping additional water in the blood is taxing to the cardiovascular system.[8,9] Frequent and careful monitoring of any patient thought to be starved prior to admission is of the utmost importance. This point cannot be overemphasized.

Refeeding syndrome can be avoided by identifying those patients at risk, and then providing them with low carbohydrate loads (2–3 gms/kg/day) and not exceeding 20 to 25 kcal/kg/day for the first week. If blood sugars are in reasonable control, the nutritional regimen can be advanced slowly. Repletion of potassium, magnesium, and phosphorus should be part of initial therapy as well.[8–10]

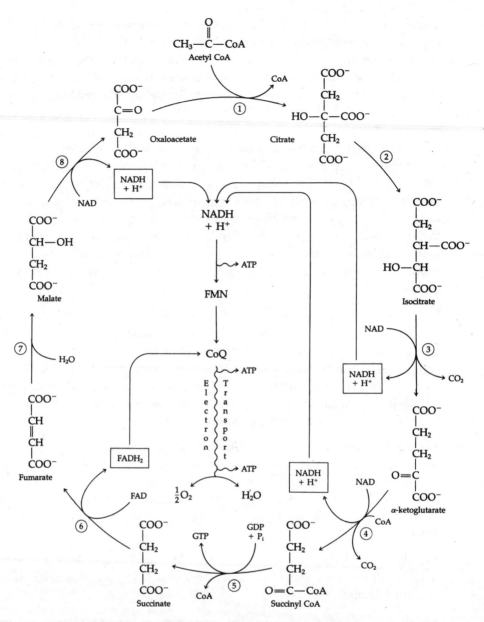

Figure 8–2 The Krebs (citric acid) cycle. This representation of the cycle is designed to emphasize the formation of reduced coenzymes and how their reoxidation by electron transport contributes to the synthesis of ATP.

MUCOSAL BARRIER AND BACTERIAL TRANSLOCATION

TPN has long been used for patients in need of bowel rest and healing of the GI tract. However, there is growing evidence to suggest positive outcomes with the initiation of early enteral feedings postoperatively in place of or in addition to TPN administration to prevent bacterial translocation.[14–19] Villi are the microscopic, hairlike projections inside the intestinal wall. This villus structure is

Table 8–1 Signs and symptoms of hypophosphatemia, hyomagnesemia, and hypokalemia

Hypophosphatemia	Hypomagnesemia	Hypokalemia
Moderate <2.5 mg/dL	Moderate <1.5 mEq/L	<3.5 mEq/L
Severe <1.0 mg/dL	Severe <1.0 mEq/L	Muscle weakness
Weakness	Muscle weakness	Leg cramps
Poor heart and respiratory	Hyperactive tendon reflexes	Nausea
muscle function	Muscle tremors	Vomiting
Acute respiratory failure	Tetany	Ileus
Poor white blood cell	Blood pressure elevation	Weak, irregular pulse
function (due to decrease	Cardiac arrhythmias	Parasthesias
in ATP)	Increased vascular resistance	
Confusion	Hypokalemia	
Seizures	Delirium	
Coma	Convulsions	

responsible for the absorption of nutrients. With the delivery of TPN, villi become flattened. Because the bowel is not being used for nutrient absorption during TPN administration, bacterial translocation may occur, allowing translocation of bacteria and endotoxin into the portal system. The factors that promote bacterial translocation are described in Exhibit 8–1.[20] The provision of nutrients via the GI tract, even in small amounts, helps to preserve the villous structure and maintain its delicate immune function in hemodynamically stable patients.[15,18,20]

DYSPHAGIA

Dysphagia is a concern when transitioning certain patient populations. Dysphagia is defined as difficulty in swallowing. It has many causes, including developmental disabilities, injuries, neurological conditions, and aging.[21] See Exhibit 8–2 for a more complete listing of diagnoses associated with dysphagia. A Speech/Language Pathologist (SLP) should be consulted to perform a swallowing study to confirm the level and degree of dysphagia. Often, a modified barium-swallow study is ordered to determine the presence of dysphagia.

Exhibit 8–1 Bacterial translocation

Three factors that promote translocation of bacteria:

1. bacterial overgrowth—oral antibiotic treatment, post-operative or opiate-induced ileus, intestinal obstruction, blind loop syndrome
2. disruption of the intestinal mucosal barrier—starvation and TPN result in gut atrophy and loss of barrier
3. altered host immune status—malnutrition, metabolic stress, sepsis, steroid treatment, chemotherapy, radiation therapy, surgery

Exhibit 8–2 Diagnoses associated with dysphagia

- Amylotrophic lateral sclerosis
- Cerebrovascular accident or stroke
- Guillain-Barré syndrome or poly-
  radiculoneuritis
- Head and neck cancers

- Multiple sclerosis
- Myasthenia gravis
- Parkinson's disease
- Radiation therapy to head, neck,
  and chest areas

A special diet is planned depending on the patient's swallowing ability.[22–29] Each facility should have dysphagia diets, outlining the level of consistency a patient can tolerate.[30]

Liquids often present the greatest problem. Liquids can be thickened to prevent aspiration using a commonly available item in food service, such as tapioca. Exhibit 8–3 demonstrates the three basic levels of thickened fluids used by many institutions. A variety of commercially available products such as Thick-enUp (Novartis Nutrition, Minneapolis, MN) are available for use by patients and caregivers. These products are designed to make thin liquids thicker while providing the patient with adequate fluid. Additional fluid by mouth, tube feedings, or IV may still be needed to prevent dehydration.[24]

UPGRADING FROM PARENTERAL TO ENTERAL OR ORAL NUTRITION

Transitioning from parenteral to enteral or oral nutrition is not feasible until GI function has returned. This includes a bowel of sufficient length for absorption of nutrients. There are multiple recommendations for what is considered adequate length and multiple means for measuring the bowel. Between 100 cm and 500 cm is considered sufficient for using intact nutrients for feeding. A normal adult small bowel (where most nutrients are absorbed) is estimated to be between 700 cm and 800 cm long with more than 2 million cm of absorptive area. To visualize this, it is equivalent to the size of a doubles tennis court. The large bowel or colon (approximately 150 cm–200 cm) absorbs fluid, electrolytes, and unabsorbed carbohydrate in addition to acting as a holding tank for fecal matter.[31] An intact ileocecal valve is usually necessary to prevent rapid transit and malabsorption of nutrients, better known as "dumping syndrome." Normal peristalsis or GI motility prevents complications of delayed gastric emptying. A

Exhibit 8–3 Levels of liquid consistency for dysphagia diets

- Level 1   Nectar consistency
- Level 2   Honey consistency
- Level 3   Pudding consistency

protected airway decreases the risk of aspiration. Once all of these systems have been checked and cleared, enteral or oral feeding can safely begin.[32–35]

Depending on the patient's digestive ability at the time of transition, and the type of tube being used, a polymeric or hydrolyzed formula may be chosen for tube feeding. See Chapter 2, Enteral Nutrition Basics, for more on formula selection. A standard isotonic feeding is best initiated between 25 and 50 cc per hour, with the usual rate being about 40 cc per hour. Advancement of tube feedings is judged by patient tolerance. If there is abdominal distention, residuals equal to 2 times the amount of formula or greater than 200 cc, nausea, diarrhea, or cramping, advancement should be delayed. If any of these symptoms are severe, stopping the feeding for 1 hour and rechecking before restarting the feeding may be required. If feedings are tolerated, advancement can proceed at 20 to 25 cc per hour increments over a 12- to 24-hour period until final volume is achieved.[1]

When the patient is tolerating the feeding at one-half to two-thirds the final volume, TPN can be decreased by half of total volume. TPN can be discontinued once the patient is tolerating tube feedings at the rate needed to meet nutritional requirements. Tapering TPN cautiously prevents rapid glucose changes and abrupt fluid shifts.[36,37] PPN does not need to be tapered because it does not provide such large amounts of dextrose or calories. If the patient is getting adequate fluid, PPN can be discontinued as tube feedings begin,[1] providing tolerance to initial feeds is established.

Transitioning from TPN directly to oral nutrition is often seen in the hospital setting and requires careful monitoring to be sure the patient is able to achieve near-normal nutrition before discontinuing the TPN. Patients moving to an oral diet after being on long-term TPN may experience transient problems with anorexia for a short time due to the high volume of calories provided in the TPN solution.[38,39] It is wise to begin with a low-fat, clear liquid diet. See Exhibit 8–4 for an example.

The clear liquid diet is intended to provide some fluid and electrolytes and is composed of clear fluids and simple carbohydrates. It provides less than 500 calories and should not be utilized for more than a few days. The patient should be instructed to consume small quantities at first (e.g., 1 to 2 ounces each half hour) and then to increase as tolerated. If this is well accepted, the diet can be advanced to full liquids (see Exhibit 8–5).

Some patients may graduate to solid foods without using full liquids. Others may have some degree of lactose intolerance and may warrant use of lactose-free products. Commercial oral supplements (see Table 8–2) or homemade varieties can be given between meals if intake is inadequate (less than two-thirds or less than 75% of calculated needs) after a few days of trial with solid foods. Lactose-sensitive patients should be instructed to read product labels, because some commercial products do contain lactose.

Tube feedings can also be used to help the patient transition to an oral diet, though they are best provided in a cyclic fashion at night or by intermittent

Exhibit 8–4 Clear liquid diet

Fruit—juices without pulp
   Apple, cranberry, grape
Fruit juices—strained
   Orange, grapefruit, pineapple
Juices—without fruit concentrate
   Lemonade, Hi-C, Kool-Aid
Non-carbonated beverages
   Ginger ale, Sprite, 7-Up

Hot beverages
   Coffee, decaffeinated coffee, tea
Soups – clear or strained
   Broth, consomme
Gelatin – without whole fruit
Popsicles – without milk
Condiments
   Sugar, salt

(between meal) feedings to encourage consumption of nutrients during the day. TPN can be discontinued by tapering to 50% in the first hour and completely stopped in the second hour. If the patient is on PPN, it can be discontinued once the patient is eating solid foods without a tapering process.[1,36,37]

UPGRADING FROM TUBE FEEDING TO ORAL NUTRITION

In order to transition from tube feeding to oral nutrition, you must have a patient who is willing and able to consume food by mouth. Force-feeding a patient orally, by syringe, is not safe and is considered by most professionals to be an unethical practice.[40] The transitional process can usually begin using a full liquid diet. Oral supplements can be given between meals or as part of a meal to achieve caloric goals. Tube feedings are decreased in relation to the amount of oral intake.[1] As previously mentioned, patients are often transitioned using cyclic feedings at night and oral feedings during the day. The formula generally runs between 8 and 20 hours and provides anywhere from 25% to 75% of requirements during the time of transition.[6,7] A calorie-dense formula may be needed to achieve this amount of calories in a shortened time frame. Flushing of the tube is crucial to maintain patency even when the tube is not in use. See Chapter 4, Nursing Care of Patients with Enteral Feeding Devices, for more on the importance of flushing the tube.

Exhibit 8–5 Full liquid diet

Any foods on the clear liquid diet
All juices and nectars
Eggnog
Milk
Soups
Cream
Milkshakes

Custard, pudding
Yogurt
Ice cream
Carbonated beverages
Condiments
   Margarine, butter, honey, sugar, salt

Table 8–2 Commercial oral supplements

Mead Johnson	Nestlé	Novartis	Ross
Boost	NuBasics	Resource	Ensure
Sustacal	Carnation Instant Breakfast	Citrotein	Ensure Plus

If appetite is not resuming, there may be several causes. First, investigate the patient's usual intake and activity prior to the initiation of tube feeding. Is it possible the patient has specific religious or ethnic preferences that are not being provided? If so, can food be delivered to the patient from outside the institutional setting? In some cases, the patient may be clinically depressed due to prolonged illness. Ensure that the food is appealing and appropriate texture for consumption. If a patient typically uses dentures, ensure that they fit properly.

If the patient continues to have difficulty getting adequate oral intake once these issues are investigated, pharmacologic agents are available to assist with appetite stimulation,[41–43] such as Megace (Bristol-Myers Squibb, New York, NY). Typically, these agents are prescribed for the period of time when a patient is experiencing anorexia or poor appetite. They are usually discontinued within a few weeks or months when the appetite has resumed normalcy.[41–43]

MONITORING TRANSITIONAL FEEDINGS

Documenting the patient's intake during the transitional phase can be cumbersome, yet it is critical in deciding when to discontinue a modality, or a feeding modality. Typically, an intake assessment of some sort is maintained by the nursing staff and calculated by nutrition services personnel. Documentation of intake is generally recorded in the patient's permanent record. There are many forms of intake assessments, more commonly referred to as "calorie counts." Some have spaces to record exactly what was consumed, others use visual cues such as a pie chart to determine percent consumed, still others require checkmarks in boxes to show percent consumed at a given meal, etc. Each institution develops these basic tools and should evaluate them on a regular basis to ensure they are useful and being completed.

Calorie counts should include all intake by mouth; therefore, if something other than what was served at a meal is consumed, it should be recorded—e.g., food brought by family from home, fast food ordered by the patient, vending machine purchase. Additionally, all beverages or liquids (e.g., juice, oral supplementation, fluids given with medications), extras (e.g., butter, sauces, gravy), and condiments (e.g., cream, sugar, mayonnaise) should be recorded as well. Calorie counts give us a clearer picture of what the patient's preferences are and may prove beneficial when trying to discontinue feedings altogether. See Exhibit 8–6 for an example of a Calorie Count form. Other intake such as tube feeding or TPN is likely to be recorded by nursing on intake and output sheets. This should be included when documenting the patient's estimated intake of calories.

A common observation in many facilities is that calorie counts are only partially recorded. Documenting part of a day's intake is no more relevant to the whole clinical picture than are partial weights or partial labs. Partial documentation could mean the difference between 10% and 90% of the total intake consumed. They may seem tedious in the day-to-day operation of patient care, but well-maintained calorie counts can have a direct effect on patient cost and avoid the delay for transition to an oral diet.

Exhibit 8–6 Calorie count

Day _____   Date_____   Patient Name _____

This calorie count was ordered to get an accurate account of what is being consumed by the patient on a daily basis. Please record all intake including meals, snacks, condiments (creamers, sugar, butter, and mayonnaise), and beverages (coffee, sodas, milk, water). If the patient is consuming oral supplements please record that as well—even if they are being recorded in another record. This is very important to the patient's outcome. We greatly appreciate your efforts in gathering this information.

The Department of Clinical Nutrition.

Meal/Snack	Portion Consumed	Dietary Use Only
Breakfast	1/4 1/2 3/4 All	
Snack		
Lunch		
Snack		
Dinner		
Snack		

REFERENCES

1. Zibrida JM, Carlson SJ. Transitional feeding. In: *Nutrition Support Dietetics Core Curriculum.* 2nd ed. Silver Spring, MD: American Society for Parenteral and Enteral Nutrition; 1993:459–465.

2. Campbell S. If the gut works, use it; the appropriate provision of medical foods can save a bundle. *Health Care Strateg Manage* 1996;14:14–15.

3. Delegge MH. Changes in Medicare reimbursement policy may restrict nutrition therapy option. *Nutrition* 1997;13:926–927.

4. American Society for Parenteral and Enteral Nutrition: Guidelines for the use of parenteral and enteral nutrition in adult and pediatric patients. *J Parenter Enteral Nutr* 1993;17(4 Suppl):1SA–52SA.

5. Krzywda EA, Edmiston CE Jr. Parenteral access and equipment. In: *The A.S.P.E.N. Nutrition Support Practice Manual.* Silver Spring, MD: American Society for Parenteral and Enteral Nutrition; 1998:4–5.

6. Forloines LS. How to smooth the way for cyclic tube feeding. *Nursing* 1996;26:57–60.

7. Hebuterne X, Broussard JF, Rampal P. Acute renutrition by cyclic enteral nutrition in elderly and younger patients. *JAMA* 1995;273:638–643.

8. Soloman SM, Kirby DF. The refeeding syndrome: a review. *J Parenter Enteral Nutr* 1990;14:90–97.

9. Apovian CM, McMahon MM, Bistrian BR. Guidelines for refeeding the marasmic patient. *Crit Care Med* 1990;18:1030–1033.

10. Weinsier RL, Krundieck CL. Death resulting from overzealous total parenteral nutrition: the refeeding syndrome revisited. *Am J Clin Nutr* 1981;34:393–399.

11. Groff JL, Hunt SM. Carbohydrates. In: *Advanced Nutrition and Human Metabolism.* St. Paul, MN: West Publishing Company; 1990:87.

12. Whitmire SJ. Fluids and electrolytes. In: Matarese LE, Gottschlich MM, eds. *Contemporary Nutrition Support Practice: A Clinical Guide.* Philadelphia, PA: WB Saunders Company; 1998:135–138.

13. Grant JP. Administration of Parenteral Nutrition Solutions. In: *Handbook of Total Parenteral Nutrition.* 2nd ed. Philadelphia, PA: WB Saunders Company; 1992:181–184.

14. Greenberg GR. Nutritional support in inflammatory bowel disease: current status and future directions. *Scand J Gastroenterol Suppl* 1992;192:117–122.

15. Sax HC, Ilig KA, Ryan CK, Hardy DJ. Low dose enteral feeding is beneficial during total parenteral nutrition. *Am J Surg* 1996;171:587–590.

16. Kudsk KA, Croce MA, Fabian TC, et al. Enteral versus parenteral feeding: effects on septic morbidity after blunt and penetrating abdominal trauma. *Ann Surg* 1992;215:503.

17. Sandstrom R, Drott C, Hyltander A, et al. The effect of postoperative intravenous feeding (TPN) on outcome following major surgery evaluated in a randomized study. *Ann Surg* 1993;217:185.

18. Nirgoitis JG, Andrassy RJ: Bacterial translocation. In: Borlase BC, Bell SJ, Blackburn GL, et al., eds. *Enteral Nutrition.* New York: Chapman & Hall; 1994:15.

19. Lowen CC, Greene LM, McClave SA. Nutritional support in patients with inflammatory bowel disease. *Postgrad Med* 1992;91:407–414.

20. Harrison LE, Fong Y. Enteral nutrition in the cancer patient. In: Rombeau JL, Caldwell MD, eds. *Enteral and Tube Feeding.* Philadelphia, PA: WB Saunders Company; 1997:300–323.

21. Whitney EN, Cataldo CB, DeBruyne LK, Rolfes SR. Nutrition and upper GI disorders. In: *Nutrition for Health and Health Care.* Minneapolis/St. Paul, MN: West Publishing Company; 1996:479–482.

22. Horner J, Massey EW. Silent aspiration following stroke. *Neurology* 1988:317–319.
23. Sizmann JV. Nutritional support of the dysphagic patient: methods, risks, and complications of therapy. *J Parenter Enteral Nutr* 1990:60–63.
24. Hester DD. Neurological impairment. In: Gottschlich MM, Matarese LE, Schronts EP, eds. *Nutrition Support Dietetics: Core Curriculum*. 2nd ed. Silver Spring, MD: American Society for Parenteral and Enteral Nutrition; 1993:238.
25. Hester DD, Kjelde JA. Nutrition support in neurologic impairments. In: Matarese LE, Gottschlich MM, eds. *Contemporary Nutrition Support Practice: A Clinical Guide*. Philadelphia, PA: WB Saunders Company; 1998:380–383.
26. Konvolinka CW, Morell VO. Nutrition in head trauma. *Nutr Clin Pract* 1991;6:251–255.
27. Gauwitz DF. How to protect the dysphagic stroke patient. *Am J Nurs* 1995;95:34–38.
28. DePippo KL, Holas MA, Reding MJ, et al. Dysphagia therapy following stroke: a controlled trial. *Neurology* 1994;44:1655–1660.
29. Mackay LE, Morgan AS, Bernstein BA. Swallowing disorders in severe brain injury: risk factors affecting return to oral intake. *Arch Phys Med Rehabil* 1999;80:365–371.
30. Pardoe EM. Development of a multistage diet for dysphagia. *J Amer Diet Assoc* 1993;(93):568–571.
31. Underhill BML. Intestinal length in man. *Br Med J* 1955;2:1243–1246.
32. Moran JR, Greene HL. Digestion and absorption. In: Rombeau JL, Caldwell MD, eds. *Enteral and Tube Feeding*. Philadelphia, PA: WB Saunders Company; 1984:20–43.3.
33. Kelly DG, Fleming CR. Physiology of the gastrointestinal tract: as applied to patients receiving tube enteral nutrition. In: Rombeau JL, Caldwell MD, eds. *Enteral and Tube Feeding*. Philadelphia, PA: WB Saunders Company; 1997:12–22.
34. Silk DB. Intestinal absorption of nutrients. In: Fischer JE, ed. *Surgical Nutrition*. 1st ed. Boston: Little, Brown and Company; 1983:19–42.
35. Caspary WF. Physiology and pathophysiology of intestinal absorption. *Am J Clin Nutr* 1992;55:299S–308S.
36. Wagman LP, Miller KB, Thomas RB, et al. The effect of acute discontinuation of total parenteral nutrition. *Ann Surg* 1986;204:524–529.
37. Skipper A, Millikan KW. Parenteral nutrition implementation and management. In: *The A.S.P.E.N. Nutrition Support Practice Manual*. Silver Spring, MD: American Society for Parenteral and Enteral Nutrition; 1998:1–9.
38. Gil KM, Skeie B, Kvetan V, et al. Parenteral nutrition and oral intake: effect of glucose and fat infusions. *JPEN* 1991;15:426–432.
39. Stratton RJ, Elia M. The effects of enteral tube feeding and parenteral nutrition on appetite sensations and food intake in health and disease. *Clin Nutr* 1999;18:63–70.
40. Soriano R. Syringe feeding: current clinical practice and recommendations. *Geriatr Nurs* 1994;15:85–87.
41. Ottery FD, Walsh D, Strawford A. Pharmacologic management of anorexia/cachexia. *Semin Oncol* 1998;25(2 Suppl 6):35–44.
42. Tchekmedyian NS. Pharmacoeconomics of nutritional support in cancer. *Semin Oncol* 1998;25(2 Suppl 6):62–69.
43. Yeh SS, Schuster MW. Geriatric cachexia: the role of cytokines. *Am J Clin Nutr* 1999;70:183–197.

SUGGESTED READINGS

Dell'Olio J, Hollenstein J, Dwyer J. Noah grows up: transitioning problems from special feeding routes to oral intake. *Nutr Rev* 2000:58:118–128.

Gottschlich MM, Fuhrman P, Hammond K, Holcombe B, Seidner D (eds) *The Science and Practice of Nutrition Support: A Case Based Core Curriculum*. Dubuque, IA: Kendall/Hunt Publishing Company, 2001.

Grant JP, ed. *Handbook of Total Parenteral Nutrition*. 2nd ed. Philadelphia, PA: WB Saunders Company; 1992.

Rombeau JL, Rolandelli RR, eds. *Parenteral Nutrition*. Philadelphia, PA: WB Saunders Company; 1998.

Supplement to *Nutrition in Clinical Practice*. Disease State Management: Dysphagia. Vol. 14, No. 5. Oct. 1999.

RESOURCES

General Resources

American Society for Parenteral and Enteral Nutrition (A.S.P.E.N.)
8630 Fenton Street
Suite 412
Silver Spring, MD 20910
800–727–4567
www.nutritioncare.org

Dysphagia Resource Center
www.dysphagia.com

Oley Foundation
Albany Medical Center
214 Hun Memorial
Albany, NY 12208
800–776–OLEY
www.wizvax.net/oleyfdn

Menu Magic Publishing Company
(317) 269–3500
Non-Chew Cookbook
(800) 843–2409

MenuDirect
(888) MENU123
Med Diet Laboratories, Inc.
3600 Holly Lane
Suite 80
Plymouth, MN 55447
(800) 633–3438

Oral Supplement Companies

Mead Johnson Nutritionals
A Bristol-Myers Squibb Company
2400 West Lloyd Expressway
Evansville, IN 47721
1–800–457–3550
www.meadjohnson.com

Nestlé Clinical Nutrition
Three Parkway North
Suite 500
PO Box 760
Deerfield, IL 60015–0760
1–800–422–2752

Novartis Nutrition
5100 Gamble Drive
St. Louis Park, MN 55416
1–800–999–9978

Ross Laboratories
Division of Abbott Laboratories
625 Cleveland Avenue
Columbus, OH 43215
1–800–544–7495
www.pedialyte.com/html/products.cfm

9

Special Considerations for the Pediatric Patient

MICHELLE HARRINGTON AND BETH LYMAN

The provision of adequate nutrition during infancy and early childhood is imperative for growth and development and may even affect long-term health.[1] The severity, age of incidence, and duration of suboptimal nutrition intake impact the extent of adverse effects on growth and cognitive development.[2] Enteral nutrition support is indicated in infants and children with functioning gastrointestinal (GI) tracts who are unable to consume or absorb adequate nutrients.[3] Tube feedings can provide supportive or primary nutrition therapy. The development of an appropriate enteral tube feeding regimen can positively affect tolerance and the duration that nutrition support is necessary, as well as the growth and development of the pediatric patient. Figure 9–1 illustrates the steps and rationale used when determining whether a child needs enteral nutrition support and the optimal technique and schedule to implement enteral feedings based on individualized parameters.

Pediatric nutrition assessment should encompass current dietary intake, medical and dietary history, physical activity, biochemical analysis, anthropometry, observable physical signs (skin, hair, lips, gums, teeth, tongue, and eyes), and feeding skills. Exhibit 9–1 is an example of a nutrition assessment form used for documenting findings of the caregiver interview as well as evaluating the patient and his or her current nutrition regimen.

Caregivers should be asked specifically about the following:

1. the child's present dietary intake
2. the child's appetite
3. who normally feeds the child
4. the duration of a typical feed
5. the position of the infant during feeds
6. perceived feeding problems
7. changes in the child's intake
8. the child's food preferences and dislikes
9. the child's history of any known food allergies and/or dietary intolerances
10. vitamin supplements or medications being provided[4]

Past growth trends, growth charts, and pubertal history, if age-appropriate, should be reviewed.[5] Tracking the growth trend of a pediatric patient over time is extremely helpful in performing an accurate nutrition assessment. This is especially true when the child's current growth parameters are considered acceptable on the growth chart but the growth velocity has slowed and the child has crossed percentiles in a downward trend. A diet history elucidates the patient's pattern of usual food intake and requires a detailed interview.[6] To better assess nutrient adequacy, caregivers are often asked to complete a 3-day

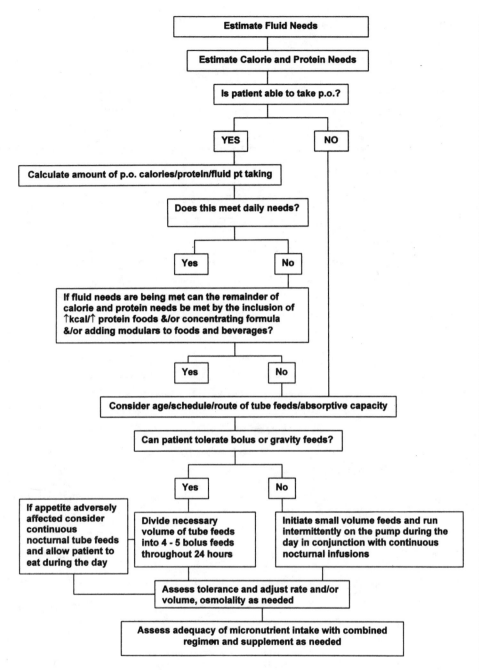

Figure 9–1 Steps in creating an enteral nutrition regimen

dietary record that includes 1 weekend day, with exact consumed portion sizes specified. If the patient is consuming formula, an exact description of how the caregiver mixes the formula is necessary to determine the caloric concentration and to ensure that the dilution is correct. A thorough interview should include questions about the child's development and the family's socioeconomic status.

Exhibit 9–1 Pediatric Nutrition Assessment

Patient's Name ————————— Date ——— D.O.B. ——— Age ——— Corrected Age —————

Diagnosis ————————————— GI ROS: Diarrhea ☐ Emesis ☐ Gastric Residuals ☐

Food Allergies ————————————— Diet History ———————————————————————

Weight —— Length/Height —— Head Circumference —— IBW —— UBW—— Ht/Age Standard ——
(——%ile/age) (——%ile/age)   (——%ile/age)   %IBW—— %UBW—— %Ht/Age Standard ——

MAC ———— (——%ile/age) TSF ———— (——%ile/age) Arm Muscle Area ———— (——%ile/age)

Arm Fat Area ———— (——%ile/age)

Medications ——

Labs ——/—/—< ——< ————————————————————————————————————

Diet: ——

Tube feeding   ☐ Yes ☐ No   NGT ☐   NJT ☐   Gtube ☐   Jtube ☐   Other ☐ ——
Formula ⎞————————— **Continuous** ☐ **Bolus** ☐ Additives —————————————
Volume ————————— cc/day = **Rate** —— cc x —— hours and/or —— cc x ——# feeds daily
Projected: cc/day or cc/kg/day ————   kcal/day or kcal/kg/day ————   gm protein/kg/day ——

TPN   ☐ Yes   ☐ No   TPN weight —— kg   Line Type ——————
% Dextrose ——   Amino Acid —— gm/kg/day Fat —— gm/kg/day TPN bag volume —— cc
Additives ——
☐ **3 in 1**   Volume —— cc/day = Rate —— cc x —— hours
☐ **Separate lipid infusion**   Dextrose/Amino Acid Volume —— cc/day = Rate —— cc x —— hours
                          20% Intralipid Volume —— cc/day = Rate —— cc x —— hours

Projected: cc/day or cc/kg/day ————   kcal/day or kcal/kg/day ————   gm protein/kg/day ————
          % calories from fat ————   carbohydrate ————   protein ————

Total projected: cc/day or cc/kg/day ————   kcal/day or kcal/kg/day ——   gm protein/kg/day ——
          % calories from fat ——   carbohydrate ——   protein ——

Estimated   **Estimated**   **Estimated**
kcal needs ——   **fluid needs** —— cc   **protein needs** —— gm (gm/kg/d)

☐ **RDA technique** —— kcal/kg × —— kg ☐ **WHO Equation** = —— × —— = ——

                              REE   Stress Factor

Assessment:
  ☐ no wasting present ☐ mildly wasted ☐ moderately wasted ☐ severely wasted ☐ obese
  ☐ no stunting present ☐ mildly stunted ☐ moderately stunted ☐ severely stunted

---

Plan: 1)

2)

3)

One should ascertain whether the child is experiencing any GI symptoms such as gastroesophageal reflux (GER), diarrhea, vomiting, constipation, or any other problems potentially resulting from underlying medical conditions. The presence of malabsorption, hypermetabolic, or hypometabolic states need to be considered when estimating daily nutrient needs. A hypermetabolic state may occur with sepsis, burns, or cardiac disease, while a hypometabolic state may occur with conditions that result in profound and global hypotonia.

The most rapid physical growth occurs between conception and the end of the first year of life. Birth weight usually doubles by 5 months of age and triples by 1 year of age. Length increases by approximately 50% during the first year of life. Head circumference reflects brain growth; generally the brain doubles its birth weight by 1 year of age and more than triples its birth weight by age 6. Infancy and the preschool years are when the most rapid postnatal brain growth occurs. Adverse conditions experienced during these periods will have the greatest effect on brain growth.[7]

Anthropometric measurements should include height (recumbent length from birth to 3 years of age), weight, head circumference (from birth to 3 years of age), triceps skinfold (TSF), and mid-upper arm circumference (MAC).[7] Well-calibrated and appropriate instrumentation, as well as correct technique and reference data, is critical in accurately obtaining and interpreting this information.[8,9]

Past nutrition status and chronic malnutrition are reflected by stature and head circumference in a child without other syndromic effects.[9] Recumbent length and stature are indicators of linear growth, primarily due to skeletal growth.[7] Weight-bearing stimulates the growth of long bones; thus non-ambulatory children may have constitutional short stature that is not nutrition-related.[9] If possible, the heights of both biological parents should be obtained and midparental stature determined to establish the child's genetic potential for linear growth.[10] Brain growth is most rapid during the first 3 years of life, and head circumference is a good reflection of this; thus a child's head circumference should be closely monitored during this time. Poor head circumference growth usually reflects severe malnutrition in children.[8] In the presence of malnutrition, head circumference is the best preserved anthropometic parameter. Generally weight, followed by stature, is adversely affected when suboptimal nutrition intake occurs. If malnutrition is prolonged, then head circumference growth will also be affected.[5] However, in patients with medical conditions that result in macrocephaly or microcephaly, head circumference cannot be used as an indicator of nutritional status. Head circumference reference data is available for children up to 18 years of age.[8]

Current nutrition status is reflected by skinfold thickness, mid-upper arm circumference, and weight. Weight indicates growth in muscle, adipose tissue, and bone. Children should be weighed at a consistent time of day, using the same scale, and wearing the same amount of clothing. Skinfold thickness measures body fat. Approximately half of the body's fat is in the subcutaneous tissue, thus TSF correlates well with the whole body fat content and is sensitive to changes in nutritional status.[5] Measuring skinfolds in an infant can be very difficult, as it may be hard to get good separation of subcutaneous adipose tissue from muscle tissue. National Center for Health Statistics (NCHS) reference data for skinfold thickness is available for Caucasian, Black, and Hispanic children older than 2 months of age.[7] Mid-upper arm circumference measures muscle, fat, and bone.[8] MAC is sensitive to current nutrition status and is used frequently in combination with TSF measurements.[5,8] National reference norms that categorize by age and gender for TSF and MAC are available to interpret measurements.[5] The upper arm muscle area and upper arm fat area that are calculated from the TSF and MAC provide an indication of total body fat mass and lean body mass.[8,11] Subscapular skinfold is a useful measure of fat stores on the trunk and is less sensitive to acute changes in nutrition status. Fat stores at this site tend to be preserved during chronic malnutrition.[8] Subscapular skinfold combined with TSF measurements are useful in assessing fat distribution and total body fat.[12] Upper arm muscle circumference reflects total muscle mass, which is an index of the body's protein stores. Serial anthropometric measurements should be repeated at established intervals to assess growth velocity and response to nutrition therapy.

Height, weight, and head circumference (if age-appropriate) should be plotted on the NCHS standard growth charts. These measurements help to determine ideal body weight, and percentiles for weight, height/length, and head circumference for age, as well as height/length for age standards compared to a reference population of other healthy American children.[2,6] There are four different NCHS growth charts: male and female birth to 36 months, and male and female 2 to 18 years of age. The birth to 36 month old growth chart uses recumbent length, while the 2- to 18-year-old growth chart uses standing height. Recumbent length is almost 1 inch greater than standing height, thus it is important to plot the measurement on the appropriate growth chart in accordance with the method it was obtained. When plotting anthropometrics on the growth charts, gestational age of the child must be established and corrected for if the infant was premature by 3 or more weeks. Correcting for prematurity or determining the patient's adjusted age is done by subtracting the weeks or months that the infant was premature from the chronological age.[2] Corrections for weight should be made until the child is 24 months of age, corrections for length until the child is 36 months of age, and corrections for head circumference until the child is 18 months of age.[13] Specialized growth charts have been developed for premature infants, low-birth weight preterm infants who are past term, children with Down syndrome, myelomeningocele, Prader-Willi and William's syndrome, to name a few. The World Health Organization (WHO) has accepted NCHS growth charts for all ethnic groups. Many practitioners feel that the NCHS growth charts should be used in conjunction with some of the special population growth charts since very small samples were used to develop many of these specialized charts. Additionally, the consensus is that serial measurements and growth trends are of much greater importance than percentile values. Pediatric growth charts using Body Mass Index (weight in kg/stature in meters^2) have been developed and are now available. Body Mass Index (BMI) is useful as a measure of the degree of obesity in children and adults.[6,7]

When using the growth charts, weight for age is often used to assess whether the child is overweight or underweight. However, weight can be skewed with the presence of edema, or can reflect altered body composition such as with increased proportions of muscle or fat.[8] Weight compared to ideal body weight (IBW), which is also referred to as the weight for length/height standard, in pediatrics can be used to determine the degree of adiposity or wasting in the patient and is independent of age.[7,8] BMI and percentage of IBW are generally used to identify obesity; however, they do not differentiate between adiposity and muscle mass. Therefore, the use of BMI combined with TSF should provide a more accurate assessment of adiposity.[8] Stunting can occur as a result of endocrine or genetic conditions, but is more commonly due to chronic malnutrition and/or illness resulting in a child who is small for his or her age but with a body weight proportional to stature. Wasting occurs when body weight is less than the weight for length/height standard as a result of acute nutritional deprivation. However, it is important to acknowledge that acute changes in weight, such as with dehydration or edema, do occur and need to be considered when evaluating the nutritional status of the patient.[4]

A thorough physical examination is an important component of a nutrition assessment in the pediatric patient because observable signs and symptoms of nutrient deficiencies in a depleted patient can be identified.[14] However, most physical findings are fairly nonspecific and therefore not conclusive for individual nutrient deficiencies without further evidence. The physical examination in combination with the diet and medical history, laboratory values, and anthropometric measurements can elucidate whether the patient has any nutrient deficiencies.[15] Table 9–1 lists observable signs and symptoms of possible nutrient deficiencies or excesses and the nutrients that could be causing these symptoms.

NUTRIENT REQUIREMENTS

Body composition measurements obtained during growth and development, in conjunction with weight and stature, can often clarify anthropometric findings and enhance the accuracy of a nutritional assessment.[6,8] The individual body compartments reflect nutrition stores. Lean body mass reflects the body's water and protein content, while fat reflects energy stores. Body composition information is important in determining estimated nutrition needs, especially in children who have requirements that are affected by disease states, medical therapy, or chronic conditions.[8] For the pediatric patient, nutrition goals are to provide adequate nutrition for growth and development and for the preservation of lean body mass.[16] Estimated nutrient requirements are determined by multiple factors, which include the patient's clinical and overall nutritional status, activity

Table 9–1 Clinical signs and symptoms of nutrient deficiency or excess

Abnormal Clinical Findings	Possible Nutrient Deficiency	Possible Excess
General		
Growth failure, emaciated, depleted fat and muscle stores	Zinc, Calories, Protein	
Hair		
Lack of shine, thin	Protein, Zinc or essential fatty acid	
Transverse depigmentation	Protein, Copper	
Easily plucked	Protein	
Alopecia	Protein, Biotin, Zinc	Vitamin A
Face		
Pallor	Iron, Folate or B_{12}	
Temporal wasting	Protein and/or calorie	
Nails		
Ridging	Protein	
Spoon shaped (Koilonychia)	Iron	
Skin		
Scaling, dry	Vitamin A, Zinc, essential fatty acids	Vitamin A
Petechiae	Vitamin C	
Purpura	Vitamin C or Vitamin K	
Pigmentation	Niacin	
Yellow pigmentation (not observed in sclera)		Carotene
Poor wound healing	Vitamin C, Zinc, Protein	
Eyes		
Pale conjunctiva	Iron, Folate or B_{12}	
Night blindness	Vitamin A	
Papilledema		Vitamin A
Dull, opaque cornea (Corneal Xerosis)	Vitamin A	
Mouth		
(Perioral)		
Angular stomatitis	Riboflavin, Pyridoxine, Niacin	
Cheilosis	Riboflavin, Pyridoxine, Niacin	
(Oral)		
Glossitis	Riboflavin, Pyridoxine, Niacin, Folate	
Swollen, bleeding, retracted gums	Viamin C	
Tongue fissures, edema	Niacin	
Magenta tongue	Riboflavin	
Smooth tongue, loss of papillae	Folate, Niacin, Riboflavin or B_{12}	
Bones		
Enlargement of epiphyses at wrist, ankle or knee	Vitamin D	
Bowed legs	Vitamin D	
Beading of ribs	Vitamin D	
Neurologic		
Peripheral neuropathy	Thiamin, Pyridoxine, Vitamin B_{12}	Pyridoxine (2,15)
Tetany	Calcium, Magnesium, Vitamin D	

level, age, gender, and requirements for growth. The Recommended Dietary Allowances (RDAs) were developed to meet the calorie and protein needs of healthy, active children and may be inappropriate to use in many of the populations that have chronic medical problems. Many practitioners feel that calculating basal metabolic rate (BMR) using the World Health Organization (WHO) equations is a more accurate method of determining estimated daily caloric requirements for children with special needs. The equations are based on data from several thousand children and provide a more individualized prediction of BMR, since they are based on weight, gender, and age.[8] A stress/activity factor needs to be applied to the BMR based on the child's level of activity, growth velocity, and current nutrition status and disease process. Tables 9–2 and 9–3 illustrate how to calculate estimated nutritional needs in pediatrics using the RDAs and the WHO equation.

Short-term nutrition support goals may include adequate nutrient provision, weight gain, and introduction or advancement of oral nutrition. Long-term goals may include achieving or maintaining adequate nutrition status, appropriate growth, and transitioning to complete oral nutrition. Ongoing assessment of growth parameters is necessary to determine the adequacy of calorie, protein, and micronutrient provision, since needs may fluctuate in conjunction with changes in medical status. Developing and implementing oral dietary modifications in patients who are able to eat is extremely important and can facilitate an increase in volitional intake and a decreased dependence on nutrition support.[17] It is just as important to continuously assess the patient's psychosocial status, making changes in the nutrition regimen as needed to accommodate individual lifestyles and to support age-appropriate activity.[18]

BREAST MILK

Human milk provides the ideal nutrient composition for appropriate growth and development during infancy. Infant formula cannot reproduce the immunological properties, digestibility, and trophic effects of human milk, although formula companies continuously strive to replicate the nutrient profile of breast

---

Table 9–2 RDAs for calories and protein

Age	Calories/Kg/day	Grams of Protein/Kg/day
0–0.5 years	108	2.2
0.5–1 years	98	1.6
1–3 years	102	1.2
4–6 years	90	1.1
7–10 years	70	1.0
Males 11–14	55	1.0
Males 15–18	45	0.9
Females 11–14	47	1.0
Females 15–18	40	0.8

Table 9–3 World Health Organization equations for basal metabolic rate (BMR)

Age	Calories/day
Males: 0–3 years	60.9 × wt in kg − 54
Males: 3–10 years	22.7 × wt in kg + 495
Males: 10–18 years	17.5 × wt in kg + 651
Females: 0–3 years	61.0 × wt in kg − 51
Females: 3–10 years	22.5 × wt in kg + 499
Females: 10–18 years	12.2 × wt in kg + 746

Estimated daily calorie needs = BMR × Activity factor × Stress factor

Activity Factor		Stress Factor	
Paralyzed	1.0	Surgery	1.2
Nonambulatory	1.1	Sepsis	1.2–1.6
Ambulatory	1.2–1.3	Trauma	1.1–1.8
		Burn	1.5–2.5
		Starvation	0.7
		Growth Failure	1.5–2.0

milk.[1] Human milk provides conditionally essential nutrients, digestive enzymes, hormones, and growth factors.[19] Breast milk is reported to have protective effects against GI infections and otitis media, as well as upper and lower respiratory infection.[20] Breast milk has also been reported to provide benefits in terms of enhanced long-term cognitive development and decreased incidence of neurologic disabilities.[19] Breast milk contains less protein than infant formula; however, the protein is of high quality and is easy to digest and absorb. Lactose is the primary carbohydrate present in breast milk. Usually infants are born with sufficient quantities of the enzyme lactase, which enables them to digest lactose.[21]

Contraindications to providing breast milk include the inborn error of metabolism, galactosemia, since the infant must not receive lactose. Other contraindications include chylothorax and severe food allergies, although concerted efforts to counsel the mother regarding a milk-free diet are usually made for the latter if a cow's milk protein allergy is suspected before breast milk is replaced with formula. In the developed world, the provision of breast milk is not recommended if the patient's mother is positive for the human immunodeficiency virus (HIV) or acquired immune deficiency syndrome (AIDS).[22] Cocaine, heroin, amphetamines, and marijuana are contraindicated when breast milk is provided but tobacco and alcohol are not considered harmful in small quantities. The American Academy of Pediatrics (AAP) Committee on Drugs suggests that alcohol intake during lactation not exceed 2.5 fluid ounces of liquor, 8 fluid ounces of wine, or 2 cans of beer per day, as alcohol appears in breast milk in proportion to blood alcohol levels.[23]

Caregivers who need to provide breast milk by bottle or tube feeding must be taught aseptic methods for collection and storage. Hand washing combined with correct cleaning and sterilization of pumping equipment is necessary to minimize bacterial contamination. Freshly pumped breast milk may be stored in the refrigerator safely for up to 5 days when used to feed a healthy, full-term infant.[24] For long-term storage, the breast milk should be frozen as soon as possible after expression, and can be stored in the freezer for up to 6 months. Freshly pumped breast milk can safely remain at room temperature for up to 8 hours.[25]

Tube feedings of breast milk can result in significant fat losses due to separation of the fat out of solution and adherence to the tubing. This can lead to a significant decrease in the amount of fat and calories that the infant actually receives. Fat losses vary in relation to the rate and method of feeding, slower rates resulting in larger fat losses. Mean fat losses are reported to be 17% for bolus feeds and 34% for continuous infusion.[26] Therefore, bolus feeds are preferred when tube-feeding breast milk and continuous feedings should only be used when absolutely necessary.

INFANT FORMULA

The caloric density of standard infant formula is 20 calories per ounce, as this is the average for human milk.[1] When the provision of breast milk is not possible or desired by the mother, iron-fortified infant formulas are appropriate for full-term infants through 12 months of age. Specialized formulas have been developed and are indicated for preterm infants.[27]

Infant formulas are often categorized by the protein source with cow's milk-based, soy, whey, casein hydrolysate, free amino acid-based, and specialized metabolic formulas available. The patient's nutrient needs, intolerances, and clinical status will determine which category of formula is indicated. The carbohydrate source in most standard infant formulas is lactose, although Lactofree (Mead Johnson, Evansville, IN) and Similac Lactose-free (Ross, Columbus, OH) are examples of lactose-free, cow's milk protein–based formulas. Rarely would an infant need a lactose-free, cow's milk protein formula, since primary lactose intolerance in infancy is unusual. However, secondary lactose intolerance following intestinal mucosal damage from acute diarrhea and gastroenteritis is more prevalent.[1] The AAP does not routinely recommend changing to a lactose-free formula when an infant has diarrhea; however, depending on the extent of the mucosal damage, the infant may require a formula where the carbohydrate, protein, and fat have been modified to enhance absorption. The amount of protein in cow's milk–based formula is greater than in breast milk in an effort to provide a high quality amino acid profile. Some formulas contain a whey-predominant protein base, since it is thought to be more comparable to the protein in human milk and to enhance gastric emptying. However, whey proteins are species-specific and the whey proteins in breast milk are different than those present in cow's milk.[27]

The soy formulas contain soy protein isolates, added corn syrup solids (glucose polymers, hydrolyzed cornstarch), sucrose, and vegetable oils.[28] All soy formulas are lactose-free and some are also sucrose-free. The total protein content of soy formulas is higher than both breast milk and cow's milk–based formulas due to the decreased biologic value of soy protein. Methionine is added to improve the quality of the protein and make it complete.[27] Indications for soy formulas include but are not limited to infants with galactosemia, mild cow's milk protein intolerance, and lactase deficiency. Infants who are allergic to cow's milk protein may also be allergic to soy protein, necessitating the use of a protein hydrolysate formula.[28] Up to 60% of infants who present with cow's milk protein-induced enterocolitis will be equally as sensitive to soy protein. Soy formulas are not recommended for low birth weight premature infants due to evidence of decreased bone mineralization and conflicting studies on growth and plasma protein levels.[29]

The majority of the protein hydrolysate formulas contain casein that is enzymatically broken down to amino acids and small peptides, which facilitate easier absorption.[27] The fat composition of these formulas is usually modified, with 60% to 86% of the fat consisting of medium-chain triglycerides (MCTs). The portal blood instead of the lymphatic system transports medium-chain triglycerides. They have a more rapid intraluminal hydrolysis than long-chain triglycerides (LCTs), and intestinal absorption can occur without pancreatic enzymes or bile salts. Protein hydrolysate formulas are indicated primarily for infants with cow's milk and soy protein intolerance and disorders of digestion and absorption. This category of formulas may also prove helpful when transitioning an infant from parenteral to enteral nutrition or in an infant who has not received enteral feeds for greater than 5 to 7 days. Protein hydrolysate formulas are generally used when an infant's GI tract has sustained damage (usually as a result of a viral or bacterial infection), after bowel resection, and when malabsorption is suspected.[28] A damaged GI tract is permeable to foreign proteins, predisposing the infant to an allergic condition. An infant with an acute infection and diarrhea that does not resolve after treatment of the infection may need a hypoallergenic formula to allow for the gut mucosa to heal. Once the mucosa is healed, the infant can generally be transitioned back to a less expensive, standard formula.[27]

Casein-based hydrolysate formulas are considered hypoallergenic.[30] β-Lactoglobulin is the main protein present in whey and the most prevalent allergenic protein in cow's milk.[31] In whey hydrolysate formula, the whey fraction of the cow's milk protein has been enzymatically broken down, yielding peptides that are less allergenic than the whole proteins of standard formula.[27] However, whey hydrolysate formula can still produce symptoms in patients with cow's milk protein allergies.[30] Whey hydrolysate formula reportedly offers the advantage of increased gastric emptying time, comparable to that observed in breast milk.[32] The carbohydrate in whey hydrolysate formula is a combination of lactose and maltodextrin, which offers the beneficial effects of lactose such as enhanced calcium absorption, but at the same time is easier to digest due to the modified carbohydrate source. Whey hydrolysates are less expensive than the casein hydrolysates and are appropriate for normal infants, infants with a family history of allergies, or those transitioning from the more elemental casein hydrolysates.

If malabsorption is suspected, it is important to identify which nutrient is being malabsorbed in order to provide appropriate diet therapy. The macronutrient sources differ among the protein hydrolysate formulas and need to be considered when selecting from this formula group.[30] If fat malabsorption is experienced, a casein hydrolysate that contains MCT oil is indicated. Loose, watery stools with a change in the pH may indicate carbohydrate intolerance, necessitating a lactose-free formula that contains an easily digested carbohydrate source.[27]

Portagen (Mead Johnson, Evansville, IN) is a modified formula that is lactose-free and contains intact cow's milk protein and a fat source that is composed primarily of MCT oil. Conditions where dietary fat is malabsorbed—such as bile acid deficiency, intestinal resection, lymphatic anomalies, pancreatic insufficiency, chylous ascites, or chylothorax—are indications for a formula containing significant amounts of MCT oil. However, it is important to monitor the patient's intake of the essential fatty acids linoleic and linolenic acid, to avoid an essential fatty acid deficiency, especially if this type of formula is the sole or primary source of nutrition.[33] In such cases, supplementation with safflower oil may be necessary to provide adequate amounts of the essential fatty acids.

The protein source of elemental infant formulas is synthetic, free amino acids. Elemental infant formulas contain glucose polymers and the fat source is 95% LCTs and 5% MCTs. This type of formula is used in the management of infants who have a severe cow's milk protein allergy or multiple food protein intolerances. Some infants reportedly have such severe protein intolerances that they are sensitive to peptide residues present in the hypoallergenic casein hydrolysate formulas, necessitating the use of an elemental formula.[30] Free amino acid–based formulas have also been used successfully in infants and children with gastroesophageal reflux (GER) and eosinophilic esophagitis who have not responded to maximal medical therapy or to formula changes.[34] Exhibit 9–2 lists the names, categories, and manufacturers of many of the commonly used infant formulas.

Infant formulas are often concentrated in an effort to meet the estimated daily nutrient needs of infants who require additional calories and/or nutrients but who are unable to consume or tolerate an increase in volume. The nutrient density of formula can be increased by adding less water to a powder or liquid concentrate formula base, or by adding modulars such as fat, carbohydrate, or protein. Infant formulas can safely be concentrated to 30 calories/ounce by adding less water. However, it may be prudent to concentrate to a maximum of 24 to 27 calories/ounce for home use to avoid dehydration that may result from a higher renal solute load (RSL) as electrolyte and protein provision increases. The caloric density of the formula could be safely increased further by adding glucose polymers or fat or products that contain both carbohydrate and fat. Concentrated infant formulas contain less free water than standard dilutions, therefore routine assessment of the patient's fluid needs and hydration status is necessary. Concentrating infant formulas by adding less water ensures that an appropriate distribution of macronutrients is maintained. When adding modulars one must be careful to avoid creating a mixture with a disproportionate

Exhibit 9–2 Infant formulas

Cow's Milk Based

Similac® (Ross)
Enfamil® (Mead Johnson)
Enfamil AR® (Mead Johnson)
Lactofree® (Mead Johnson)
Similac Lactose-free® (Ross)
Similac PM 60/40® (Ross)

Cow's Milk Based with MCT Oil

Portagen® (Mead Johnson)

Soy Based

Isomil® (Ross)
Isomil DF® (Ross)
Isomil SF® (Ross)
Prosobee® (Mead Johnson)
Carnation Alsoy® (Nestlé)

Casein Hydrolysates

Alimentum® (Ross)
Nutramigen® (Mead Johnson)
Pregestimil® (Mead Johnson)

Whey Hydrolysate

Carnation Good Start® (Nestlé)

Elemental

Neocate® (Scientific Hospital Supplies)

Premature Transitional

Neosure® (Ross)
EnfaCare® (Mead Johnson)

Store brand/private label, and premature formulas are not listed

---

macronutrient percentage[28] or deficiencies of vitamins, minerals, trace elements, or electrolytes. The suggested distribution of calories in infant formulas is 7% to 16% protein, 35% to 55% fat, and 35% to 65% carbohydrate.[23] The recommended distribution of calories in pediatric formulas is 10% to 20% protein, 30% to 40% fat, and 40% to 60% carbohydrate. Providing greater than 60% of calories from fat may induce ketosis.[28] Modulars are often used in infants who either cannot tolerate a significant increase in formula osmolality or RSL, or who require a restricted intake of certain nutrients but at the same time additional calories. When adding modulars to infant or pediatric formulas, clinical conditions must be considered. Modulars such as fat or carbohydrate do not change the renal solute load of the formula; however, the addition of fat may decrease gastric emptying time, a contraindication in patients at risk for aspiration or who already have delayed gastric emptying.[3] The addition of carbohydrate or protein may affect the formula osmolality. Hyperosmolar formulas may result in nausea, vomiting, diarrhea, and delayed gastric emptying.[35] The osmolality of standard infant formulas (20 kcal/oz) ranges from 150 to 380 mOsm/kg. The American Academy of Pediatrics recommends that infant formulas have osmolalities of less than 460 mOsm/kg.[3] Exhibit 9–3 lists the names, categories, and manufacturers of some of the commonly used modulars.

PEDIATRIC ENTERAL FORMULAS

Pediatric formulas are 30 calories per ounce and contain a nutrient composition that is appropriate for children 1 to 10 years of age. Standard pediatric formulas

Exhibit 9–3 Examples of modulars

Carbohydrate	Polycose® (Ross)
	Moducal® (Mead Johnson)
Fat	Microlipid® (Mead Johnson)
	Vegetable Oil
	MCT Oil® (Mead Johnson)
Protein	Promod® (Ross)
	Casec® (Mead Johnson)
Carbohydrates & Fat	Duocal® (Scientific Hospital Supplies)

are nutritionally complete, are lactose- and gluten-free, are isotonic, can be provided orally or via tube, and contain intact protein and a fat source with both LCTs and MCTs for improved absorption.[30] Fiber-containing, intact formulas are also available and may prove beneficial with bowel management in a child with chronic constipation and/or diarrhea who is receiving adequate fluid.

Pediatric hydrolyzed protein formulas are lactose-free and contain protein in the form of short-chain peptides and/or amino acids. The fat source is a combination of polyunsaturated fat and MCT oil, and the carbohydrate consists of intermediate starch-hydrolysis products such as maltodextrins and glucose oligosaccharides.

Pediatric elemental formulas contain free amino acids, and a combination of polyunsaturated fat and MCT oil. Both pediatric hydrolysates and elemental formulas are used in children with compromised digestive or absorptive capacities, such as those with short gut syndrome, cystic fibrosis, inflammatory bowel disease (IBD), or chronic diarrhea. Pediatric elemental formulas are useful in managing patients with severe food allergies. Usually a protein hydrolysate formula is prescribed first, except in the case of severe food allergies; if tolerance is poor, then an elemental formula is provided. Pediatric elemental products are seldom used for patients requiring very low fat diets, such as those recovering from pancreatitis, since the fat content is significantly greater than that of adult elemental products.

For children between the ages of 1 and 6, enteral nutrition products should contain less protein and electrolytes than adult formulas to reduce the renal solute load and should contain higher levels of vitamins and minerals to meet the increased requirements for growth.[16] There are no disease-specific pediatric formulas (e.g., hepatic, renal, or trauma) and no hypercaloric pediatric enteral formulas (e.g., 1.5 cal/cc), so occasionally adult products will be selected if the characteristics of these formulas are believed to be advantageous. Ongoing assessment of the patient's hydration status, tolerance of the formula, and adequacy or excess of protein and micronutrient provision must be performed routinely.[30] Exhibit 9–4 lists the names, categories, and manufacturers of many of the commonly used pediatric formulas.

Exhibit 9–4 Toddler and pediatric formulas

Toddler Formulas	Pediatric Formulas
Intact Enfamil Next Step® (Mead Johnson) Carnation Follow-Up® (Nestlé)	**Intact** Pediasure® (Ross) Pediasure with fiber® (Ross) Kindercal® (Mead Johnson) Nutren Junior® (Nestlé) Nutren Junior with fiber® (Nestlé) Resource Just for Kids® (Novartis)
Soy Based Enfamil Nest Step Soy® (Mead Johnson) Carnation Follow-Up Soy® (Nestlé)	
	Hydrolyzed Whey Peptamen Junior® (Nestlé)
	Elemental Pediatric Vivonex® (Novartis) Neocate One Plus® (Scientific Hospital Supplies) Elecare® (Ross)
	Blenderized Compleat Pediatric® (Novartis)

Store brand/private label formulas are not listed

FORMULA SELECTION

The enteral formula selected for home use should be appropriate for any underlying disease processes; be compatible with medications, other therapies, the access route; and meet nutrient-provision goals.[36] Factors to consider when selecting an enteral formula are summarized in Exhibit 9–5.

Formula changes and modifications may be necessary if the patient demonstrates intolerance. However, caution should be exercised in changing formulas too quickly without observing the effects of the new formula and investigating other etiologies for intolerance, such as concurrent illness, medications, formula concentration, osmolality, incorrect formula preparation, or patient having volume sensitivity.

Exhibit 9–5 Factors to consider when selecting an enteral formula

- Child's age
- Daily fluid and nutrient requirements
- History of formula tolerance
- Food allergies
- GI function
- Diagnosis
- Whether the formula is intended to be provided orally
- Child's activity level
- Formula osmolality
- Formula viscosity
- Formula cost
- Availability in the home setting
- Ease of formula preparation
- Adequacy of insurance coverage

The daily volume of formula to be provided via tube is determined by the child's daily nutrition needs, the nutrient density of the selected formula, and the amount of fluid, formula, and solids being consumed orally. Additional free water may be needed to meet fluid requirements, although the volume of daily flushes with medications should be quantified, as the total can be significant. Vitamin and mineral supplementation may also be required. Nutritional assessment in the outpatient or home setting is an ongoing process. The nutrition support regimen is constantly undergoing revisions based on the patient's progress with volitional intake, tolerance of current dietary regimen, growth, laboratory values, and caregiver feedback.[37]

Initiation of tube feeds in children is usually with full-strength formula at low volumes. If the tube feeding is not tolerated, either the volume or strength should be decreased and the child allowed adequate time to tolerate the lower volume or strength before advances are attempted. After the child achieves, tolerates, and becomes accustomed to the goal regimen, changes to the feeding schedule may be made to better accommodate for lifestyle.

ACCESS SELECTION

Selection of the access device and infusion method for enteral tube feeds should be based on efficacy, safety, cost-effectiveness, and ability to meet daily estimated nutrient requirements. Volume to be infused, anticipated daily duration of enteral nutrition support, type of regimen (cyclic, continuous, intermittent), and activity level of the patient should also be considered.

Types of tubes include nasogastric (NG), orogastric (OG), nasoduodenal (ND), oroduodenal (OD), nasojejunal (NJ), percutaneous endoscopic gastrostomy (PEG) or jejunostomy (PEJ), surgically placed gastrostomy (G-tube) or jejunostomy (J-tube), or a jejunal tube placed through a gastrostomy (G-J tube). Each tube and provision type has advantages and disadvantages.

NASOGASTRIC FEEDING TUBES

The nasogastric tube (NGT) is inserted through the nose with the tip in the stomach. NGT feeding remains the most common method for short-term enteral feeding or supplementation for a child. Indications for using an NGT are summarized in Exhibit 9–6.

Essentially, any child that cannot or will not consume adequate fluid to maintain hydration and/or calories to promote normal growth and development but has a functional (albeit marginally functional at times) GI tract is a candidate for NGT feeding. Typically, the anticipated need is for no more than 4 to 6 weeks, but for children with chronic liver failure where portal hypertension is anticipated, an NGT may be preferred over a gastrostomy tube. It is possible to

Exhibit 9–6 Indications for nasogastric tube feeding

- Short-term enteral feeding trial to assess if a child needs a gastrostomy tube
- Severe failure to thrive with feeding aversion or avoidance
- Malabsorption
- Infantile diarrheal syndrome
- Post severe gastroenteritis with failure to tolerate oral diet
- Need for a non-palatable enteral formula or refusal to drink enteral formula
- Chronically ill, malnourished child who cannot consume sufficient calories to achieve or maintain adequate nutrition status
- No weight gain or weight loss for 3 consecutive months
- Total feeding time greater than 4 to 6 hours per day
- Oral aversion and mechanical problems with chewing, swallowing, or peristalsis

---

teach parents and adolescents to administer NGT feedings in the home, as oftentimes the reasons for needing NGT feedings are chronic in nature.

Medical conditions that often require the provision of enteral nutrition support in pediatric patients include critical illness, inflammatory bowel disease, cystic fibrosis, renal disease, congenital heart disease, certain inborn errors of metabolism, short-bowel syndrome, cancer, and chronic liver disease.[16]

SIZE OF TUBE

When using an NGT for a pediatric patient, an important consideration is the size of the tube in relation to the size of the child. The goal is to use the smallest tube possible, but at the same time one that is large enough to accommodate the needs of the child. The prevalence of gastroesophageal reflux in pediatric patients has been reported to increase as the size of the NGT increases.[38] Neonatal feeding tubes are only indicated for small or premature infants. Should the need for NGT feeding continue longer than expected, a larger tube should be considered as the neonate grows. Neonatal feeding tubes require more diligence regarding medication administration and flushing to prevent tube clogging. A commonly used NGT for children up to 1 year of age is a 5 French (Fr) NGT. (French is a term used to describe the diameter of an enteral feeding tube.) Fiber-containing formulas do not flow easily through a 5 Fr tube. For children older than 1 year, a 6 Fr tube is typically used. The length of the tube can vary but choosing a longer length is helpful, as the tube can be looped around the ear of the child and taped to his/her back to keep it out of reach. Adolescents also can use a 6 Fr NGT, as it will allow high rates of formula to be infused. However, if a fiber-containing formula is being provided, an 8 Fr tube is probably necessary for the viscous formula to flow easily.

TEACHING/PARENT EDUCATION

Use of a preprinted teaching sheet is helpful for parents and patients who will be doing home NGT placement. (See Figure 9–2, Nasogastric feeding tube inser-

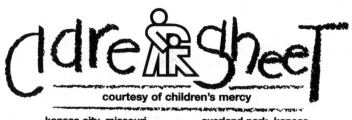

courtesy of children's mercy

kansas city, missouri   overland park, kansas

Nasogastric Feeding Tube Insertion

Insert _____ feeding tube as follows:
(Name and size of tube)

1. Wash your hands with soap and water.

2. Gather all supplies:
   - Feeding tube
   - Piece of tape
   - Small cup of water
   - Skin protector to place on face under tape (Stomahesive, Duoderm, Tegaderm)
   - ____ cc syringe
   - Stethoscope (optional)

3. Remove feeding tube from package.

4. Measure tube for correct length to insert it:
   1) Hold the tip of the feeding tube at the end of your child's nose where it will be inserted.
   2) Extend the tube to the earlobe, and then bend it down toward the stomach, to a point halfway between the tip of the breastbone and the belly button.
   3) Put a piece of tape on or around the tube to mark this length. If the tube is marked with black dots, note the dot closest to the piece of tape.

5. Dip the tip of the tube in water to moisten and make it slippery.

6. Gently insert the tube in the child's nose and continue to push it in until it reaches the tape mark on the tube. If your child starts coughing, or you see the tube curling in the mouth, pull it out. Let your child rest a minute. Then start again.

7. Place a piece of skin protector on your child's face and tape the tube to it. You may put the tape directly on the skin.

8. Check the tube to make sure it is in the proper place:
   1) Attach the syringe to the open end of the tube.
   2) Pull back on the plunger. If stomach contents appear in the tube, it is in the correct place. Push the stomach contents back into the stomach with the syringe.

CMH-02-206S

_____

continues

Figure 9–2 Nasogastric feeding tube insertion care sheet

Figure 9–2 continued

3) Another way to check the tube for proper placement is by listening with a stethoscope over the stomach while pushing 1 to 2 cc of air into the tube with a syringe. You should hear a whooshing sound. Remove the air after pushing it in by pulling back on the plunger.
4) If no stomach contents can be drawn back into the tube, and/or injected air cannot be heard with a stethoscope, advance the tube a short distance and check again.

9. Close off the end of the tube until it is needed for feeding.

Safety precautions:
- Only insert the feeding tube when your child's stomach is empty, since it can cause gagging and vomiting.
- If the child starts choking or coughing while putting in the tube, take it out. Let your child rest and then try again.
- If no stomach contents can be drawn back into the tube, and/or injected air cannot be heard with a stethoscope, advance the tube a short distance and check again.
- Always check the tube for proper placement before giving any feeding through it.

Call your child's doctor or the Children's Mercy Information Line at (816) 234-3188 if:
- you are not able to insert the feeding tube.
- you do not think your child's feeding tube is in the proper place.
- you are unable to get the feeding to flow into the tube. (The tube is clogged.)
- your child's abdomen (belly) becomes swollen.
- you have questions or concerns regarding your child's feeding tube or condition.

Call 911 if:
- your child has difficulty breathing after putting in the tube.

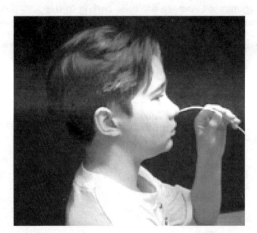
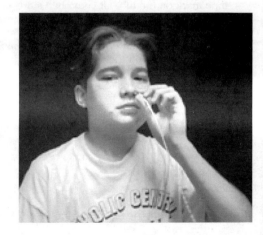

Exhibit 9–7 Placement of an NGT in an infant

1. Place a 3 cm × 1.5 cm oval thin pectin wafer on the cheek near the nare. (The pectin wafer serves as a protective barrier for the child's skin as the tape is actually placed over the pectin wafer.)
2. Cut a piece of transparent dressing the size of the pectin wafer to be used for securing the tube.
3. Immobilize the infant. It may be helpful to raise the child's arms up over the head and hold them with one hand while cupping the head with the other hand. (This is especially helpful when the child has respiratory difficulties, as raising the arms expends the lungs.)
4. Position the head in the anatomically correct position. Even a modest tilt backward can allow the tube to enter the lungs.
5. Advance the tube and blow in the infant's face just as he/she starts to gag to facilitate swallowing.
6. Keep advancing the tube until the placement marking tape is within 1 cm of the nare.
7. Have the infant suck on a pacifier after the tube is inserted.
8. Secure the tube with the transparent dressing on top of the pectin wafer.
9. Verify placement.
10. Use arm splints to prevent an older infant from removing the tube. This is most important the first few days and during the night at home. After that, the infant tends to not bother the tube as often.

---

tion care sheet.) It is important to consider the specific developmental needs of each pediatric age group when inserting the NGT or teaching NGT placement. In general, the older the child, the more detailed the verbal and written information should be—for the benefit of the caregiver and so the child can prepare mentally for the procedure.[39] These considerations are summarized in Exhibits 9–7, 9–8, and 9–9. It is best to use a treatment room to place the NGT for a toddler and older child so they can have the sense that the hospital room is a safe place.

Bedside placement of transpyloric feeding tubes has been reported to be very successful in critical care settings.[40] Often these children receive small amounts

---

Exhibit 9–8 Placement of an NGT in a toddler

1. Explain the procedure to the child.
2. Get someone to distract/comfort the child. (Sometimes the parent may not want to be that person.)
3. Place a 3 cm x 1.5 cm oval thin pectin wafer on the cheek near the nare. (The pectin wafer serves as a protective barrier for the child's skin as the tape is actually placed over the pectin wafer.)
4. Cut a piece of transparent dressing the size of the pectin wafer to be used for securing the tube.
5. Immobilize the child by holding him/her in a lap or lying him/her on a treatment table.
6. Control the head from sideways movement.
7. Reinforce how well-behaved the child is being.
8. Advance the tube.

Exhibit 9–9 Placement of an NGT in an adolescent

1. Explain the procedure to the adolescent. Appeal to body image issues of not having a "permanent fixture" such as a gastrostomy tube to contend with.
2. Teach the teenager to self-insert a pre-measured tube.
3. Have patient stand in front of a mirror if possible.
4. Some adolescents prefer to drink water while advancing the tube. Offer both approaches (drinking, not drinking) and let him/her choose.
5. Secure the tube with hypoallergenic tape so that no tape marks show when tape is removed.
6. Verify placement.
7. Stress flexibility with schedules when using an NGT—i.e., taking nights off for social events, hooking up later on weekends, etc.
8. Do not have a parent in the room. Stress that this is the adolescent's responsibility and that the parents will be taught tube placement. Stress that this is an opportunity for the adolescent to take control over one aspect of his/her health.

(trophic feedings) of enteral formulas as tolerated and then the rate is advanced as the patient's condition allows. While this method is not expected to be commonplace in pediatric care, it is a viable option in a subset of patients. Any child who has serious respiratory compromise should be on an oxygen saturation monitor during this procedure, as children more commonly arrest from respiratory rather than cardiac events. Reports in the literature have documented episodes of desaturation in very low birth weight infants who have an NGT in place.[41] OG feeding tube placement has been described in the literature in premature neonates, as they are obligate nose-breathers, and in other populations, such as cystic fibrosis patients.[42,43]

MEASUREMENT

Appropriate measurement of the NGT is essential for safe placement. Using an estimate of tube insertion length that is extrapolated from a formula based on height has been described. The use of the nose-ear-xiphoid process is known to be somewhat short in estimating NGT placement, so an additional 3 to 4 cm can be added to the insertion distance in larger children.[44] For an older child, use the same procedure as in Exhibit 9–6 but explain the process in more depth. Outline the expected behaviors (holding still, swallowing, trying not to gag) and stress that cooperating with the procedure will minimize any potential discomfort. Older children tend to think that they did something wrong and that the NGT is punishment, so it is important to clearly state that the NGT is an attempt to improve the child's health. Children often admit that the tube is smaller than most of the candy they eat. This helps alleviate some of the fear of swallowing the tube. In this age group, having the parent remain in the room during the procedure can prove helpful. It is also prudent to bring all of the supplies into the room immediately after obtaining the child's assent to do the procedure. Prolonging the time from assent to insertion tends to escalate feelings of anxiety. This potentially tends to cause more crying, which results in swelling of the nasal mucous membranes, making the tube more difficult to pass. Using guided imagery where the parent calmly talks about something the child enjoys remembering is very helpful during this procedure. Tubes may also be passed during sedation for another procedure to help eliminate the cause for anxiety.

It must be readily apparent that the developmental age of the child is a crucial factor in the success of NGT placement. Since NGTs must be replaced periodically due to accidental dislodgment, etc., it is important that nurses and other caregivers appropriately address the child's physical, mental, and emotional needs during this procedure. In many instances patients and parents will view NGT placement as more invasive than central line placement. Toddlers and small children must feel safe, loved, and respected by nurses and caregivers so that they do not view the tube placement as a form of abuse. Older children need to have clear messages conveyed regarding the need for the tube so that they can use their limited reasoning skills to understand correctly. Adolescents need to have issues of control placed as much as possible with themselves and not their parents. Both older children and adolescents do have the right to refuse NGT placement, which is something that is often not communicated to them. No adolescent or parent should ever be sent home to perform this task without being supervised in a return demonstration in the health care setting. A final point that is important is to alternate the nares when a NGT is replaced to avoid excoriation of the sensitive tissue.

NASOGASTRIC TUBE MANAGEMENT

Once the NGT is successfully placed, the goal of safe and effective enteral feeding becomes the priority. This can be a challenge in pediatrics, as an adult does not typically watch children 24 hours per day. Nurses and other caregivers need to be vigilant about securing the tube, placement verification, flushing, and prevention of complications.

Securing the NGT properly is critical for a pediatric patient. Infants may be able to partially dislodge the tube by unwittingly hooking their little fingers around the tube as it enters the nare. It may also be dislodged during episodes of sneezing, coughing, or vomiting. Placement needs to be verified after any of these occurrences if there is any question of tube dislodgment. Infants and children tend to be sensitive to many of the adhesives currently used to tape NGTs. It is important to use a pectin wafer for young children and hypoallergenic tape for adolescents to avoid skin excoriation.

Tube placement verification remains a clinical dilemma in all age groups. A study evaluating the prevalence of NGT placement errors in children found that 20.9% had some sort of placement error.[45] While none of the errors involved placement into the trachea or lungs, many of the tubes were placed in the esophagus. Abdominal distention, vomiting, and altered level of consciousness were correlated with placement error. While this was not an outcomes study, it is important to realize that NGT misplacement may put a child at increased risk for aspiration or infusion of enteral formula into the pulmonary tree. Typically, pediatric patients do not have x-rays performed to verify placement of an NGT. It is not cost effective or clinically feasible to obtain an x-ray for this purpose in a population who may require tube replacement several times per day. If the patient is exclusively tube-fed, prompt tube replacement is extremely important in order to prevent dehydration or a lengthy duration of fasting, especially in small infants whose glycogen stores are not yet well developed. It is important to be consistent in the hospital and home setting with feeding tube verification. Pediatric nurses and parents are taught to aspirate for gastric contents and then to instill air via a syringe into the tube and auscultate for the air bubble. X-ray verification of feeding tube placement may be done in special circumstances, particularly in critical care areas, but bedside verification remains the standard in other settings.

As with adults, flushing an NGT to prevent clogging is important, especially since many patients receive medications as well as enteral formulas via tube. In pediatric patients, it is important to consider the size of the child when flushing an NGT. An infant should only need to be flushed with 3 to 5 ml of tap water before and after medication administration. This population does not need, nor do they tolerate, large amounts of calorie-free fluid. Older toddlers and adolescents are also often provided small volumes of flushes with medications, as they too may be intolerant of fluid excesses. In general, most pediatric NGTs are not routinely flushed with water to prevent clogging unless an institution has experienced a problem with clogged tubes. See Chapter 7, Enteral Nutrition Complications, for more on unclogging enteral feeding tubes. It is also not common to use any other fluid besides water to flush a pediatric NGT.

Parents who take their child home with an NGT must be adequately prepared before assuming this responsibility. Parents will often want a nurse to come to the home for the first time he or she needs to replace the tube. Understandably, parents report a tremendous amount of anxiety at first when performing this task independently at home. Helping the parents identify a neighbor or relative who could assist them is often necessary. As with any procedure, parental comfort increases with practice as their skill level increases. Assuring parents that they are doing this so that their child can grow and develop makes it easier to justify what feels like an abusive task. The caregiver should receive clear and consistent education and training on the proper preparation and administration of the prescribed formula. Instruction should include specific formula characteristics, aseptic technique for measuring and providing proper volumes, use and maintenance of the equipment, specific instruction on the infusion method(s), potential drug-nutrient interactions, medication administration, and problem management. Refer to Figure 9–3 (the nasogastric tube feeding care sheet) for various methods to teach parents bolus feedings. The caregiver's knowledge and skills should periodically be reassessed and retraining provided as needed.[9] Any hint that the parent will be noncompliant in the home needs to be shared with the child's physician and documented in the medical record.

It is a fairly common occurrence for a pediatric patient to have a dislodged NGT, either accidentally (as a result of sneezing, coughing, or vomiting), or intentionally (because the patient pulled it out). Nurses and parents need to be vigilant in monitoring for this, as the tube can be coughed up into the esophagus or pharynx without the child being able to communicate that there is a problem. Parents are taught that any sudden change in respiratory status (grunting, blue around the lips, substernal retractions, increased work of breathing, etc.) warrants immediate discontinuation of the enteral tube feedings and notification of the physician. The more severe or sudden the onset of problems, the more urgent a call for emergency medical services becomes. Here again, respiratory arrest is much more common in pediatrics than cardiac arrest.

Otitis media and sinusitis on the NGT ipsilateral side has been reported in the literature.[46,47] This is attributed to the movement of the NGT (from swallowing) against the eustachian tube. Nurses and parents should observe for the classical signs of otitis media, which include fussiness, pulling on the affected ear, and fever. Routine assessments by nurses should include palpating the ear and checking for tenderness. The NGT should be rotated between the right and left nare when replaced to avoid unnecessary irritation of one side and in an effort to prevent sinusitis. It is not as common to find sinusitis in a pediatric patient but it can be identified by the appearance of mucopurulent drainage from the nares, low-grade fever, and, sometimes, tenderness under the eye. Treatment of otitis media and sinusitis should involve avoiding the affected side for NGT placement during antibiotic therapy.

Infants and young children who receive exclusive NGT feedings may experience feeding problems when oral feedings are introduced. The loss of a normal pattern of suck, swallow, and breathe has been reported in infants who have received exclusive NGT feedings.[48] For toddlers and preschoolers, oral aversion may occur as the child is either afraid to place food in his/her mouth or simply does not feel the need to eat.[49] Both of these situations can be best treated or prevented with the help of an occupational therapist who prescribes a regimen of oral stimulation. Home visits by an occupational therapist can be very helpful to work with the child and parents in their own environment. Frequently these problems are chronic in nature and can last for a prolonged time. Parents can become discouraged by the fact that their child has accomplished much by being fed via tube but lost a vital skill in the process. It may be helpful to contact a parent who was in a similar situation and has had a successful outcome to offer support to a struggling parent during this time. Behavioral issues regarding feeding tube replacement are easier to prevent than to treat. It is best to send clear messages to the child regarding needed cooperation with the procedure. Reinforcing positive behaviors with praise and rewards will help the child learn to cooperate during the procedure. Even toddlers are capable of learning to cooperate with this procedure. Rewards need to be developmentally appropriate. Nurses might develop a treasure box for children to pick out a small toy, sticker, or book as a reward. Prompt tube replacement followed by a consequence is the typical response when cooperation fails. In the home, power struggles will continue as long as the child senses that the parent is ambivalent or overly anxious about the replacement of the NGT.

A clogged NGT is typically removed, cleaned, and replaced in a pediatric patient. It tends to be too time-consuming to try and unclog a tube compared to replacement. It may become necessary to use a new tube if the previous tube remains clogged after an unsuccessful attempt to clean it. Use of pancreatic enzymes for tube unclogging has been reported in adult studies and is discussed elsewhere. This option has not been widely used in pediatrics, but many pediatric centers do use commercially available products to dissolve clogs. The best way to approach clogged feeding tubes is to prevent clogs from occurring by flushing before and after medications, flushing routinely when using fiber-containing formulas, and careful preparation of powdered formulas. Exhibit 9–10 summarizes potential complications of NGT placement.

GASTROSTOMY TUBES

G-tubes pass directly into the stomach and are the preferred route for long-term enteral tube feeding. They are lower maintenance than an NGT and are not readily visible to the general public. Many parents will opt for a gastrostomy tube so that their child can go out in public without "looking different" or to deal with the chronic challenge of trying to provide adequate nutrition to a developmentally delayed child. Gastroesophageal reflux may be a concurrent problem that needs to be evaluated. It may develop after a percutaneous endoscopic gastrostomy tube (PEG) is inserted.[50] Several reports in the literature caution that cancer patients may be at risk for significant cellulitis when G-tubes are used.[51–53] However, all of these authors do acknowledge that nutrition support can be effectively accomplished by using G-tube feeding. Indications for G-tube placement are summarized in Exhibit 9–11.

Commonly used pediatric G-tubes are the PEG tube, surgically placed G-tube, and a low-profile device such as the Button (Bard Interventional Products, Billerica, MA), which can be placed surgically or endoscopically. The sizes of G-tubes frequently used in pediatrics range from 8 Fr to 18 Fr. PEG tubes are

---

Exhibit 9–10 Complications of NGT placement

- Tube dislodgment
- Otitis media
- Sinusitis
- Loss of suck/swallow/breathe
- Oral aversion
- Possible nasal, esophageal, or tracheal irritation
- Behavioral issues related to tube replacement
- Clogged tube

Exhibit 9–11 Indications for gastrostomy placement

- Profound developmental delays with inability to safely ingest adequate nutrients, including fluid
- Profound developmental delays with inability to ingest enough nutrients to achieve or maintain adequate nutrition status
- Chronic illness with malnutrition and inability to ingest enough nutrients to achieve or maintain adequate nutrition status
- Chronic malabsorption requiring continuous feeding
- Organic failure to thrive
- Need for enteral feeding tube for greater than 2–3 months

more cost effective to insert than surgically placed tubes.[54] One report in the literature documents an 88% success rate in a series of 224 consecutively placed PEGs. The authors reported serious complications such as the deaths of two children with known cardiac conditions, one episode of intestinal obstruction, and five gastrocolic fistulae. The authors stress the importance of appropriate patient selection for this procedure versus a surgically placed G-tube. They also acknowledge that some complications were less common as their surgical team's skill level increased.[55] A Canadian study, which evaluated a low profile gastrostomy device in 19 children over a 6-month time period, reported relatively minor complications such as disconnection of the feeding tubing from the device. The authors found that this type of tube was preferred over the traditional G-tube by families and that there were fewer reports of skin irritation.[56] Another group reported problems with anti-reflux valve failure in 23 of the 31 devices placed in children.[57] Low-profile devices are often the replacement tube of choice for pediatric patients. The tract should be approximately 12 weeks old before changing tubes.[54] For low-profile devices, the length of the device is an important consideration for replacement.

GASTROSTOMY TUBE MANAGEMENT

Skin Care

Good skin care is essential to keep the gastrostomy site healthy. Refer to the button gastrostomy and percutaneous endoscopic gastrostomy tube care cards in Figures 9–3 and 9–4, respectively, for details regarding routine skin care. In general, the use of hydrogen peroxide at a gastrostomy skin site is contraindicated as it can oxidize (damage) the cell membranes that help make the tract. Parents are advised to assess the skin at the site carefully and notify the inserting physician if attempts to treat any problems at home are unsuccessful. It is recommended that the child sit in a bath with water below the level of the G-tube or take a shower. For swimming and boating outings, the G-tube should be covered with a transparent, waterproof dressing. Children are discouraged from sitting in hot tubs.

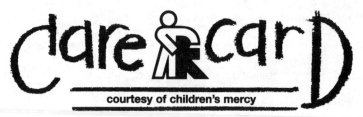

Button Gastrostomy

A button gastrostomy has been inserted into your child's stomach to provide the nutrition that he is unable to get by mouth. A special formula will be given through the button by a feeding tube.

Your child has a _____ french ____ cm button gastrostomy.

Skin care:
It is important to take care of the skin around your child's button gastrostomy. Skin care needs to be done at least 2 times each day. The area around the button gastrostomy needs to stay clean and dry at all times Talk to your child's doctor about bathing and swimming instructions.

1) Wash the skin around the button gastrostomy with soap and water.
2) Rotate the button gastrostomy to fully clean all of the skin around it.
3) Rinse the area well with warm water.
4) Dry the area well, especially the skin around the button gastrostomy.
5) Turn the button gastrostomy so it is not sitting on the incision.

Feeding tube adaptors: There are only 3 types of feeding tubes that can be used with your child's button gastrostomy. **DO NOT put anything else into the button gastrostomy**—including syringes.

1) Continuous Feeding Tubes: This type of tube gives feedings slowly to prevent diarrhea, cramping and bloating.
2) Bolus Feeding Tubes: This type of tube gives fluids and medications rapidly.
3) Decompression Tube: This type of tube helps relieve bloating and excess gas.

Care of the feeding tube during feedings:
• Tape the tube to your child's stomach during the feeding to prevent it from being accidentally pulled out.

• Flush the button gastrostomy before and after each feeding or medication. Use _____ cc of warm tap water.

Cleaning the feeding tubes:
1) Clean the feeding tube with soapy water and rinse well after each feeding.

CMH-99-114

_____

continues

Figure 9–3 Button gastrostomy tube care card

Figure 9–3 continued

2) Let the feeding tube air dry between feedings.
3) Feeding tubes should be thrown away every 4 weeks, **or** sooner if they begin to look cloudy or become cracked.

To reorder supplies:
1) Bring a list of needed supplies with you to your child's clinic appointment.
or
2) You may call the supply company _____
    at _____.

When reordering supplies, be sure to know the size of your child's button gastrostomy. This can be found on the button gastrostomy or at the top of this card.

Call your child's doctor at (816) 234-3000 and ask for him or the GI-doctor-on-call if you notice any of the following:
• your child's stomach remains bloated for more than one hour.
• any redness, swelling, drainage or skin breakdown around the button gastrostomy.
• you are unable to give feeding or medication.
• your child has pain, diarrhea, vomiting or unexplained fever.
• you have questions or concerns about your child's button gastrostomy.

Take your child to the Emergency Room if the button gastrostomy:
• is difficult to turn.
• becomes dislodged (slips out of place).

Flushing

Some low-profile devices have an anti-reflux valve that prevents gastric contents from popping the cap off the tube during times of increased gastric pressure. These valves can become "stuck open" when viscous formula and medications are routinely administered. Parents are advised to flush the tube with a carbonated beverage (seltzer) periodically if this happens. Some parents start doing this routinely, upon beginning the use of the tube, as this can be a good preventive measure. Volumes of 5 to 10 ml for infants and up to 30 to 60 ml for adolescents are usually well tolerated. The more viscous the solution (such as fiber-containing formulas) or the more medications that are administered by tube, the more likely it is that the anti-reflux valve will stick open on occasion. PEG tubes and surgically placed G-tubes rarely clog, but when this occurs, provision of the carbonated beverage is usually successful.

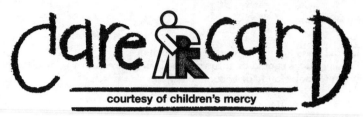

courtesy of children's mercy

kansas city, missouri   overland park, kansas

Percutaneous Endoscopic Gastrostomy Tube (PEG)

A PEG tube has been inserted into your child's stomach to provide the nutrition he is unable to get by mouth.

Your child has a _____ french PEG tube.

Skin Care:
It is important to take care of the skin around your child's PEG. Skin care needs to be done at least 2 times each day. The area around the PEG needs to stay clean and dry at all times. Talk to your child's doctor about bathing and swimming instructions. There is a bolster (crossbar) on your child's PEG. The bolster keeps the tube in place. It needs to be rotated with each cleaning. Rotating the bolster with each cleaning prevents skin irritation. The bolster should remain at the number _____.

1) Wash the skin around the PEG tube with soap and water.
2) Rotate the bolster to fully clean the PEG tube site.
3) Rinse the area well with warm water.
4) Dry the area well, especially the skin around the PEG tube.
5) Turn the bolster so it is not sitting on the incision.
6) After cleaning the skin, tape the feeding tube to your child's stomach.

Care of the feeding tube during feedings:
• Flush the PEG tube before and after each feeding or medication. Use __ cc of warm tap water to flush the feeding tube.

To reorder supplies:
1) Bring a list of needed supplies with you to your child's clinic appointment or call _____
or
2) You may call the supply company
   at _____.

CMH-99-111

continues

Figure 9–4 Percutaneous endoscopic gastrostomy tube care card

Figure 9–4 continued

Call your child's doctor at (816) 234-3000 and ask for him or the GI-doctor-on-call if you notice any of the following:
- your child's stomach remains bloated for more than one hour.
- there is any redness, swelling, drainage or skin breakdown around your child's PEG tube.
- you are unable to give feedings or medications.
- your child has pain, diarrhea, vomiting or unexplained fever.
- you have any questions or concerns about your child's PEG tube.

Connection for Feeding and Venting

When a low-profile device is inserted, parents are given two adapters. There is a feeding adapter for bolus or continuous drip feedings and medication administration. To prevent accidental disconnection, the feeding tubing should be taped to the low-profile device unless the device has a locking mechanism, such as with the MIC-KEY (Medical Innovations Corporation, Santa Clara, CA). This tubing should be cleaned with hot water between uses and stored dry on a counter or in a bag in the refrigerator. If a residue builds up inside the tubing, overnight soaking in a dilute vinegar solution should dissolve it. The other tubing given to parents is a decompression tube that is used for venting or "burping" the child during times of abdominal distension. The tube is attached to a syringe and placed in the G-tube so that air and formula can flow up into the syringe. The air escapes into the atmosphere and the gastric contents flow back into the stomach. Parents should be discouraged from "routinely" doing this and should only use the decompression tube when significant abdominal distension is observed. The tube is then rinsed off and stored in open air.

Administration of Medications

Medication administration via G-tube is a challenge. The caregiver should always consult with the primary health care provider and/or a pharmacist before administering medications with tube feedings. Many medications are incompatible with formula and can cause tube clogging or adversely affect the child's tolerance of the regimen. Crushing solid medications such as tablets or capsules may accelerate the drug absorption time, resulting in undesirable elevations of blood levels, and most syrups will cause tube clogging. Compressed tablets, elixirs, and suspensions can usually be provided via tube. Gastric residuals should always be checked before administering medications. Residual volumes exceeding half of a bolus feed or half of 1 hour's volume for continuous infusions may result in inadequate drug absorption, depending on the drug. The feeding tube should be flushed with water before and after medication administration.[58] However, gastrostomy tubing is long enough that a significant volume of water may be required to flush the medication(s) down the tube and a small infant may not tolerate the additional volume. Rather than using excessive water flushes, medications are often given before bolus feedings or a small water flush (3 to 5 ml) is used and then the feeding pump is restarted. For low-profile devices, nurses should not use syringes to administer medications directly into the device, as this can cause damage to the anti-reflux valve. This is especially important as caregivers watch nurses for the "proper" method of delivering feedings, medications, flushes, etc. Parents need to be taught that the appropriate method for medication administration is by using a syringe to measure the medication (if appropriate) and then instilling the medication down the feeding adapter.

Gastrostomy Tube Complications

G-tubes tend to be easier to manage in the home than other feeding tubes and are associated with a low incidence of complications. Complications with G-tubes are usually related to skin problems. Exhibit 9–12 summarizes complications associated with G-tubes.

Many of these complications can be treated at home without notifying the health care provider if parents have been provided good post-insertion instruction. It is still necessary to give parents a resource person to contact if problems persist. In a hospital, nutrition support nurses or enterostomal therapists are good resources for treatment of these problems.

To begin developing a common language for health care providers to describe problems encountered at the gastrostomy site, an assessment tool was developed that incorporated the variables documented from signs and symptoms of inflammation and infection. Also included were variables commonly encountered at gastrostomy sites of granulation tissue and erosion. The Gastrostomy Skin Assessment Tool was first tested in a small pediatric population (see Figure 9–5). The data from the first test of its validity resulted in a revision of the tool. Variables that did not demonstrate significance were eliminated and defining criteria for the remaining variables were clarified. Currently, work is being

---

Exhibit 9–12 Gastrostomy tube complications

- Inflammation at site
- Drainage
- Granulation tissue
- Bacterial infection

- Yeast infection
- Dislodged into tract
- Accidental removal

Gastric tube _____ Low profile device _____
Date _____

LEGEND	OPERATIONAL DEFINITION	SCORE
Skin Redness		
0 = None	No signs of redness	
1 = Redness	Pink or red skin	
2 = Severe redness	Very red skin	
Drainage		
0 = None	No secretions from site	
1 = Serous Drainage	Watery drainage, clear	
2 = Drainage with color	Red, creamy, tan, or green drainage	
3 = Purulent drainage	Drainage containing pus from site	
	(Multiply × 2 indicating probable site infection)	
Erosion		
0 = None	No erosion of the skin at the site	
1 = Mild	Small area of breakdown	
2 = Severe	Significant skin breakdown	
Granulation Tissue		
0 = None	No new protruding pink, moist tissue from site	
1 = Mild	Fleshy tissue, pink, moist tissue, patchy around site	
2 = Moderate	Fleshy tissue, pink, moist tissue, partially surrounding the site	
3 = Severe	Fleshy tissue, pink, moist tissue, completely surrounding the site	
Discomfort		
0 = None	No pain reported or observed	
1 = Mild	Mild pain reported by the patient, the caregiver, or observed during examination, such as movement with assessment, verbal response as "ow" or "that hurts," *pain intermittent*	
2 = Moderate	Moderate pain reported by the patient, caregiver, or observed during examination, such as pushing examiner's hand away, more intense loud verbal response or initiation of crying, *pain intermittent*	
3 = Severe	Severe or intense pain as reported by the patient, caregiver, or observed during examination, may be combative when assessed, may elicit extreme verbal response, crying or screaming, *pain constant*	
TOTAL GASTROSTOMY	**ASSESSMENT SCORE**	

Figure 9–5 Gastrostomy Skin Assessment Tool

done to reevaluate the tool for validity. Problems encountered with skin assessment are associated with the subjectiveness of the variables in question, especially skin redness. Once refined, a valid assessment tool can provide a common language to communicate problems and measure change. Then interventions can be initiated that will benefit both patients and health care providers.

Most patients who have a G-tube will experience an occasional bout of inflammation at the site. There may not always be an identified etiology for this problem. Sometimes the bolster for the PEG tube is too tight on the skin, and when it is loosened up, inflammation resolves. This can occur when a child has gained a lot of weight after tube insertion and the parents were not advised to periodically move the bolster. It can also occur in children who experience intermittent distension, such as with pseudo-obstruction. When an inflammatory reaction occurs at a G-tube site, nurses and parents should stop using soap and simply wash the site 2 or 3 times daily with water. Soap can be more irritating to the skin than water alone. It is important for parents to be advised that inflammation is not always associated with an infection. Routine culturing of the gastrostomy site is not recommended when only inflammation is present.[57] Limited use of over-the-counter topical antibiotic ointment is permissible, but is not advised for more than 2 days. New onset inflammation that does not resolve after 3 days warrants a visit to the inserting physician's office. Often a nurse in the office can assess the tube site and offer other solutions.

Drainage around a G-tube site is often difficult to assess. One should try and establish whether the drainage is caused by leakage of formula from the stomach or is a mucous exudate. Any drainage at a G-tube site puts the patient at risk for infection. Drainage should be cleaned with water and a gauze pad. Although it is not usually a good idea to place a slit gauze pad between the skin and the bolster, it may be necessary to do this when drainage is present to wick the moisture away from the site. Absorptive dressings are available if the drainage is more than a small amount. Drainage that seems to be from leakage of gastric contents can be especially caustic to the skin. Every effort should be made to be sure there is a snug fit between the internal and external fixation apparatus. Drainage that seems to be mucoid in nature indicates an acute inflammatory response. Culturing the site is indicated if the drainage is purulent; otherwise, an over-the-counter topical antibiotic ointment may be used for up to 3 days to see if it helps resolve the inflammation. Rarely is the drainage actually blood, but if this occurs, it could be indicative of recent trauma to the tract such as accidental pulling. The physician should be notified if direct pressure for a minute or two does not stop the bleeding or if the tube does not function well after the episode. Granulation tissue is a friable tissue that forms in the tract in response to movement or irritation by a foreign body.[59] Some children have chronic problems with granulation tissue formation and other children may never experience a problem. G-tubes that are allowed to migrate in and out of the tract tend to cause more cellulitis than those tubes that fit snugly to the skin. It is important for nurses and parents to report granulation tissue so that it can be adequately treated. A silver nitrate stick generally is used to cauterize the tissue. Untreated granulation tissue is painful, bleeds easily, and increases the risk of gastrostomy site infection.

Infection at a G-tube site is very painful for the child and may result in loss of tube function. Bacterial infections with a known organism may be treated with oral antibiotics. It is important for the child to be seen by the prescribing physician after the course of antibiotics has been completed to assure that the infection has been adequately treated. Use of prescription antibiotic ointments should be limited to 10 days with a follow-up visit so that parents do not abuse the topical ointment, setting the stage for resistant organisms.

A yeast infection at the G-tube site is fairly common in pediatrics, especially among infants and toddlers in diapers. The most likely source of Candida infection in PEG tubes is thought to be from the patient's mouth. One report in the literature found that 20 malnourished patients compared to 10 controls had significantly higher fungal counts in the antrum of the stomach (13 of 20 versus 1 of 10).[60] This can be initially treated with a dilute vinegar and water (1/4 c vinegar and 3/4 c water) solution poured over the site 3 times per day. It is important that some of the vinegar water flows down the tract, as the yeast tends to grow in the gastrostomy site tract, skin, and tube. The skin should be allowed to air dry and then a topical antifungal cream should be applied. Leaving the child's abdomen open to the air and sunlight for part of the day is helpful as well. Nurses should evaluate the lumen of the tube as well as the skin when a yeast infection is suspected. The fungus may adhere to the internal lumen of the tube, causing the tube to weaken, which could result in it falling out.[61] Pouring 15 ml of the dilute vinegar water down the tube when skin care is done may adequately treat the luminal yeast infection. Occasionally, the tube has to be replaced because the yeast cannot be effectively removed from the internal lumen of the tube. This is often the case when parents report the tube is "bumpy" on the inside.

Accidental removal of a G-tube is a fear of nurses and parents alike. If the G-tube has an internal bolster, it may have damaged the tract when it was removed so the child needs to be observed for bleeding. If the G-tube has a balloon, the parents should have a replacement tube at home. They need to be taught how to check the balloon and replace the tube if the balloon is leaking. If the parent is confident that the tube replacement was successful and gastric contents can be aspirated, feedings can proceed as ordered. For any other type of accidental G-tube removal, immediate notification of the inserting physician is indicated. A Foley catheter can be placed in the ostomy site to keep it from closing until an appropriate tube can be placed.

A rare and serious complication associated with G-tubes is dislodgment into the tract. The child typically experiences tremendous pain when the tube is touched or used. Parents report that the formula will either flow slowly or not at all. A well-defined area of induration is often present. This problem requires hospitalization, tube removal, and parenteral antibiotics. Children who have had their G-tube for many years and have grown a lot are at risk for this, as are children who do not understand that they should not pull on the tube.

JEJUNOSTOMY TUBES

A J-tube bypasses the stomach and pylorus, entering directly into the jejunum. J-tubes can be placed nasojejunally, percutaneously (PEJ), or surgically. A G-J tube allows for transpyloric feeds and gastric decompression. In pediatrics, the most common indications for jejunal feeding are severe gastroesophageal reflux, severely delayed gastric emptying, and chronic aspiration. Clinical problems such as persistent vomiting after tube placement and accidental dislodgment still plague J-tubes. In general, older and larger children tend to have fewer complications than younger children with J-tubes.[62] J-tubes require the closest monitoring of all the enteral feeding routes. Insertion of these tubes requires a great deal of skill on the part of the nurse or physician. They tend to be labor intensive to insert; therefore, significant effort is put forth by nurses and parents to keep the tubes in place and patent. It is very important that parents have thorough teaching before taking a child with a J-tube home.

JEJUNOSTOMY TUBE MANAGEMENT AND COMPLICATIONS

J-tube management is primarily directed at preventing complications. Therefore, this section will consider the two together. Potential disadvantages of using J-tubes include increased risk of bacterial overgrowth, inability to check residuals, necessity of continuous infusions, possible abdominal distention due to gas and poor motility, and diarrhea if formula volume or osmolality exceeds patient's threshold for tolerance.[63] Nursing management is directed at site care, maintaining patency, and securing the tube to prevent cellulitis, clogging, and dislodgment. Site care for a PEJ or surgically placed J-tube is the same as for G-tubes. Refer to Figure 9–6 for the care card information for jejunostomy tubes.

The internal diameter of a J-tube tends to be smaller than that of a G-tube, so the risk for clogging increases when viscous formulas and liquid medications are provided. J-tubes should be routinely flushed every 6 to 8 hours with at least 10 ml of water. The older child will tolerate flush volumes of up to 60 cc. Flushing with 10 ml of water before and after medications is essential to prevent clogging. Most centers have some sort of commercial tube declogger to use for instances of clogging. Pancreatic enzymes activated with sodium bicarbonate or a miniature brush stylet are some of the available products. Only a nurse or physician familiar with J-tubes should attempt to unclog a tube using a device such as a brush, for obvious safety reasons.

The best method of securing a J-tube depends on the type of tube. An NJ tube is secured the same way as an NGT. A PEJ has an internal balloon and external

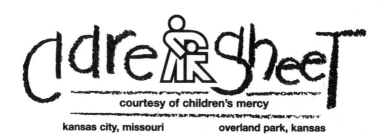

courtesy of children's mercy

kansas city, missouri   overland park, kansas

Jejunostomy Tube Care

On _____ your child had a _____ jejunostomy tube placed by _____ in _____ department. This was because your child's medical treatment plan includes using a jejunostomy tube for nutrition and/or medications. Children who go without nutrition for a long time can have serious problems, especially if they have metabolic disorders. The tube bypasses the stomach and is placed in the second part of the small intestine. It is important to know how the jejunum works so that you can understand what to watch for when feeding your child. It is also important to prevent complications with the jejunostomy tube so it does not need to be replaced frequently. This care sheet will tell you what you need to know to use the jejunostomy tube correctly.

Jejunum

The second part of the small intestine is called the jejunum. It is several feet long in older children and adults. The jejunum digests and absorbs nutrients from liquid food it receives from the stomach and duodenum (first part of the small intestine). Large amounts of fluid or food at one time in the jejunum can cause diarrhea. The jejunum cannot stretch and hold onto liquid food until digestion is complete. This is why a feeding pump is necessary for your child to get a set amount of formula per hour. Also very concentrated fluids, such as liquid medicines, need to be diluted so that the medicine does not irritate the jejunum and cause diarrhea.

Jejunostomy tube

Your child's jejunostomy tube may go through the nose and stomach and into the small intestine or it may go through an opening in the abdomen. In both cases, it is VERY important that the tube not be pulled out of place. Please make every effort to make sure the tube is secure with tape (if appropriate) and that your child cannot easily get at the tube. This is especially important for children who are too young or unable to understand that the tube must not be disturbed.

Gastro-jejunostomy tube

Your child's feeding tube may have an opening into his stomach and jejunum. This type of tube is called a gastro-jejunostomy. It is important to find out from your child's PCP (primary care provider who normally treats your child) where medicines are to be given. Some medicines may be put down the gastric port (opening into the stomach). It is also very important to make sure that the feeding pump tubing does not get connected to the gastric port. When giving medicines, it is important to flush before and after with waterregardless of whether the medicine goes into the stomach or jejunum. There is a

CMH-99-111

_____

continues

Figure 9–6 Jejunostomy tube care sheet

Figure 9–6 continued

third port for the balloon that keeps the tube in your child's stomach. Please do not try to put any fluid or medicine down that port.

Tube care

Since this tube can be difficult to replace, it is important that it not become clogged. A clogged jejunostomy tube usually takes a long time to get open and may have to be replaced by the doctor. Your child may miss several hours of nutrition, fluids or medicines. Prevention of a clogged jejunostomy tube is very important. **The following procedures should help keep the tube open:**

1. Flush the jejunostomy tube at least 4 times per day with at least 10 cc (2 tsp) of tap water.
2. If the tube becomes hard to flush, put 1–2 ounces of cola down the tube. Cola acts as a mild acid that will clean the tube.
3. If the tube often becomes hard to flush, use cola at least once a day to prevent clogging.

The following procedures should help avoid diarrhea:

1. Do not give more than 4–5 ounces of fluid at any one time.
2. When giving a medicine, flush before and after the medicine with at least 10 cc of tap water.
3. It is best to dilute medicines with up to _____ ounces of water.

Other suggestions:

1. Clean the skin around an abdominal jejunostomy tube with soap and water everyday. If the skin becomes red, stop using soap. Clean the skin with water only. If any drainage, pain, or swelling are present, call your PCP.
2. It is a good idea to put the pump backpack in a small shopping cart or doll carriage for toddlers who are on 24 hour feedings.

Possible problems:

As with any medical therapy, problems can occur that may or may not be associated with the therapy. The following problems will need to be reported as they can affect jejunostomy tube functioning or the health of your child.

1. Diarrhea and/or cramping: To prevent either of these it is best to:
   * Make sure the pump rate is correct
   * Dilute all medicines with water before putting down the tube.
   * Make sure the formula and medicines are at room temperature.
   * Use only very clean supplies and formula that have been prepared within the last 24 hours.

Call your child's PCP if diarrhea lasts longer than 24 hours or for any vomiting.

2. **Call the Nurses line at 816-234-3188 if the tube becomes clogged.**

3. Dislodged or misplaced tube: Replace the tube into the opening. Tape the tube in place. **DO NOT USE THE REPLACED TUBE UNDER ANY CIRCUMSTANCES.** Call the department that placed the tube at 8 am to schedule replacement.
   (Gastroenterology Department 816-234-3704)
   (Radiology Department 816-234-3270)

Special Instructions:

_____
_____
_____

For further assistance call: _____

CMH-99-114
© The Children's Mercy Hospital
This card is provided as a public education service. The information does not replace instructions your physician gives you. If you have questions about your child's care, please call your physician.

contents expire 12/31/2003

bolster, so the primary nursing action is to assure the external bolster is not loose or too tight. A surgically placed J-tube may be sutured in place, and care must be taken to make that sure the sutures are replaced if they come out of the skin. Occasionally, cellulitis develops at the suture site requiring topical antibiotic ointment or, more commonly, removal and replacement of sutures.

Occasionally, a J-tube will migrate into the stomach. When this happens, the child typically starts vomiting. If the tube has a gastric port, attempting to aspirate enteral formula from that port can help the nurse determine whether the tube has migrated. An x-ray can conclusively confirm tube displacement. Nurses and parents should not use a J-tube that they suspect has become dislodged without a physician order.

Medication administration for a child with a J-tube may require careful thought. Some medications must be administered via the gastric port. Before giving any medication via J-tube, it is necessary to verify what port the medication should be provided through. This information should be verbally communicated and clearly written out for parents in discharge instructions. Dilution of medications given via J-tube is absolutely essential as nearly all liquid medications are hyperosmolar. Whenever possible, the medication should be diluted with equal parts of water, and multiple medications should not be administered at one time.

ADMINISTRATION TECHNIQUE AND SCHEDULE

Patient's type of access, tolerance, amount of volitional intake, absorptive capacity, volume requirements, and lifestyle will determine the method and duration of daily tube feedings.[18] Tube feedings may be administered using bolus, intermittent gravity, or continuous infusion technique. There are advantages and disadvantages to each type of administration of enteral tube feedings.

Pediatric nutrition support practitioners are creative in the methods they use to enterally feed a child. Continuous nocturnal tube feedings are often provided to children who are able to eat in an effort to preserve or stimulate appetite during the day while meeting daily nutrition requirements. A child may receive a continuous drip feeding at night and bolus feedings during the day, with a combination of bottle and tube feedings. It is important for nurses to carefully follow the prescribed directions for enteral feeds. It is also important to assess the tolerance of the feeding delivery method. Episodes of vomiting, diarrhea, abdominal distension, pain, irritability, reflux, etc., need to be documented in relation to feeding time and volume. It is also important for nurses to monitor and document how long it takes an infant to take a bottle-feeding to avoid excessive caloric expenditure from extended periods of feeding. On the other extreme, an infant may be taking the bottle too quickly, which can result in irritability, discomfort, and abdominal distension afterward.

CONTINUOUS DRIP FEEDINGS

Continuous infusions are delivered via stationary or ambulatory pump from 8 to 24 hours at a prescribed rate without interruption.[18] Continuous feedings are indicated when there is a high risk for aspiration or volume sensitivity, with transpyloric feedings, and sometimes in patients with delayed gastric motility. Continuous feedings allow for improved nutrient absorption and tolerance. Disadvantages of continuous feedings include the need for a pump and for the child to be connected to the feeding apparatus for lengthy periods.[58] It is best to use an enteral pump that is specially designed for pediatric patients because it has been tested with powdered and fortified formulas and found to be accurate using these products. These pumps also come with a backpack for the parent or child to carry. Ideally, the pump would only be used at night, but many pediatric patients have conditions that require around-the-clock feedings. This means developmental milestones such as turning, crawling, cruising, and walking must be facilitated. Small children use a play shopping cart or doll stroller to push their backpack around. For outdoor mobility, a tricycle with a basket on the front serves the same purpose. Enteral tubing needs to be long enough to allow a crawler some room to navigate freely. Parents often express concern that the enteral tubing will become wrapped around the child's neck during the night. This is a valid concern and should be addressed in teaching sessions. Extending the tubing down the bottom of a sleeper and then placing it under a blanket that is tucked under the mattress can enhance the child's safety. Finally, it is again important to stress the need to work on oral stimulation during this time period. Use of a pacifier during continuous drip feedings helps the infant associate the acts of sucking, swallowing, and breathing with a full sensation in the stomach.[64]

GRAVITY FEEDINGS

Gravity feeding is a slow, manually controlled infusion of formula. A specific volume of formula is hung in a formula bag or bottle on an IV pole above the insertion site of the feeding tube. A roller clamp on the tubing is used to regulate the flow rate of the formula. Feedings may be provided over several minutes to hours depending on patient tolerance. The flow rate of the formula may fluctuate throughout the feeding in accordance with the patient's positional changes or if gastric pressure rises.[18]

BOLUS FEEDINGS

Bolus feedings are typically provided several times a day, each lasting from 15 to 45 minutes.[63] Bolus feedings should take into consideration the child's age, gastrointestinal function, type of formula, and volume to be delivered. Bolus feedings are the preferred method of tube-feeding delivery for children who can tolerate the increased volume, since they are the easiest and least expensive method and are more physiologic because they mimic normal feedings. A pump is not usually required, and the patient is allowed breaks from feeding, which enhances mobility. Potential disadvantages of bolus feedings include increased risk of aspiration, poor tolerance of volume, emesis, or delayed gastric emptying. Bolus feedings are preferred for children who are receiving breast milk, are physically active, or are transitioning to oral feeds.

In a study of premature infants in a neonatal intensive care unit, bolus feedings were associated with better weight gains than continuous drip feedings. Investigators divided 171 premature infants into 4 groups based on gestational age and diet (breast milk versus preterm formula). Neonates were evaluated for the amount of time required to reach full oral feedings. While no difference was observed between groups for this outcome, the bolus-fed group had fewer feeding tolerance problems and gained weight faster than the continuously fed group.[65] When bottle feedings are introduced to an infant, it is common for the baby to suck for a predetermined amount of time (typically 10 to 15 minutes) and then receive the remainder of the formula via slow gravity drip. In time the volume taken by bottle-feeding tends to increase to the goal amount. For older children, nurses and parents can gauge the adequacy of oral intake of solids and liquids and augment it with the necessary volume enteral formula via tube. Bolus feedings are typically not provided throughout the night. A combination of daytime bolus and continuous drip nocturnal feedings allows parents to receive much-needed rest and gives the child the nutrition he or she needs. Since infants tend to sleep 10 to 12 hours at night, it is best to run the pump for that time interval and give bolus feedings during waking hours.

Feedings can be delivered in several ways, as described on the nasogastric tube feeding care sheet. Nurses and parents tend to try several methods and settle on one that best meets the needs of the child. A method not mentioned on the care sheet is intermittent feeds. This technique involves placing the formula in an enteral feeding bag and connecting it to an enteral pump. This is a safe and effective method for children who require longer than 30 minutes for a bolus feeding. In pediatrics, a bolus feeding should last approximately as long as a normal bottle-feeding would—or for larger volumes of 6 to 8 ounces, 20 to 30 minutes. It is not common for a child to receive over 8 ounces per bolus feeding unless he or she is an older adolescent. In that case, adult volumes of bolus feedings are appropriate to try.

NOCTURNAL FEEDINGS

Nocturnal continuous feedings are often provided as adjunct support to oral nutrition in an effort to preserve the child's appetite and promote oral intake during the day. Some children only need enteral feedings at night for treatment of conditions such as feeding aversion, inflammatory bowel disease, cystic fibrosis, or some metabolic disorders, to name a few. These children are often school-aged, so the formula can only realistically infuse over 10 to 14 hours per night. Many patients willingly place their own NGT nightly rather than have a G-tube placed. They view an NGT as less invasive to their body image. Older children and adolescents may self-insert their tube 6 or 7 nights per week. It is common to give these individuals a night off to go to a sleepover or other social event as long as they do not have a metabolic disorder and/or can keep adequately hydrated by mouth. Making an effort to accommodate for the child's lifestyle will greatly help with compliance with the nutrition support regime. Nocturnal feedings are an excellent method of augmenting a diet but are not intended to serve as the sole source of nutrition for a child. Rates of up to 125 ml per hour for gastric feeds are generally well tolerated by children over the age of 12.

INITIATION AND ADVANCEMENT OF TUBE FEEDINGS

Initiation of tube feedings in children usually involves provision of full-strength formula at low volumes. Bolus feedings may be started with 25% of the goal volume divided into the desired number of daily feedings. Formula volume may be increased by 25% per day as tolerated, divided equally between feedings.[3] Bolus feedings may need to be delivered by gravity over 15 to 20 minutes in some patients. In a critically ill child, continuous feeding is preferred, as the slower infusion is believed to enhance tolerance. For continuous gastric feedings provided via pump, an isotonic formula can be started at 1 to 2 cc/kg/hour and advanced by 0.5 to 1 cc/kg/hour every 6 to 24 hours until goal volume is achieved. Preterm, very sick, or malnourished children with an extended NPO (nothing by mouth or *non per os*) status may require a lower initial volume of 0.5 to 1 cc/kg/hour.[30] During feeding advancement, only one change should be made at a time to allow for assessment of tolerance. If the child demonstrates poor tolerance of the enteral regimen, the formula volume or strength should be decreased and adequate time should be allowed for good tolerance of the reduced volume or strength to be achieved before further advances are attempted. Occasionally, it becomes necessary to change the formula to achieve improved feeding tolerance. After the child achieves the goal regimen and demonstrates good tolerance, modifications to the feeding schedule may be implemented to better accommodate the patient and family's lifestyle.

PATIENT MONITORING

New home enteral nutrition support patients should be reassessed 1 week after discharge or outpatient initiation of tube feedings and monthly thereafter. Once the regimen is well tolerated and the child demonstrates adequate growth and weight gain, reassessment may be needed only every 3 to 4 months.[58] Parameters that should be routinely monitored in follow-up assessments of pediatric patients receiving enteral tube feedings are summarized in Exhibit 9–13.

Some practitioners also check trace elements every 6 to 12 months.[16] The enteral feeding regimen should be calculated and modified as needed at every follow-up visit to account for growth, changes in oral intake, and clinical status. Working with speech and occupational therapists who assess oral-motor func-

Exhibit 9–13 Parameters that should be routinely monitored in follow-up assessments of pediatric patients receiving enteral tube feedings

1. Reassessment of the underlying medical condition(s) to evaluate feasibility of transitional feeding
2. Nutrient intake
3. Medications
4. Tolerance of enteral nutrition regimen
5. Growth parameters
6. Daily intake and output
7. Stool characteristics
8. Gastric residuals (if applicable)
9. Biochemical and hematological indices[16]
   a. complete blood count
   b. electrolytes, blood urea nitrogen, creatinine, glucose
   c. liver function tests
   d. calcium, magnesium, phosphorous
   e. total protein and albumin[37]

---

tion and make recommendations for certain food textures and feeding techniques can prove extremely helpful in optimizing feeding skills while prioritizing the nutrition support interventions necessary to achieve or maintain optimal weight gain and growth.[9] It is equally important to continuously monitor the caregiver and patient's psychosocial status and lifestyle changes.[18]

COMMON COMPLICATIONS OF TUBE FEEDINGS

Children receiving tube feedings are at risk for both dehydration and fluid overload. Fluid needs increase with warm weather, diarrhea, emesis, and fever. Medical conditions such as bronchopulmonary dysplasia, renal disease, and cardiac disease may predispose the patient to fluid retention and may necessitate a daily fluid restriction. Any factors causing increased insensible water losses or fluid retention should be considered and the child's fluid needs estimated accordingly. Additional free water can be added to feedings, be provided between feedings, or be given as flushes to rinse the feeding tubes. Caregivers should be instructed on their child's minimum and maximum fluid needs over 24 hours. Table 9–4 provides maintenance fluid needs for pediatrics.

Instruction should include possible signs of dehydration, such as constipation, polydipsia, crying without tears, decreased urine output or number of wet diapers, concentrated strong smelling urine, dry lips, poor skin turgor, sunken eyes, dark circles around eyes, and rapid weight loss. Conversely, caregivers need to be aware that signs of fluid overload include rapid weight gain, edema, and quick, uncomfortable breathing. If the child exhibits any of these symptoms, the child's physician should be contacted immediately.[66]

Table 9–4 Maintenance fluid requirement calculations

Weight	cc fluid/day
1–10 kg	100 cc/kg/day
11–20 kg	1000 cc + 50 cc/kg for each kg > 10 kg
>20 kg	1500 cc + 20 cc/kg for each kg > 20 kg

Nausea, vomiting, and diarrhea may occur in children receiving enteral nutrition support. Possible etiologies include rapid infusions of formula, hyperosmotic formulas, medications, air in stomach or intestine, tube migration from stomach to small intestine, infection, cold formula, bacterial contamination, lactose intolerance, and fat intolerance. Changes in gut microflora due to bacterial overgrowth or antibiotic use can also cause diarrhea. Formula changes are often implemented to treat GI symptoms when the cause is actually nonnutritional. Formula intolerance should only be suspected after other possible etiologies have been ruled out.

Gastroesophageal reflux (GER) may occur with oral or gastric feedings. Strategies used to manage GER include providing small, frequent feedings; elevating the child's head to a 30- to 45-degree angle during and for 1 hour after feeds, and checking gastric residuals prior to each feeding. If these interventions do not prove effective, motility agents as well as continuous and/or transpyloric feedings may be necessary.[3]

Children receiving tube feedings occasionally experience constipation. Possible dietary causes of constipation include inadequate intake of fiber, fluid, or calories. Interventions to prevent or alleviate constipation include increasing free water intake, providing fiber-containing formulas, and/or providing prune juice.

Checking residuals before intermittent feeds or every 4 hours with continuous feeds is a way to assess gastric tube feeding tolerance. Residuals are checked by aspirating gastric contents through the feeding tube using a syringe, and returning aspirate to the stomach after checking the volume. The amount of residual is dependent on the volume and timing of the last feeding and/or medications, as well as the child's activity and positioning, since both may affect the rate of gastric emptying. Residuals may be clear, which indicates the presence of gastric juices, or may contain partially digested formula.[63] If the gastric residuals are equal to half of the patient's bolus feeding or exceed 1 hour's volume of continuous feeds, the tube feedings should be held for 30 to 60 minutes.[67] Residuals should be rechecked and if they are still high, the health care provider needs to be contacted for instructions. Once the residuals decrease, feedings can be restarted at the previous rate and strength. Large gastric residuals may be a result of decreased gastric motility, hypertonic formula, or medications. Residuals cannot be obtained when transpyloric tubes are in the correct place.[63] Tolerance of small bowel feedings may be evaluated by observing for abdominal distention and diarrhea. If intolerance develops, hold feeds for 30 to

60 minutes. Resume previously tolerated formula strength or volume and gradually advance as tolerated.[16]

CARE OF THE FEEDING SYSTEM

While no standard exists for how to care for the pediatric feeding system, there are some general guidelines to follow. All supplies and the space used to prepare the formula need to be clean. Only 24 hours of formula should be prepared at one time. Commercially prepared formulas may be safely hung for 8 to 12 hours; breast milk and homemade formulas, prepared under good sanitation, should not remain in a feeding container for more than 4 hours.[3] Enteral feeding bags are typically used for one 6- to 8-hour hang time only in the hospital and then discarded. If a bag is used for an entire 24-hour period, it should be thoroughly rinsed with hot water before refilling. In the home, feeding bags are rinsed with hot water and stored either in open air with the cap open or in the refrigerator in a plastic bag. Some institutions use a special auxiliary bag that allows air and enteral formula to flow retrograde into the bag and for the air to escape and the formula to flow back into the stomach. These bags are used for 24 hours only.

NUTRITION SUPPORT TRANSITIONING

Before beginning the process of weaning from enteral nutrition support, the child should have an adequate nutrition status. Transitioning a child from continuous drip feedings to bolus feedings is typically done by stopping the feeding for 2 to 3 hours several times during the day and offering a bottle or giving a bolus in an amount equivalent to the usual 2- to 3-hour volume. The rationale for this intervention is to try and have the feeds resemble meals in an effort to stimulate hunger and have the child associate feeds with a feeling of satiety.[63] Gradually, the interval off of the pump increases as the child's ability to tolerate bolus feeds increases. The smaller the child, the more likely it is that the intervals will be no longer than 3 hours. The more gastrointestinal dysfunction the child has, the more likely the bolus feedings will be mostly for oral stimulation or psychological benefit, as the child's ability to digest and absorb nutrients can be greatly diminished in conditions such as short bowel syndrome and Crohn's disease. Initially, oral intake is often minimal and supplemental feedings provided via tube after each meal will continue to provide the majority of the nutritional intake. It is important to keep in mind that some types of formula may not be a good choice to offer orally due to the taste. As oral intake increases and provides a greater proportion of energy needs, the tube-feeding volume should be decreased accordingly, keeping the combined regimen isocaloric.[68] If the patient is receiving elemental tube feedings or if weight gain is inadequate, additional calories may be needed via tube. However, it is often difficult to meet the child's nutrition needs to achieve weight gain, while simultaneously preserving the child's appetite and increasing intake of solids. The nutrition regimen should be routinely scrutinized to ensure that the patient's fluid and micronutrient needs are being met during the transitional phase. When the child is able to consume approximately 75% of daily nutrition needs orally, tube feedings are usually discontinued but the tube is left in place. After the child demonstrates the ability to consume enough calories, protein, and fluid orally and achieve adequate growth, the feeding tube can be removed. This should be a decision made by the health care team and the primary caregiver(s). Factors to be considered when determining future necessity of the feeding tube include any underlying medical condition(s) that caused the child to originally need the tube, whether the child can meet fluid needs orally, and whether medications can be administered without it.[63]

PSYCHOSOCIAL AND DEVELOPMENTAL ISSUES

Nurses tend to be very helpful in guiding parents through the process of enteral feeding on an emotional level. Feeding one's child is a basic responsibility for a parent, and many times there is a grieving process associated with the realization that chronic enteral tube feeding is going to be required. Encouraging the parent to hold the child during bolus feedings will keep the parent bonded to the child. Having the child in an infant seat in the kitchen during mealtime keeps the child connected to the family. Teaching a parent that kissing on the face, tickling the child's face with a feather, and offering to let the child play with spoons are all good forms of oral stimulation that can be done anywhere. Finally, it is helpful to encourage parents to focus on non-food-related traditions.

Nurses can model appropriate responses when an older child resists having an NGT replaced. They can also show the adolescent respect when needs for autonomy play out as refusal to insert an NGT until a certain program on television is completed. Nurses teach parents what to expect and watch for at different developmental stages. For example, an infant may suck on the enteral pump tubing when teething. A toddler may become curious about the pump and change the settings. A school-aged child may turn off the pump if it alarms at night to stop the noise.

CONCLUSION

Pediatric practitioners have made great advances in the development of enteral solutions and feeding tubes that meet the unique needs of this population. With these clinical strides, enteral nutrition support of the infant, child, and adolescent is safer, easier, and more effective. While supporting growth and development remain the goals for enteral nutrition interventions, there are many options available to help a child attain that goal. This process remains multidisciplinary in nature, with pediatricians, family practice physicians, subspecialists, nurses, nutrition support specialists, and dietitians collaborating on the best way to meet a child's nutritional needs.

The nurse is pivotal in this process as the observer of the patient's response to therapy and the caregiver's reaction, and as a direct care provider. The nurse is a role model for parents to emulate when feedings are provided, tubes placed, site care performed, etc. The nurse is a teacher who prepares parents and children for discharge. The nurse is a person who lends moral support when parents and children get discouraged.

REFERENCES

1. Klish W. Special infant formulas. *Pediatr in Rev* 1990;12:55–62.
2. Ekvall SW. Nutritional assessment and early intervention. In: Ekvall SW, ed. *Pediatric Nutrition in Chronic Diseases and Developmental Disorders—Prevention, Assessment, and Treatment.* New York: Oxford University Press, Inc; 1993:41–76.
3. Nevin-Folino N, Miller M. Enteral nutrition. In: Samour PQ, Helm KK, Lang CE, eds. *Handbook of Pediatric Nutrition.* 2nd ed. Gaithersburg, MD: Aspen Publishers, Inc; 1999:513–549.
4. American Academy of Pediatrics, Committee on Nutrition. Assessment of nutritional status. In: Kleinman RE, ed. *Pediatric Nutrition Handbook.* Elk Grove Village, IL: American Academy of Pediatrics; 1998:165–184.
5. Stallings VA, Fung EB. Clinical nutrition assessment of infants and children. In: Shils ME, Olson JA, Shike M, Ross CA, eds. *Modern Nutrition in Health and Disease.* 9th ed. Philadelphia, PA: Lippincott Williams & Wilkins; 1998:885–893.
6. Bessler S. Nutritional assessment. In: Samour PK, Helm KK, Lang CE, eds. *Handbook of Pediatric Nutrition.* 2nd ed. Gaithersburg, MD: Aspen Publishers, Inc; 1999:17–42.
7. Chumlea WC, Guo SS. Physical growth and development. In: Samour PQ, Helm KK, Lang CE, eds. *Handbook of Pediatric Nutrition.* 2nd ed. Gaithersburg, MD: Aspen Publishers, Inc; 1999:3–15.
8. Zemel BS, Riley EM, Stallings VA. Evaluation of methodology for nutritional assessment in children: anthropometry, body composition, and energy expenditure. *Annu Rev Nutr* 1997;17:211–235.
9. Bora MT, Harris AB. Pediatric nutrition assessment: identifying children at risk. *J Am Diet Assoc* 1997;97:S107–S115.
10. Himes JH, Roche AF, Thissen D, Moore WM. Parent-specific adjustments for evaluation of recumbent length and stature of children. *Pediatrics* 1985;75:304–313.
11. Frisancho AR. New norms of upper limb fat and muscle areas for assessment of nutritional status. *Am J Clin Nutr* 1981;34:2540–2545.
12. Zemel B. Anthropometric assessment of nutritional status. In: Altshuler SM, Liacouras CA, eds. *Clinical Pediatric Gastroenterology.* Philadelphia, PA: Churchill Livingstone; 1998:597–606.
13. Brandt I. Growth dynamics of low birth weight infants with emphasis on the perinatal period. In: Falkner F, Tanner JM, eds. *Human Growth: A Comprehensive Treatise.* Vol. 2. New York: Plenum Press; 1978:557–617.
14. McLaren DS. Clinical manifestations of human vitamin and mineral disorders: a resume. In: Shils ME, Olson JA, Shike M, eds. *Modern Nutrition in Health and Disease.* 8th ed. Philadelphia, PA: Lea & Febiger; 1994:909–922.

15. Gianino S, St. John RE. Nutritional assessment of the patient in the intensive care unit. *Crit Care Nurs Clin of North Am* 1993;5:1–15.
16. Marian M. Pediatric nutrition support. *Nutr Clin Pract* 1993;8:199–209.
17. Position of the American Dietetic Association: Nutrition monitoring of the home parenteral and enteral patient. *J Am Diet Assoc* 1994;94:664–666.
18. Weckwerth J, Nelson JK, O'Shea R. Home nutrition support. In: Gottschlich MM, Matarese LE, Shronts EP, eds. *Nutrition Support Dietetics Core Curriculum.* 2nd ed. Silver Spring, MD: American Society for Parenteral and Enteral Nutrition; 1993:467–473.
19. Kunz C, Rodriguez-Palmero M, Koletzko B, Jensen R. Nutritional and biochemical properties of human milk, part I: general aspects, proteins, and carbohydrates. *Clin Perinatol* 1999;26:307–330.
20. Lawrence RA, Howard CR. Given the benefits of breast-feeding, are there any contraindications? *Clin Perinatol* 1999;26:479–490.
21. Fletcher A. Nutrition. In: Avery GB, Fletcher M, eds. *Neonatology: Pathophysiology and Management of the Newborn.* Philadelphia, PA: J.B. Lippincott Company; 1994:330–353.
22. Morrison P. HIV and infant feeding: to breastfeed or not: the dilemma of competing risks, part 2. *Breast-feeding Rev* 1999;7:11–19.
23. American Academy of Pediatrics Committee on Drugs. The transfer of drugs and other chemicals in human milk. *Pediatr* 1994;93:137–150.
24. Sosa R, Barness L. Bacterial growth in refrigerated human milk. *AJDC* 1987;141:111–112.
25. Hamosh M, Ellis L, Pollock D, Henderson T, Hamosh P. Breast-feeding and the working mother: effect of time and temperature of short-term storage on proteolysis, lipolysis and bacterial growth in milk. *Pediatr* 1996;97:492–498.
26. Stocks RJ, Davies DP, Allen F, Sewell D. Loss of breast milk nutrients during tube feeding. *Arch Dis Child* 1985;60:164–166.
27. Tatum Hattner J. Pediatric formula update. *Nutr Focus* 1998;13:1–8.
28. Davis A. Indications and techniques for enteral feeds. In: Baker SB, Baker RD, Davis A, eds. *Pediatric Enteral Nutrition.* New York: Chapman & Hall; 1994:67–94.
29. American Academy of Pediatrics, Committee on Nutrition. Soy protein-based formulas: recommendations for use in infant feeding. *Pediatr* 1998;101:148–153.
30. Akers SM, Groh-Wargo SL. Normal nutrition during infancy. In: Samour PQ, Helm KK, Lang CE, eds. *Handbook of Pediatric Nutrition.* 2nd ed. Gaithersburg, MD: Aspen Publishers, Inc; 1999:65–97.
31. Klawitter BM. Pediatric enteral nutrition support. In: Parkman Williams C, ed. *Pediatric Manual of Clinical Dietetics.* Chicago: The American Dietetic Association; 1998:479–502.
32. Blecker U. Role of hydrolyzed formulas in nutritional allergy prevention in infants. *South Med J* 1997;90:1170–1174.
33. American Academy of Pediatrics, Committee on Nutrition. Formula Feeding of Term Infants. In: Kleinman RE, ed. *Pediatric Nutrition Handbook.* Elk Grove Village, IL: American Academy of Pediatrics; 1998:29–42.
34. Kelly KJ, Lazenby AJ, Rowe PC, Yardley JH, Perman JA, Sampson HA. Eosinophilic esophagitis attributed to gastroesophageal reflux: improvement with an amino acid-based formula. *Gastroenterol* 1995;109:1503–1512.
35. Davis A, Baker S. The use of modular nutrients in pediatrics. *J Parenter Enteral Nutr* 1996;20:228–236.
36. American Society for Parenteral and Enteral Nutrition. Standards for home nutrition support. *Nutr Clin Pract* 1999;14:151–162.
37. Yowell Warman K. Enteral nutrition: support of the pediatric patient. In: Hendricks KM, Walker WA, eds. *Manual of Pediatric Nutrition.* Philadelphia, PA: B.C. Decker Inc; 1990:72–109.

38. Noviski N, Yehuda YB, Serour F, Gorenstein A, Mandelberg A. Does the size of nasogastric tubes affect gastroesophageal reflux in children? *J Pediatr Gastroenterol Nutr* 1999;29:448–451.

39. Holden CE, MacDonald A, Ward M, et al. Psychological preparation for nasogastric feeding in children. *Br J Nurs* 1997;6:376–381, 384–385.

40. Chellis MJ, Sanders SV, Webster H, Dean JM, Jackson D. Bedside transpyloric tube placement in the pediatric intensive care unit. *JPEN* 1996;20:88–90.

41. Shiao SY, Brooker J, DiFiore T. Desaturation events during oral feeding with and without a nasogastric feeding tube in very low birth weight infants. *Heart Lung* 1996;25:236–245.

42. Daga SR, Lunkad NG, Daga AS, Ahuja VK. Orogastric versus nasogastric feeding of newborn babies. *Trop Doct* 1999;29:242–243.

43. Asfaw W, Miles A, Caplan D. Orogastric enteral feeding: an alternative feeding access. *Nutr Clin Pract* 2000;15:91–93.

44. Ellett M, Beckstrand J, Welch J, Dye J, Games C. Predicting the distance for gavage tube placement in children. *Pediatr Nurs* 1992;18:119–121, 127.

45. Ellett ML, Maahs J, Forsee S. Prevalence of feeding tube placement errors and associated risk factors in children. *Am J Maternal Child Nurs* 1998;23:234–239.

46. Vento BA, Derrant JD, Palmer CV, Smith EK. Middle ear effects secondary to nasogastric intubation. *Am J Otol* 1995;16:820–822.

47. Wald ER. Microbiology of acute and chronic sinusitis in children and adults. *Am J Med Sci* 1998;316:13–20.

48. Huggins PS, Tuomi SK, Young C. Effects of nasogastric feeding tubes on the young, normal swallowing mechanism. *Dysphagia* 1999;14:157–161.

49. Dello Strologo L, Principato F, Sinibaoldi D, et al. Feeding dysfunction in infants with chronic renal failure after long-term nasogastric tube feeding. *Pediatr Nephrol* 1997;11:84–86.

50. Isch JA, Rescorla FJ, Scherer LR 3rd, West KW, Grosfeld JL. The development of gastroesophageal reflux after percutaneous endoscopic gastrostomy. *J Pediatr Surg* 1997;32:322–333.

51. Fox VL, Abel SD, Malas S, et al. Complications following percutaneous endoscopic gastrostomy and subsequent catheter replacement in children and young adults. *Gastroenterol Endosc* 1997;45:64–71.

52. Matthew P, Bowman L, Williams R, et al. Complications and effectiveness of gastrostomy feedings in pediatric cancer patients. *J Pediatr Hematol/Oncol* 1996;18:81–85.

53. Aquino VM, Smyrl LB, Hagg R, et al. Nutrition support by gastrostomy tube in children with cancer. *J Pediatr* 1995;127:58–62.

54. Mascarenhas MR, Redd D, Bilodeau J, Peck S, Liacouras CA. Pediatric enteral access center: a multi-disciplinary approach. *Nutr Clin Pract* 1996;11:193–198.

55. Gauderer MWL. Percutaneous endoscopic gastrostomy: a 10-year experience with 220 children. *J Pediatr Surg* 1991;26:288–294.

56. Malki TA, Langer JC, Thompson V, et al. A prospective evaluation of the button gastrostomy in children. *Can J Surg* 1991;34:247–250.

57. Gauderer MWL, Olsen MM, Stellato TA, Dokler, ML. Feeding gastrostomy button: experience and recommendations. *J Pediatr Surg* 1988;23:24–28.

58. Detamore Lingard C. Enteral nutrition. In: Queen PM, Lang CE, eds. *Handbook of Pediatric Nutrition.* Gaithersburg, MD: Aspen Publishers, Inc; 1993:249–273.

59. Barry D, Beyers J, Lyman B, Hafeman C. *Gastrostomy Skin Assessment: Preliminary Data from Staff versus Expert Nurses* [unpublished master's project]. Kansas City: UMKC School of Nursing; 1999.

60. Gauderer MWL, Stellato TA. Gastrostomies: evolution, techniques, indications and complications. *Curr Probl Surg* 1986:661–719.
61. Hagelgans NA, Janusz HB. Pediatric skin care issues for the home care nurse: part 2. *Pediatr Nurs* 1994;20:69–76.
62. Gottlieb K, Iber FL, Livak A, et al. Oral candida colonizes the stomach and gastrostomy feeding tubes. *J Parenter Enteral Nutr* 1994;18:264–267.
63. Smith BC, Pederson AL. Nutrition focus tube feeding update. *Nutr Focus* 1990;5:1–6.
64. Gottlieb K, Mobarhan S. Review: microbiology of the gastrostomy tube. *J Am Coll Nutr* 1994;13:64–71.
65. Peters JM, Simpson P, Tolia V. Experience with gastrojejunal feeding tubes in children. *Am J Gastroenterol* 1997;97:476–480.
66. Nardella MT. Practical tips on tube feedings for children. *Nutr Focus* 1995;10:1–8.
67. Keller G. Clinical assessment. In: Groh-Wargo S, Thompson M, Cox J, eds. *Nutritional Care for High Risk Newborns.* Chicago: Precept Press, Inc; 1994:15–20.
68. Reimers KJ, Carlson SJ, Lombard KA. Nutritional management of infants with bronchopulmonary dysplasia. *Nutr Clin Pract* 1992;7:127–132.

Enteral Nutrition in Alternate Sites: Home Care and Institutional Care

Marcia Silkroski

Providing enteral nutrition support for consumers in settings outside the hospital usually means long-term management. The general term "alternate site" in this chapter refers to home care, as well as out-of-hospital "institutional" care, such as extended care in nursing homes, rehabilitation centers, assisted living facilities, skilled nursing facilities, and subacute care centers. According to statistics of the Oley Foundation's North American Home Parenteral and Enteral Nutrition Patient Registry, as of 1992 there were 152,000 patients receiving enteral nutrition therapy (ENT) in their homes.[1,2] It is estimated that there is an equal number of patients receiving enteral nutrition in the out-of-hospital institutions described above. Although this information is dated, it gives us some idea of the significance of ENT.

The fastest growing population in the United States is the elderly. In the early 1900s, approximately 1 in 25 adults was over the age of 65. According to 1998 census statistics, more than 44 million people are over the age of 60.[3] That number has dramatically changed to include 1 in 5 adults over the age of 65 in the year 2000. The elderly are the greatest consumers of health care today and will no doubt continue to be so in the future. Undernutrition is common among the elderly population. Associated with undernutrition are increased infection rates, pressure ulcers, cognitive problems, decreased wound healing, and increased length of hospital stays. There are now more "outpatient" centers than acute care facilities in this country to accommodate this growing population of individuals. Although statistics have not been defined to date, it appears that the elderly are the largest users of enteral nutrition as well.

Administration techniques and indications for tube feedings do not change in alternate sites. Rather, long-term care of tube-fed patients presents a special subset of considerations. Along with clinical considerations, this chapter will address reimbursement and financial points that are an integral part of this subset. While similarities exist throughout feeding provision, issues specific to home care and institutionalized care will be identified separately.

DISCHARGE PLANNING/ PATIENT SELECTION

To facilitate an expedient transition, discharge planning should begin when a patient is admitted to the hospital. Once the patient is ready for discharge from the acute care setting, the setting for rehabilitation or living should be clearly defined. Hospital case managers usually direct discharge planning. Case managers perform several tasks in relation to ENT (see Exhibit 10–1).[4,5]

Once the needs of the patient have been assessed and approved by the patient, caregivers, and the entire health care team, the discharge plan can be put into action. Fewer complications are seen in patients where a greater emphasis has been placed on education prior to discharge.

Exhibit 10–1 Scope of practice for case managers and enteral nutrition therapy

- Determine the treatment plan and patient's needs
- Investigate insurance benefits for alternate site care and nutrition support therapy
- Anticipate ancillary needs—e.g., speech pathology, physical therapy, wound management, specialized nursing care, respiratory therapy, and approximate number of visits necessary
- Anticipate equipment needs—e.g., pump, pole, feeding supply kit, syringe, enteral tubes—as well as prescribed formula
- Communicate patient needs to the health care team
- Analyze potential interventions and predict if outcomes will be met
- Enhance the quality of life and satisfaction of patients and their families

---

The clinical selection guidelines (A.S.P.E.N.) for enteral nutrition therapy are the same in alternate sites as they are in the acute setting.[6–8] See Chapter 2, Enteral Nutrition Basics, for a more detailed description of these selection criteria. The main difference in provision of tube feeding in all sites lies within reimbursement issues, readiness of the health care team, patient ability to learn, and support availability.

REIMBURSEMENT AND DOCUMENTATION

Diagnosis-related groups (DRGs) refer to the capitated rate allowed by insurance carriers according to the patient's primary diagnoses. Since 1983, when Congress put DRGs into place, there has been an emphasis on moving patients out of the hospital environment and into alternate settings to better control costs. Congress started the Medicare program in 1965. Medicare is now administered by the Health Care Financing Administration (HCFA), an agency within the Department of Health and Human Services (HHS). Consumer demand has also played a role in bringing the patient home for treatment. To help understand the financial aspects of providing ENT to patients, several issues need to be clarified.

Unfortunately, there is no national repository for data collection on home ENT patients. In addition to the statistics maintained by the Oley Foundation, Medicare houses the largest working database available. It is a primary payer for ENT, accounting for about 48% of all claims.[2] Most commercial insurance companies follow the guidelines posed by Medicare for payment of parenteral and enteral nutrition (PEN) therapy alike. With appropriate documentation, commercial insurance companies are more likely to be flexible on a case-by-case basis than is Medicare. Other payment systems such as the Department of Veterans Affairs (VA) and individual state Medicaid programs exist but, for simplicity, they are not discussed in this chapter.

Medicare is divided into three main categories: Parts A, B, and C. Medicare Part A covers inpatient hospital costs such as nursing care, home care nursing visits, and hospices. Part C is the Medicare Plus Choice Program, an HMO equivalent. Part B covers non-hospital costs such as medical equipment and supplies, and physician services. The PEN benefit falls under Part B of Medicare. Oddly enough, PEN is covered under the "prosthetic device" benefit. The rationale behind this classification is due to there being a malfunctioning body part—i.e., the digestive tract. PEN therapy is a prosthesis in a sense, replacing a portion of the gastrointestinal (GI) tract. The controversy surrounding the prosthetic device benefit is that it explicitly recognizes only the provision of *direct costs* (e.g., supplies, equipment, and nutrient)—no *services* are allotted. In other words, nursing and other professional costs are not figured into the equation of total necessary expenses for patient care.[5]

The patient's physician must complete and sign a Certificate of Medical Necessity (CMN) describing the functional impairment rendering the need for PEN therapy. See Figure 10–1 for an example of a CMN for enteral nutrition. Medicare states that the patient must have a *permanently* inoperative condition—which is understood to be greater than 90 days. Sufficient documentation to support the diagnosis and related need for ENT in order to sustain patient well-being must accompany the CMN. Many state Medicaid programs also require that a physician order for enteral therapy be provided with the CMN. Documentation by a nutrition health professional must be provided if the patient is receiving ENT less than 20 calories per kilogram per day or more than 35 calories per kilogram per day.

Nutrients provided to patients are broken down into 6 HCFA Common Procedure Coding Categories (HCPCS) according to calories, product specialty, and composition, plus a category for modular products (see Table 10–1).[5] Medicare reimburses for these Nutrient Categories on the basis of units of enteral product used—each unit is defined as 100 calories. The physician's written prescription must include the nutrient product name and/or Nutrient Category, number of calories per day, method of administration (e.g., nasointestinal, jejunostomy, percutaneous endoscopic gastrostomy), and frequency of feedings per day.

Additional documentation must be submitted with the claim for any specialty formula (i.e., proof of specific organ failure, or metabolic disorder, for any specialty product). Further documentation is needed if the patient will require a pump for administration of feedings. Justifiable reasons for a pump include a diagnosis of "dumping syndrome," congestive heart failure, elevated blood glucose, risk of aspiration, or any condition where uncontrolled volume might present a harmful risk. Medicare pays for only 1 month's supply of nutrients at a time. Oral nutritional supplements are not covered under normal circumstances.

A revised certification is required if there is a change in tube feeding Nutrient Category or number of days per week administered; if calories are increased/decreased; if the method of infusion changes; or if the patient transitions from enteral to parenteral nutrition therapy. Likewise, if a patient progresses from one Nutrient Category to a more specialized Category, substantial documentation is required to justify necessity for the change before payment of claim takes place.

Reimbursement

U.S. DEPARTMENT OF HEALTH & HUMAN SERVICES
HEALTH CARE FINANCING ADMINISTRATION

FORM APPROVED
OMB NO. 0938-0679

CERTIFICATE OF MEDICAL NECESSITY

DMERC 10.02B

ENTERAL NUTRITION

SECTION A Certification Type/Date: **INITIAL** __/__/__ **REVISED** __/__/__ **RECERTIFICATION** __/__/__

PATIENT NAME, ADDRESS, TELEPHONE and HIC NUMBER	SUPPLIER NAME, ADDRESS, TELEPHONE and NSC NUMBER
(__)___-____ HICN _____	(__)___-____ NSC# _____

PLACE OF SERVICE ____ NAME and ADDRESS of FACILITY if applicable (See Reverse)	HCPCS CODE _____ _____ _____ _____	PT DOB __/__/__ ; Sex ___ (M/F); HT.___ (in.); WT.___(lbs.) PHYSICIAN NAME, ADDRESS (Printed or Typed) PHYSICIAN'S UPIN: _____ PHYSICIAN'S TELEPHONE #: (__) ___-____

SECTION B Information in this Section May Not Be Completed by the Supplier of the Items/Supplies.

EST. LENGTH OF NEED (# OF MONTHS):
____ 1-99 (99=LIFETIME)

DIAGNOSIS CODES (ICD-9): ____ ____ ____ ____

ANSWERS	ANSWER QUESTIONS 7, 8, AND 10–15 FOR ENTERAL NUTRITION (Circle **Y** for Yes, **N** for No, or **D** for Does Not Apply, Unless Otherwise Noted) Questions 1–6, and 9, reserved for other or future use.
Y N	7. Does the patient have permanent non-function or disease of the structures that normally permit food to reach or be absorbed from the small bowel?
Y N	8. Does the patient require tube feedings to provide sufficient nutrients to maintain weight and strength commensurate with the patient's overall health status?
A) _____ B) _____	10. <u>Print</u> product name(s).
A) _____ B) _____	11. Calories per day for each product?
_____	12. Days per week administered? (Enter 1–7)
1 2 3 4	13. Circle the number for method of administration. 1 - Syringe 2 - Gravity 3 - Pump 4 - Does not apply
Y N D	14. Does the patient have a documented allergy or intolerance to semi-synthetic nutrients?
	15. Additional information when required by policy:

NAME OF PERSON ANSWERING SECTION B QUESTIONS, IF OTHER THAN PHYSICIAN (Please Print):
NAME: _____ TITLE: _____ EMPLOYER:_____

SECTION C Narrative Description Of Equipment And Cost

(1) <u>Narrative</u> description of all items, accessories and options ordered; **(2)** Supplier's charge; and **(3)** Medicare Fee Schedule Allowance for <u>each</u> item, accessory, and option. (*See Instructions On Back*)

SECTION D Physician Attestation and Signature/Date

I certify that I am the physician identified in Section A of this form. I have received Sections A, B and C of the Certificate of Medical Necessity (including charges for items ordered). Any statement on my letterhead attached hereto, has been reviewed and signed by me. I certify that the medical necessity information in Section B is true, accurate and complete, to the best of my knowledge, and I understand that any falsification, omission, or conceal-ment of material fact in that section may subject me to civil or criminal liability.

PHYSICIAN'S SIGNATURE _____ DATE __/__/__

(SIGNATURE AND DATE STAMPS ARE NOT ACCEPTABLE)

FORM HCFA 853 (4/96)

Figure 10–1 Certificate of Medical Necessity for enteral nutrition (front)

SECTION A:	(May be completed by the supplier)
CERTIFICATION TYPE/DATE:	If this is an initial certification for this patient, indicate this by placing date (MM/DD/YY) needed initially in the space marked "INITIAL." If this is a revised certification (to be completed when the physician changes the order, based on the patient's changing clinical needs), indicate the initial date needed in the space marked "INITIAL," and also indicate the recertification date in the space marked "REVISED." If this is a recertification, indicate the initial date needed in the space marked "INITIAL," and also indicate the recertification date in the space marked "RECERTIFICATION." Whether submitting a REVISED or a RECERTIFIED CMN, be sure to always furnish the INITIAL date as well as the REVISED or RECERTIFICATION date.
PATIENT INFORMATION:	Indicate the patient's name, permanent legal address, telephone number and his/her health insurance claim number (HICN) as it appears on his/her Medicare card and on the claim form.
SUPPLIER INFORMATION:	Indicate the name of your company (supplier name), address and telephone number along with the Medicare Supplier Number assigned to you by the National Supplier Clearinghouse (NSC).
PLACE OF SERVICE:	Indicate the place in which the item is being used, i.e., patient's home is 12, skilled nursing facility (SNF) is 31, End Stage Renal Disease (ESRD) facility is 65, etc. Refer to the DMERC supplier manual for a complete list.
FACILITY NAME:	If the place of service is a facility, indicate the name and complete address of the facility.
HCPCS CODES:	List all HCPCS procedure codes for items ordered that require a CMN. Procedure codes that do not require certification should not be listed on the CMN.
PATIENT DOB, HEIGHT, WEIGHT AND SEX:	Indicate patient's date of birth (MM/DD/YY) and sex (male or female); height in inches and weight in pounds, if requested.
PHYSICIAN NAME, ADDRESS:	Indicate the physician's name and complete mailing address.
UPIN:	Accurately indicate the ordering physician's Unique Physician Identification Number (UPIN).
PHYSICIAN'S TELEPHONE NO:	Indicate the telephone number where the physician can be contacted (preferably where records would be accessible pertaining to this patient) if more information is needed.
SECTION B:	(May not be completed by the supplier. While this section may be completed by a non-physician clinician, or a physician employee, it must be reviewed, and the CMN signed (in Section D) by the ordering physician.)
EST. LENGTH OF NEED:	Indicate the estimated length of need (the length of time the physician expects the patient to require use of the ordered item) by filling in the appropriate number of months. If the physician expects that the patient will require the item for the duration of his/her life, then enter 99.
DIAGNOSIS CODES:	In the first space, list the ICD9 code that represents the primary reason for ordering this item. List any additional ICD9 codes that would further describe the medical need for the item (up to 3 codes).
QUESTION SECTION:	This section is used to gather clinical information to determine medical necessity. Answer each question which applies to the items ordered, circling "Y" for yes, "N" for no, "D" for does not apply, a number if this is offered as an answer option, or fill in the blank if other information is requested.
NAME OF PERSON ANSWERING SECTION B QUESTIONS:	If a clinical professional other than the ordering physician (e.g., home health nurse, physical therapist, dietician). or a physician employee answers the questions of Section B, he/she must print his/her name, give his/her professional title and the name of his/her employer where indicated. If the physician is answering the questions, this space may be left blank.
SECTION C:	(To be completed by the supplier)
NARRATIVE DESCRIPTION OF EQUIPMENT & COST:	Supplier gives (1) a narrative description of the item(s) ordered, as well as all options, accesssories, supplies and drugs; (2) the supplier's charge for each item, option, accessory, supply and drug; and (3) the Medicare fee schedule allowance for each item/option/accessory/supply/drug, if applicable.
SECTION D:	(To be completed by the physician)
PHYSICIAN ATTESTATION:	The physician's signature certifies (1) the CMN which he/she is reviewing includes Sections A, B, C and D; (2) the answers in Section B are correct; and (3) the self-identifying information in Section A is correct.
PHYSICIAN SIGNATURE AND DATE:	After completion and/or review by the physician of Sections A, B and C, the physician must sign and date the CMN in Section D, verifying the Attestation appearing in this Section. The physician's signature also certifies the items ordered are medically necessary for this patient. Signature and date stamps are not acceptable.

According to the Paperwork Reduction Act of 1995, no persons are required to respond to a collection of information unless it displays a valid OMB control number. The valid OMB number for this information collection is 0938-0679. The time required to complete this information collection is estimated to average 15 minutes per response, including the time to review instructions, search existing resources, gather the data needed, and complete and review the information collection. If you have any comments concerning the accuracy of the time estimate or suggestions for improving this form, please write to HCFA, P.O. Box 26684, Baltimore, Maryland, 21207 and to the Office of Information and Regulatory Affairs, Office of Management and Budget, Washington, DC 20503.

Figure 10–1 Certificate of Medical Necessity for enteral nutrition (back)

Table 10–1 HCPCS payment categories and codes

Category	Code	Description
I	B4150	**Semi-synthetic Intact Protein Isolates** (e.g., Attain, Choice dm, Ensure, Ensure HN, Ensure with Fiber, Entrition HN, Fiberlan, Fibersource, Fibersource HN, Glytrol, Isocal, Isocal HN, Isolan, Isosource, Isosource HN, Jevity, Nitrolan, NuBasics, NuBasics with Fiber, NuBasics VHP, Nutren 1.0, Nutren 1.0 with Fiber, Nutrilan, Osmolite, Osmolite HN, Probalance, Profiber, Promote, Promote with Fiber, Resource, Resource Diabetic, Sustacal, Basic, Sustacal Liquid, Sustacal with Fiber, Ultracal)
I-B	B4151	**Natural Intact Protein/Protein Isolates** (e.g., Compleat B, Compleat B Modified)
II	B4152	**Intact Protein/Protein Isolates** **(Calorically dense)** (Comply, Deliver 2.0, Ensure Plus, Ensure Plus HN, Isosource 1.5 Cal., Magnacal, Nutren 1.5, Nutren 2.0, NuBasics Plus, Resource Plus, Respalor, Sustacal Plus, TwoCal HN Ultralan)
III	B4153	**Hydrolyzed Protein/Amino Acids** (e.g., Criticare HN, Isotein HN, Reabilan, Travasorb HN, Vital HN, Vivonex Pediatric)
IV	B4154	**Defined Formula for Special Metabolic Need** (e.g., Accupep HPF, Advera, Alitraq, Crucial, Diabetisource, Glucerna, Hepatic-Aid, Impact, Impact 1.5, Impact with Fiber, Isosource VHN, Lipisorb, Nepro, Nutrihep, NutriVent, Peptamen, Peptamen VHP, Perative, Protain XL, Pulmocare, Reabilan HN, Replete, Replete with Fiber, Sandosource, Suplena, TraumaCal, Travasorb Hepatic, Travasorb MCT, Travasorb Renal Diet, Vivonex Plus, Vivonex T.E.N.)
V	B4155	**Modular Components** (e.g., Propac, Promix, Casec, Moducal, Controlyte, Polycose liquid or powder, Sumacal, Microlipid, MCT Oil, Nutri-source
VI	B4156	**Standardized Nutrients** (e.g., Travasorb STD, Tolerex)

Insurance claims are submitted to HCFA using the HCFA-1500 form (see Figure 10–2). HCFA divided the country into four regions and assigned a regional carrier to each to decrease the complication of processing Medicare claims for ENT. These four Durable Medical Equipment Regional Carriers (DMERCs) each have technical, medical criteria and specialized guidelines. See Exhibit 10–2 for a listing of the DMERCs by region.[9] Among other mandates for appropriate patient selection, the DMERCs state that coverage will be denied

PLEASE
DO NOT
STAPLE
IN THIS
AREA

APPROVED OMB-0938-0008

HEALTH INSURANCE CLAIM FORM

← CARRIER →

← PATIENT AND INSURED INFORMATION →

☐☐☐ PICA   PICA ☐☐☐

1. MEDICARE   MEDICAID   CHAMPUS   CHAMPVA   GROUP HEALTH PLAN   FECA BLK LUNG   OTHER   1a. INSURED'S I.D. NUMBER   (FOR PROGRAM IN ITEM 1)

☐ (Medicare #)   ☐ (Medicaid #)   ☐ (Sponsor's SSN)   ☐ (VA File #)   ☐ (SSN or ID)   ☐ (SSN)   ☐ (ID)

2. PATIENT'S NAME (Last Name, First Name, Middle Initial)

3. PATIENT'S BIRTHDATE
MM   DD   YY   SEX
M ☐   F ☐

4. INSURED'S NAME (Last Name, First Name, Middle Initial)

5. PATIENT'S ADDRESS (No., Street)

6. PATIENT RELATIONSHIP TO INSURED
Self ☐   Spouse ☐   Child ☐   Other ☐

7. INSURED'S ADDRESS (No., Street)

CITY   STATE

8. PATIENT STATUS
Single ☐   Married ☐   Other ☐
Employed ☐   Full-Time Student ☐   Part-Time Student ☐

CITY   STATE

ZIP CODE   TELEPHONE (Include Area Code)
( )

ZIP CODE   TELEPHONE (Include Area Code)
( )

9. OTHER INSURED'S NAME (Last Name, First Name, Middle Initial)

10. IS PATIENT'S CONDITION RELATED TO:

11. INSURED'S POLICY GROUP OR FECA NUMBER

a. OTHER INSURED'S POLICY OR GROUP NUMBER

a. EMPLOYMENT? (CURRENT OR PREVIOUS)
☐ YES   ☐ NO

a. INSURED'S DATE OF BIRTH
MM   DD   YY   SEX
M ☐   F ☐

b. OTHER INSURED'S DATE OF BIRTH
MM   DD   YY   SEX
M ☐   F ☐

b. AUTO ACCIDENT?   PLACE (State)
☐ YES   ☐ NO   ( )

b. EMPLOYER'S NAME OR SCHOOL NAME

c. EMPLOYER'S NAME OR SCHOOL NAME

c. OTHER ACCIDENT?
☐ YES   ☐ NO

c. INSURANCE PLAN NAME OR PROGRAM NAME

d. INSURANCE PLAN NAME OR PROGRAM NAME

10d. RESERVED FOR LOCAL USE

d. IS THERE ANOTHER HEALTH BENEFIT PLAN?
☐ YES   ☐ NO   *If yes*, return to and complete item 9 a-d.

READ BACK OF FORM BEFORE COMPLETING & SIGNING THIS FORM.

12. PATIENT'S OR AUTHORIZED PERSON'S SIGNATURE I authorize the release of any medical or other information necessary to process this claim. I also request payment of government benefits either to myself or to the party who accepts assignment below.

13. INSURED'S OR AUTHORIZED PERSON'S SIGNATURE I authorize payment of medical benefits to the undersigned physician or supplier for services described below.

SIGNED _____   DATE _____

SIGNED _____

PHYSICIAN SUPPLIER INFORMATION

14. DATE OF CURRENT: ILLNESS (First symptom) OR INJURY (Accident) OR PREGNANCY (LMP)
MM DD YY

15. IF PATIENT HAS HAD SAME OR SIMILAR ILLNESS GIVE FIRST DATE MM DD YY

16. DATES PATIENT UNABLE TO WORK IN CURRENT OCCUPATION
FROM MM DD YY TO MM DD YY

17. NAME OF REFERRING PHYSICIAN OR OTHER SOURCE

17a. I.D. NUMBER OF REFERRING PHYSICIAN

18. HOSPITALIZATION DATES RELATED TO CURRENT SERVICES
FROM MM DD YY TO MM DD YY

19. RESERVED FOR LOCAL USE

20. OUTSIDE LAB?
☐ YES ☐ NO
$ CHARGES

21. DIAGNOSIS OR NATURE OF ILLNESS OR INJURY. (RELATE ITEMS 1,2,3 OR 4 TO ITEM 24E BY LINE)

1. |___.___|
2. |___.___|
3. |___.___|
4. |___.___|

22. MEDICAID RESUBMISSION
CODE   ORIGINAL REF. NO.

23. PRIOR AUTHORIZATION NUMBER

24.
A DATE(S) OF SERVICE						B Place of Service	C Type of Service	D PROCEDURES, SERVICES, OR SUPPLIES (Explain Unusual Circumstances) CPT/HCPCS MODIFIER	E DIAGNOSIS CODE	F $ CHARGES	G DAYS OR UNITS	H EPSDT Family Plan	I EMG	J COB	K RESERVED FOR LOCAL USE
From			To												
MM	DD	YY	MM	DD	YY										
1															
2															
3															
4															
5															
6															

25. FEDERAL TAX I.D. NUMBER   SSN ☐ EIN ☐

26. PATIENT'S ACCOUNT NO.

27. ACCEPT ASSIGNMENT?
(For govt. claims, see back)
☐ YES ☐ NO

28. TOTAL CHARGE
$

29. AMOUNT PAID
$

30. BALANCE DUE
$

31. SIGNATURE OF PHYSICIAN OR SUPPLIER INCLUDING DEGREE OR CREDENTIALS
(I certify that the statements on the reverse apply to this bill and are made a part thereof.)
SIGNED   DATE

32. NAME AND ADDRESS OF FACILITY WHERE SERVICES WERE RENDERED (If other than home or office)

33. PHYSICIAN'S, SUPPLIER'S BILLING NAME, ADDRESS, ZIP CODE & PHONE #

PIN#   GRP#

(APPROVED BY AMA COUNCIL ON MEDICAL SERVICE 8/88)   *PLEASE PRINT OR TYPE*

FORM HCFA-1500 (12-90)   FORM RRB-1500
FORM OWCP-1500
FORM AMA OP0506092

Figure 10–2 Health Insurance Claim Form—HCFA-1500

- **Region A:** Metrahealth (Traveler's) – Connecticut, Delaware, Maine, Massachusetts, New Hampshire, New Jersey, New York, Pennsylvania, Rhode Island, Vermont.

- **Region B:** AdminaStar Federal, Inc. – District of Columbia, Illinois, Indiana, Maryland, Michigan, Minnesota, Ohio, Virginia, West Virginia, Wisconsin.

- **Region C:** Palmetto Government Benefits Administrators – Alabama, Arkansas, Colorado, Florida, Georgia, Kentucky, Louisiana, Mississippi, New Mexico, North Carolina, Oklahoma, Puerto Rico, South Carolina, Tennessee, Texas, Virgin Islands.

- **Region D:** CIGNA – Alaska, Arizona, California, Guam, Hawaii, Idaho, Iowa, Kansas, Missouri, Montana, Nebraska, Nevada, North Dakota, Oregon, South Dakota, Utah, Washington, Wyoming.

for patients with lack of appetite (anorexia), or organic brain syndrome (e.g., Alzheimer's disease, senile dementia) unless there is a malfunctioning gastrointestinal tract in conjunction with these disorders. A major criticism regarding the DMERCs is that they are not consistent across the regions (i.e., what is considered standard fare in one region is not necessarily so in another). Preauthorization becomes an important aspect of discharging a patient into an alternate care site.

Medicare requires that a patient be informed what the costs will be if therapy is not covered. This is known as a Medicare Waiver and protects the patients from liability if they have not been informed of the costs up front. The Medicare Waiver also contains a statement about the appropriate appeal process should that become necessary.

READINESS OF THE HEALTH CARE TEAM

Once the patient's medical condition is stabilized, and the preauthorization process for payment reimbursement has been completed, alternate site nutrition support can be considered and discharge plans put into full motion. It is important for the case manager and others to communicate with the staff overseeing the discharge site prior to the transition. The Joint Commission on Accreditation of Healthcare Organizations (JCAHO) emphasizes the importance of continuity of care from hospital to home or alternate site.[10] For more information on JCAHO standards, consult the information listed at the end of this chapter in the Resources section. In the case of home care, this entails communicating with intake personnel at the home care agency; with institutional management, it refers to either nursing staff or the admissions director. Either way, it is important to provide the discharge site with as much clinical information regarding the patient's nutritional needs as possible. This includes a copy of the pertinent materials from the inpatient record and contact personnel and phone numbers where appropriate.

In cases where the home care agency or skilled nursing facility is affiliated with the hospital, the transition can be very smooth. Some staff may even have responsibilities in both facilities, such as case managers, physicians, nurses, or dietitians. More likely, the patient will be managed by one or more outside agencies, which makes good communication essential.

ISSUES SPECIFIC TO HOME CARE

CHOOSING A PROVIDER

According to a letter published in 1993, there were over 13,000 Medicare-certified nursing agencies in the United States and Puerto Rico[11] and the number of home care visits increased more than 72% between 1988 and 1991.[12] These numbers reflect only Medicare usage; therefore, the total number may have been roughly 50% higher when considering commercial insurance companies as well.[13]

Choosing a provider to supply medical equipment and nutrients is an important decision for the patient. JCAHO mandates that a patient be given freedom of choice to select a home care provider. The hospital case manager is often the best resource for assisting the patient in "wading through the waters" to choose an infusion provider or home care agency that will be able to supply goods as well as professionals trained in initiating and monitoring home nutrition support. For example, some providers offer a full range of goods and services while others offer only equipment; some "farm out" or subcontract consultants for specialties like nutrition or mental health. Examples of the range of services offered by providers are listed in Exhibit 10–3. Other issues to consider are access to care over a prolonged period, and reassessment of nutritional status or follow-up care.[14]

Once a company is selected, a home care nurse completes an evaluation with the patient and a primary caregiver in attendance. The home should be

---

Exhibit 10–3 List of services provided by home health agencies

- **Staffing** (nurse, dietitian, physician, mental health, physical therapy, speech therapy, occupational therapy, pharmacist, billing specialist)
- **Equipment** (pump, pole, syringe, feeding set, tubes, nutrient availability)
- **Services** (management, follow-up, education, 24-hour contact, delivery schedule, billing resources, geographical coverage)

inspected for safe/clean storage ability, adequate refrigeration if necessary, overall sanitation, acceptable telecommunications, ease of delivery, and minimal potential for pets or other family members to provide a source of bacteria or tamper with equipment.[15] A summary of this screening information is shown in Table 10–2.[16]

Home enteral patients often have a gastrostomy or jejunostomy tube for long-term access and easy administration of the feedings. Unlike the hospital setting where tube feedings are typically administered on a continuous basis, tube feedings in the home are often given by intermittent method or in a cyclic fashion. This allows the patient freedom to perform other activities and leave the house without a pump or other cumbersome equipment. See Chapter 5, Tube Feeding Administration, for a thorough list of delivery methods.

PATIENT EDUCATION

Preparing a patient to receive ENT at home requires more training and education than a patient in the institutionalized setting, due to caregivers involved in administering care. Instructors need to be respectful of patients by meeting them at their baseline learning level and understanding what they emphasize as important and acceptable. Instructors should evaluate which approach will best enable the patient to learn. Some individuals learn best through short repetitive sessions; others may learn best by using the hands-on approach very early. It is equally important to ensure the patient has a support system to rely on at home.

Table 10–2 Screening parameters prior to home care education

Status	Assess/Evaluate
Physical	Mobility Dexterity Strength Vision
Mental	Depression Medications that alter cognitive ability Senility Preoccupation with illness Fear of death
Medical	Appropriateness of enteral nutrition therapy Rate and type of formula Tube placement
Pharmacological	Type of medications given via tube Unclogging methods
Environmental	Supportive home environment Safe and appropriate conditions for storage Adequate utilities (e.g., running water, electricity)

This support network can be any number of individuals or direct caregivers, nurses and other health professionals as well as family, clergy, friends, neighbors, and peers.[15-17]

In the past, health care practitioners have been criticized for taking the "steamroller" approach to teaching. Educators need to ensure that the patient is instructed what to do, and to follow up to ensure additional questions are answered and techniques are reviewed. This will help the patient and/or caregiver feel well prepared for self-care.

Written guidelines should accompany education since it is common to forget 80 percent of what is taught by oral means alone. Professional nutrition journals occasionally list available home nutrition support teaching materials, free of charge or for purchase, to be used by hospitals.[18] Diagrams and photographs are a "gold mine" to many patients after the health care team has completed education and they are to manage their tube feeding at home. Generic patient education materials often do not have details on equipment care. Therefore, equipment should be accompanied by specific guidelines for use.

Assuring ease of readability of instruction materials is important. Flesch Reading Ease Score is the most recognized readability standard available.[19] According to Flesch, education materials are best understood at the 6th to 8th grade reading level. The popular *USA Today* newspaper is written at this level, which might explain why it is widely accepted by the general population. Pictures or other graphic means may be helpful for those with low literacy.

Patients can be instructed in the hospital or home setting by a clinician. The goal should be to have the patient or caregiver provide care independently. Therefore, after reviewing materials, patients and caregivers should effectively demonstrate their knowledge and ability with the health care team to ensure complete understanding.[20,21] Questions will still arise after discharge, but patients and caregivers should feel comfortable and any glaring safety issues should be eliminated by the time of discharge.

Patients should be trained how to inspect their feeding containers for leaks, visible contaminants, non-emulsified product, and expiration dates. Additional training may include: contingency planning in case of emergency; proper handwashing and aseptic technique; routine maintenance of equipment; recognizing signs of infection, abnormal intake and output, extreme fluctuations in body weight, and elevated temperature; and dealing with medication changes or interactions.[15,22,23] See Exhibit 10–4 for a sample of instructional topics appropriate for home enteral nutrition patients.

Occasionally, patients receive homemade tube feeding preparations. Any number of concoctions can be blenderized from a normal diet and considered nutritionally balanced if made properly. After blenderizing, the product should be strained well to prevent clogging the tube. A larger-bore feeding tube may be used to prevent clogging. Stringent flushing regimes should be employed for the same reason. Preparing homemade tube feedings requires diligence on the

Exhibit 10–4 Instructing home enteral nutrition patients

Feeding preparation

- Position of patient during administration
- Aspiration precautions
- Measuring formula
- Addition of medications
- Determining placement of tube
- Temperature of feeding
- Storage of unused feeding
- Expiration dates
- Position of IV pole
- Flushing before and after administration
- Hydration management
- Proper taping techniques
- Pump controls

Care of equipment

- Administration set and feeding container
- Pump
- Tube
- Replacing equipment

Personal care

- Mouth care
- Site care
  –Nose and nostrils
  –Abdominal wall

- Bathing with a tube
- Exercise
- Dealing with sick days
- Missed feedings
- Accurate use of home scale for weights
- Guidelines for oral intake where appropriate

Gastrointestinal problems

- Diarrhea
- Constipation
- Stomach discomfort/distension
- Vomiting
- Nausea

Mechanical problems

- Flow obstruction
- Pump alarms
- Accidental removal or displacement of tube

Who to call when problems arise

- Identify routine versus emergent situations
- Hospital emergency room
- Home care agency
- Clinic

---

part of the "chef," with food safety techniques heavily emphasized to prevent illness. For example, raw egg or undercooked protein foods should never be included in the recipe. Whether the patient is preparing homemade tube feedings or receiving commercial formulas, additional fiber is usually required, modeling the normal diet. Many homemade formulas include legumes (beans) or commercial fiber powders to promote bowel regularity. Products such as Uni-Fiber (Niche Pharmaceuticals, Roanoke, TX), and Benefiber (Novartis Nutrition, Minneapolis, MN) are commonly used as effective daily fiber sources.

FOLLOW-UP IN HOME CARE

Since inception of the JCAHO guidelines for home care, recommendation for follow-up by qualified professionals has been suggested for home care recipients.[10] Not every payer gives value to the JCAHO standards. Services such as 24-hour-a-day availability and trained clinical staff are costly issues most enteral suppliers are not able to justify. Therefore, quality care of ENT at home often suffers. Most enteral suppliers are not able to provide the nutrition follow-up that they would like, but some have been compelled to come up with creative solutions in order to provide the care needed. An example of JCAHO Home Care Standards is shown in Table 10–3.

Follow-up is critical, both by phone and in-person visits. The nurse or dietitian should conduct routine follow-up visits to observe firsthand the technique that is being used to deliver feedings. Patients or well-meaning families may be withholding medications, improperly administering tube feeding formula, or administering any number of unknown items via the tube.[24] Reports of such high-risk behaviors are important to convey to all staff involved in order to improve patient management. Re-educating the patient and caregivers to appropriate techniques is usually successful.

With advances in technology, some patients have been able to be monitored by closed-circuit television. A small television is placed in both the home and nursing agency. This allows the observer to visualize technique and provides the aura of a face-to-face visit that is lost with phone contact alone. This service is just beginning to be offered—usually for patients in remote geographical locations, for high-risk therapies, or for cases where very close observation is necessary. Additional advances in practice include use of the World Wide Web or Internet to send and receive reports, and electronic mail correspondence with both professionals and patients.

DOCUMENTATION IN HOME CARE

There is no widely accepted or necessary format for documentation of home care patients. Many clinicians follow the same standards as they would in the hospital. Issues such as weight changes, tolerance to feeding, tube site, and

Table 10–3 JCAHO home standards

Documentation	Comments
Screening and assessment	Timeliness/Frequency
Education	Detailed written and verbal guidelines in readable and understandable language
Care planning	Outlines the frequency of visitation to be expected, delivery and preparation of nutrients
Goals for therapy	Short- and long-term goals—includes transitioning the patient to the most normal possible diet
Rights and responsibilities	Includes an explanation to the patient about the agency policy on withdrawal of life-sustaining services

need for further education are some important items to document. Standardized forms are available from many home care organizations connected with hospitals such as the Mayo Clinic and the Cleveland Clinic, for use by any agency. Forms can be created to meet the needs of a particular home care agency or supplier. These records should be maintained at the primary agency as well as in the patient's home for other practitioners to utilize when visiting the patient. Updates should be made on a regular basis. Documentation of any procedures performed and response to such is especially useful to visiting staff.

ISSUES SPECIFIC TO INSTITUTIONALIZED SETTINGS

Home care is the preferred arena for patients to receive therapy, according to patient satisfaction surveys. However, due to severity of illness, individual preference, or lack of support systems, patients may be better managed in a nursing home environment. Patients in these institutional settings are often referred to as *residents*. Most nursing home facilities accept tube-fed residents, but it is wise to clarify this for each patient prior to discharge. Most of the daily care for residents is managed by nurses or certified nursing assistants (CNAs).

County, state, and federal agencies govern most institutions. Although advisory rather than mandatory, JCAHO's Standards[25] and the Best Practice Guidelines[26] are instituted in many facilities for continuity of care. The American Society for Parenteral and Enteral Nutrition (A.S.P.E.N.) has developed Standards for Nutrition Support for this population, as well, which identify specifics in relation to assessment, care planning, implementation, monitoring, reassessment and termination of therapy.[8]

Much like the hospital, nutrition screening and assessment are completed upon admission to determine current nutritional concerns. Many nutrition professionals use the Mini-Nutritional Assessment tool[27] or other standard tools such as Subjective Global Assessment (see Chapter 1, Nutrition Screening and Assessment)[28] in long-term care facilities. The information gathered from these and other assessments from nursing and ancillary staff is recorded on the Minimum Data Set (MDS) 2.0 form. The MDS is the basic assessment form required by HCFA that must be completed on every resident. HCFA mandates that they are initially completed at day 5 of admission. They are then updated and signed by all staff on days 14, 30, 60, and 90. There are 18 areas listed on the trigger legend at the end of the assessment, and many of these areas impact nutrition status. Once an area has been triggered as a nutritional concern, a resident assessment protocol (RAP) module may or may not be completed, depending on whether the issue is addressed in the care plan.[29] Examples of Section K – Oral/Nutritional Status from the MDS form and RAP Summary Sheet are shown in Figures 10–3 and 10–4, respectively.

Congress in the Balanced Budget Act of 1997 created the Prospective Payment System (PPS) for Skilled Nursing Facilities (SNF). PPS was designed to keep SNFs more accountable and have them share in the risk of cost control. The major change in SNFs is that they are now paid at a per diem prospective case-mix adjusted rate. The basic allocation for reimbursement is based on patient classification system termed RUG-III or Resource Utilization Groups. The MDS is what determines the RUG level, which is primarily driven by a patient's ability to perform activities of daily living (ADLs). The PPS system has a Special Care section that addresses areas such as enteral nutrition, dehydration, and skin lesions. In the case of enteral nutrition, a resident must receive at least 501 ml and 26% of total caloric requirement through the tube per day to be eligible for enteral nutrition payment through PPS.[30]

Proper and timely documentation on the MDS form is essential to ensure payment by HCFA. Due to the high acuity level of patients being admitted to facilities in this crunch-time of health care dollars, a resident rarely utilizes the full 100 Medicare days eligible to him or her. It is common for a patient's status to change, causing the patient no longer to be eligible to receive Medicare benefits. If there is a significant change in a patient's status (e.g., weight loss of 5% in 30 days, feeding tube inserted), another form of payment is usually applied, such as a state Medicaid grant or payment from a secondary commercial carrier. In addition, an entirely new MDS form needs to be completed and the cycle regenerated.

If a resident does not have Medicare, the MDS form is still completed but within 14 days of admission. The follow-up schedule reverts to the one originally developed by the Omnibus Budget Reconciliation Act (OBRA) in 1987. This is a quarterly and annual schedule maintained by the Registered Nurse Assessment Coordinator (RNAC) in most nursing facilities.

EDUCATION IN INSTITUTIONALIZED SETTINGS

The nursing and/or nutrition staff employed by the institution conducts the nutrition education for residents. However, some minimal education may be conducted at the hospital level in order to prepare the patient for discharge, particularly if the tube feeding is brand new. It goes without saying that a resident should be alert and oriented in order to learn discharge tube feeding instructions and perform the tasks associated with instruction. For those residents with dementia or who are unable to comprehend instruction, family members should be informed of the diet/tube feeding order. Federal regulations mandate that a resident has the right to be fully informed about treatment, and the resident has the right to refuse any treatment. As with home care, written and oral tools should be used to prepare the patient for transfer, as well as returned demonstration of learned tasks.

CLINICAL MONITORING OF ENT: HOME CARE OR OUT OF HOSPITAL SETTINGS

Clinical monitoring is critical to all patients regardless of their setting. Monitoring patients for metabolic and nutritional outcomes is essential to their well-being. Typically, follow-up does not take place as often outside of the hospital setting as in the acute setting. For example, labs may be monitored daily in the

SECTION M. SKIN CONDITION

			Number at Stage
1.	ULCERS (Due to any cause)	(Record the number of ulcers at each ulcer stage—regardless of cause. If none present at a stage record "0" (zero). Code all that apply during last 7 days Code 9 = 9 or more.) (Requires full body exam.)	
		a. **Stage 1.** A persistent area of skin redness (without a break in the skin) that does not disappear when pressure is relieved.	
		b. **Stage 2.** A partial thickness loss of skin layers that presents clinically as an abrasion, blister, or shallow crater.	
		c. **Stage 3.** A full thickness of skin is lost, exposing the subcutaneous tissues—presents as a deep crater with or without undermining adjacent tissue.	
		d. **Stage 4.** A full thickness of skin and subcutaneous tissue is lost, exposing muscle or bone.	
2.	TYPE OF ULCER	(For each type of ulcer, code for the highest stage in the last 7 days using scale in item M1—i.e., 0 = none; stages 1, 2, 3, 4)	
		a. Pressure ulcer—any lesion caused by pressure resulting in damage of underlying tissue 1 = **16**; 2, 3, or 4 = **12, 16**	
		b. Stasis ulcer—open lesion caused by poor circulation in the lower extremities	
3.	HISTORY OF RESOLVED ULCERS	Resident had an ulcer that was resolved or cured in LAST 90 DAYS 0. No 1. Yes **16**	
4.	OTHER SKIN PROBLEMS OR LESIONS PRESENT	(Check all that apply during last 7 days)	
		Abrasions, bruises	a.
		Burns (second or third degree)	b.
		Open lesions other than ulcers, rashes, cuts (e.g., cancer lesions)	c.
		Rashes—e.g., intertrigo, eczema, drug rash, heat rash, herpes zoster	d.
		Skin desensitized to pain or pressure **16**	e.
		Skin tears or cuts (other than surgery)	f.
		Surgical wounds	g.
		NONE OF ABOVE	h.
5.	SKIN TREATMENTS	(Check all that apply during last 7 days)	
		Pressure relieving device(s) for chair	a.
		Pressure relieving device(s) for bed	b.
		Turning/repositioning program	c.
		Nutrition or hydration intervention to manage skin problems	d.
		Ulcer care	e.
		Surgical wound care	f.
		Application of dressings (with or without topical medications) other than to feet	g.
		Application of ointments/medications (other than to feet)	h.
		Other preventative or protective skin care (other than to feet)	i.
		NONE OF ABOVE	j.

2.	PAIN SYMPTOMS	(Code the highest level of pain present in the last 7 days)
		a. FREQUENCY with which resident complains or shows evidence of pain	b. INTENSITY of pain
		0. No pain (skip to J4)	1. Mild pain
		1. Pain less than daily	2. Moderate pain
		2. Pain daily	3. Times when pain is horrible or excruciating
3.	PAIN SITE	(If pain present, check all sites that apply in last 7 days)
		Back pain	a.	Incisional pain	f.
		Bone pain	b.	Joint pain (other than hip)	g.
		Chest pain while doing usual activities	c.	Soft tissue pain (e.g., lesion, muscle)	h.
		Headache	d.	Stomach pain	i.
		Hip pain	e.	Other	j.
4.	ACCIDENTS	(Check all that apply)
		Fell in past 30 days 11, 17*	a.	Hip fracture in last 180 days 17*	c.
		Fell in past 31–180 days 11, 17*	b.	Other fracture in last 180 days 11, 17*	d.
				NONE OF ABOVE	e.
5.	STABILITY OF CONDITIONS	Conditions/diseases make resident's cognitive, ADL, mood or behavior patterns unstable—(fluctuating, precarious, or deteriorating)	a.
		Resident experiencing an acute episode or a flare-up of a recurrent or chronic problem	b.
		End-stage disease, 6 or fewer months to live	c.
		NONE OF ABOVE	d.

SECTION K. ORAL/NUTRITIONAL STATUS

1.	ORAL PROBLEMS	Chewing problem	a.
		Swallowing problem 17*	b.
		Mouth pain 16	c.
		NONE OF ABOVE	d.
2.	HEIGHT AND WEIGHT	Record (a.) height in inches and (b.) weight in pounds. Base weight on most recent measure in last 30 days; measure weight consistently in accord with standard facility practice—e.g., in a.m. after voiding, before meal, with shoes off, and in nightclothes.	
		a. HT (in.)	b. WT (lb.)
3.	WEIGHT CHANGE	a. **Weight loss**—5% or more in last 30 days; or 10% or more in last 180 days 0. No 1. Yes 12	
		b. **Weight gain**—5% or more in last 30 days; or 10% or more in last 180 days 0. No 1. Yes	
4.	NUTRITIONAL PROBLEMS	Complains about the taste of many foods 12	a.	Leaves 25% or more of food uneaten at most meals 12	c.
		Regular or repetitive complaints of hunger 12	b.	NONE OF ABOVE	d.
5.	NUTRITIONAL APPROACHES	(Check all that apply in last 7 days)	
		Parenteral/IV 12, 14	a.	Dietary supplement between meals	f.
		Feeding tube 13, 14	b.	Plate guard, stabilized built-up utensil, etc.	g.
		Mechanically altered diet 12	c.	On a planned weight change program	h.
		Syringe (oral feeding) 12	d.	NONE OF ABOVE	i.
		Therapeutic diet 12	e.		

6.	FOOT PROBLEMS AND CARE	(*Check all that apply during last 7 days*)	
		Resident has one or more foot problems—e.g., corns, calluses, bunions, hammer toes, overlapping toes, pain, structural problems	a.
		Infection of the foot—e.g., cellulitis, purulent drainage	b.
		Open lesions on the foot	c.
		Nails/calluses trimmed during last 90 days	d.
		Received preventative or protective foot care (e.g., used special shoes, inserts, pads, toe separators)	e.
		Application of dressings (with or without topical medications)	f.
		NONE OF ABOVE	g.

SECTION N. ACTIVITY PURSUIT PATTERNS

1.	TIME AWAKE 10B only if BOTH N1a = ✓ and N2 = 0	(*Check appropriate time periods over last 7 days*) Resident awake all or most of time (i.e., naps no more than one hour per time period) in the:		
		Morning 10B	a.	Evening	c.
		Afternoon	b.	*NONE OF ABOVE*	d.
		(IF RESIDENT IS COMATOSE, SKIP TO SECTION O)		

2.	AVERAGE TIME INVOLVED IN ACTIVITIES	(When awake and not receiving treatments or ADL care)
		0. Most—more than 2/3 of time 10B 2. Little—less than 1/3 of time 10A
		1. Some—from 1/3 to 2/3 of time 3. None 10A

3.	PREFERRED ACTIVITY SETTINGS	(*Check all settings in which activities are preferred*)		
		Own room	a.		
		Day/activity room	b.	Outside facility	d.
		Inside NH/off unit	c.	*NONE OF ABOVE*	e.

4.	GENERAL ACTIVITY PREFERENCES (Adapted to resident's current abilities)	(*Check all PREFERENCES whether or not activity is currently available to resident*)		
		Cards/other games	a.	Trips/shopping	g.
		Crafts/arts	b.	Walking/wheeling outdoors	h.
		Exercise/sports	c.	Watching TV	i.
		Music	d.	Gardening or plants	j.
		Reading/writing	e.	Talking or conversing	k.
		Spiritual/religious activities	f.	Helping others	l.
				NONE OF ABOVE	m.

Form 17339RHH   © 1998 Briggs Corporation, Des Moines, IA 50306   (800) 247-2343   PRINTED IN U.S.A.
Copyright limited to addition of trigger system.

6.	PARENTERAL OR ENTERAL INTAKE	(*Skip to Section L if neither 5a nor 5b is checked*)
		a. Code the proportion of total calories the resident received through parenteral or tube feedings in the last 7 days)
		0. None 3. 51% to 75%
		1. 1% to 25% 4. 76% to 100%
		2. 26% to 50%
		b. Code the average fluid intake per day by IV or tube in last 7 days
		0. None 3. 1001 to 1500 cc/day
		1. 1 to 500 cc/day 4. 1501 to 2000 cc/day
		2. 501 to 1000 cc/day 5. 2001 or more cc/day

SECTION L. ORAL/DENTAL STATUS

1.	ORAL STATUS AND DISEASE PREVENTION	Debris (soft, easily movable substances) present in mouth prior to going to bed at night 15	a.
		Has dentures or removable bridge	b.
		Some/all natural teeth lost—does not have or does not use dentures (or partial plates) 15	c.
		Broken, loose, or carious teeth 15	d.
		Inflamed gums (gingiva); swollen or bleeding gums; oral abscesses; ulcers or rashes 15	e.
		Daily cleaning of teeth/dentures or daily mouth care—by resident or staff Not ✓ /—15	f.
		NONE OF ABOVE	g.

TRIGGER LEGENDS

10A – Activities (Revise)   13 – Feeding Tubes   17* – Psychotropic Drugs
10B – Activities (Review)   14 – Dehydration/Fluid Maintenance   (*For this to trigger, O4a, b,
11 – Falls   15 – Dental Care   or c must = 1-7)
12 – Nutritional Status   16 – Pressure Ulcers

Figure 10–3 Minimum data set 2.0 Section K, Oral/Nutritional Status

SECTION V. RESIDENT ASSESSMENT PROTOCOL SUMMARY   Numeric Identifier _____

Resident's Name:	Medical Record No.:

1. Check if RAP is triggered.
2. For each triggered RAP, use the RAP guidelines to identify areas needing further assessment. Document relevant assessment information regarding the resident's status.
   - Describe:
     - —Nature of the condition (may include presence or lack of objective data and subjective complaints).
     - —Complications and risk factors that affect your decision to proceed to care planning.
     - —Factors that must be considered in developing individualized care plan interventions.
     - —Need for referrals/further evaluation by appropriate health professionals.
   - Documentation should support your decision making regarding whether to proceed with a care plan for a triggered RAP and the type(s) of care plan interventions that are appropriate for a particular resident.
   - Documentation may appear anywhere in the clinical record (e.g., progress notes, consults, flowsheets, etc.).
3. Indicate under the <u>Location of RAP Assessment Documentation</u> column where information related to the RAP assessment can be found.
4. For each triggered RAP, indicate whether a new care plan, care plan revision, or continuation of current care plan is necessary to address the problem(s) identified in your assessment. The Care Planning Decision column must be completed within 7 days of completing the RAI (MDS and RAPs).

A. RAP Problem Area	(a) Check if Triggered	Location and Date of RAP Assessment Documentation	(b) Care Planning Decision— check if addressed in care plan
1. DELIRIUM			
2. COGNITIVE LOSS			
3. VISUAL FUNCTION			
4. COMMUNICATION			
5. ADL FUNCTIONAL/ REHABILITATION POTENTIAL			
6. URINARY INCONTINENCE AND INDWELLING CATHETER			
7. PSYCHOSOCIAL WELL-BEING			
8. MOOD STATE			
9. BEHAVIORAL SYMPTOMS			
10. ACTIVITIES			
11. FALLS			
12. NUTRITIONAL STATUS			

Figure 10–4 Resident Assessment Protocol Summary

Figure 10–4 continued

13. FEEDING TUBES			
14. DEHYDRATION/FLUID MAINTENANCE			
15. ORAL/DENTAL CARE			
16. PRESSURE ULCERS			
17. PSYCHOTROPIC DRUG USE			
18. PHYSICAL RESTRAINTS			

B.

1. Signature of RN Coordinator for
   RAP Assessment Process

2. ☐☐ – ☐☐ – ☐☐☐☐
   Month   Day   Year

3. Signature of Person Completing
   Care Planning Decision

4. ☐☐ – ☐☐ – ☐☐☐☐
   Month   Day   Year

acute setting and only monthly, quarterly, or yearly in some outpatient settings. This varies depending upon the severity of the case, reimbursement, patient willingness/compliance, and allowable visits. Weights, too, are often monitored more frequently in the acute setting. Patients with certain conditions such as diabetes, congestive heart failure, AIDS, etc., should have specific care plans to follow. Exhibit 10–5 is provided as an example for clinical patient monitoring. It is the responsibility of the health care team to develop protocols for frequency and appropriateness of clinical monitoring.

The most common complications of tube feeding were discussed in Chapter 7, Enteral Nutrition Complications. Chronic complications may easily be overlooked due to the infrequent follow-up that seemingly stable, long-term ENT patients may receive. Some problems to be mindful of, then, when reassessing patients are dehydration; vitamin, mineral, and trace element imbalances; diarrhea; constipation; aspiration potential; drug-nutrient interactions; and likelihood for contamination.[31] Also notable are over- and underfeeding, hyperglycemia, and potential for skin breakdown.[13,16] These should be addressed at each follow-up to ensure that a patient's nutritional status is not neglected and nutrition goals are met.

HOSPICE CARE

Hospice is a unique form of nursing care and other services provided for very ill individuals. This program allows dying persons to live in dignity and be as comfortable as they can until their death ensues. Hospice care can be provided

Exhibit 10–5 Clinical monitoring of patients in alternate sites

Anthropometrics
Weight
Height
Body composition measurements

Nutrient Intake
Oral
Enteral
Parenteral
Combination of feeding methods

Output
Urine
Fistula
Stool
Gastric contents

Laboratory Parameters

Sodium	Complete Blood Count with Differential
Potassium	Albumin
Chloride	Iron
Carbon Dioxide	Total Iron Binding Capacity
Blood Urea Nitrogen	Alanine Aminotransferase
Creatinine	Aspartate Aminotransferase
Glucose	Alkaline Phosphatase
Magnesium	Prothrombin Time
Calcium	Partial Thromboplastin Time
Phosphate	Platelets
Cholesterol	Triglyceride

in the patient's home, in alternate sites, and in the hospital-based setting. Hospices receive special funds from Medicare and commercial carriers, which, unlike home care, includes the cost of both direct and indirect services. However, the rate is very minimal, so directors of hospice care must be frugal with the allotted amount to best serve the individual patient.

Because hospice is regarded as a holistic practice, nutrition objectives are very different than those imposed in other areas. Nutrition, whether provided orally or by feeding tube, is one of the last things a patient may be able to control. All patient directives are honored within reason and financial feasibility. Hospice staff is trained to monitor and promote adequate hydration, electrolyte balance, and maximum calorie intake where indicated, and above all to allow for patient comfort. For more information on hospice care, consult the Resources section at the end of this chapter.

LEGAL AND ETHICAL ISSUES IN ALTERNATE SETTINGS

The decision to forgo or to withdraw life-sustaining services such as nutrition support from a patient is not an easy one for family or staff. The Patient Self-

Determination Act (effective December 1, 1991) specified that all Medicare- or Medicaid-certified hospitals or nursing facilities provide information on advance directives to all staff and patients. These should include the wishes of the resident with regard to feeding and hydration.[32] Advance directives are instructions for medical treatment given by a patient while he or she has decisional capacity to do so. These instructions are to be carried out in case of the loss of decisional capacity. The "living will" is part of an advance directive in that it specifies those interventions not desired by the patient under certain conditions. These would include items such as mechanical ventilation, blood transfusion, and resuscitation.[32,33]

A landmark case from the 1970s in New Jersey recognized the right to withdraw life-sustaining medical treatment that they felt their family member would not have wanted.[34] There are a few notable cases since this time, but possibly the most prominent is the *Cruzan* case decided by the Supreme Court in 1991.[35] For more on ethics and clinical practice specifically relating to nutrition support, there is an excellent text noted in the Suggested Readings section of this chapter.

Without clear directives, the decision is left up to the family and/or the facility where the patient resides, depending on the state. Family members having to face this decision alone struggle with the "right" thing to do in terms of the patient's best interest. Facilities should appoint an ethics committee to establish policies and procedures for dealing with these delicate situations.[33,36]

CONCLUSION

Nutrition support in alternate site situations is more prevalent today and will likely remain so into the 21st century. The increasing number of elderly people combined with consumer demand for alternate services and the drive to lower costs is the reason for the paradigm shift from hospital and traditional care.

Health care is a business. Reimbursement is paramount to the industry if it is to survive. Nurses need to be aware of financial aspects and strive to understand the intricacies of the health care market, particularly the legislative areas.

Organizations such as JCAHO develop standards that must be adhered to if agencies and facilities are to remain in business. Nurses must remain sharp, efficient, and more compassionate than ever before. The ability of nurses to juggle all of the tasks that the "new world" of health care has to offer will depend on their desire to stay current and flexible, without compromising patient care or integrity.

REFERENCES

1. North American Home Parenteral and Enteral Nutrition Patient Registry. Annual Reports 1985–1992. Albany, NY: Oley Foundation; 1988–1994.
2. Howard L, Ament M, Fleming CR, et al. Current use and clinical outcome of home parenteral and enteral nutrition therapies in the United States. *Gastroenterol* 1995;109: 355–365.

3. Robbins J. Old swallowing and dysphagia: thoughts on intervention and prevention. *Nutr Clin Pract* 1999;14:S21–S26.

4. McKinnon BT, Wolfson MK, George P. Managed care. In: Rombeau JL, Rolandelli RH, eds. *Clinical Nutrition—Enteral and Tube Feeding*. 3rd ed. Philadelphia, PA: WB Saunders Company; 1997:599–611.

5. Parver AK, Lubinsky CA. Reimbursement issues in nutrition support. Part 1: public sector parenteral and enteral nutrition coverage and reimbursement. In: *A.S.P.E.N. Nutrition Support Practice Manual*. Silver Spring, MD: American Society for Parenteral and Enteral Nutrition; 1998:chap. 36:1–19.

6. American Society for Parenteral and Enteral Nutrition (A.S.P.E.N.) Board of Directors. Guidelines for the use of parenteral and enteral nutrition in adult and pediatric patients. *JPEN* 1993;17:1SA–4SA.

7. American Society for Parenteral and Enteral Nutrition (A.S.P.E.N.) Board of Directors. Standards for home nutrition support. *Nutr Clin Pract* 1999;14:151–162.

8. American Society for Parenteral and Enteral Nutrition (A.S.P.E.N.) Board of Directors. Standards for nutrition support for adult residents of long term care facilities. *Nutr Clin Pract* 1997;12:284–293.

9. *Durable Medical Equipment Regional Carrier Supplier Manual—Region B*. Indianapolis, IN: Health Care Financing Administration; 1994.

10. Joint Commission on Accreditation of Healthcare Organizations. *1999–2000 Comprehensive Accreditation Manual for Home Care*. Oakbrook Terrace, IL: Joint Commission on Accreditation of Healthcare Organizations; 1998.

11. SMG Marketing Group, Inc. *SMG Market Letter*. Chicago: SMG Marketing Group, Inc.; 1994;8.

12. Viall CD, Crocker KS, Hennessy KA, Orr ME. High tech home care: surviving and prospering in a changing environment. *Nutr Clin Pract* 1995;10:32–36.

13. Howard L, Malone M, Wolf BM. Home enteral nutrition in adults. In: Rombeau JL, Rolandelli RH, eds. *Clinical Nutrition—Enteral and Tube Feeding*. 3rd ed. Philadelphia, PA: WB Saunders Company; 1997:510–522.

14. Hermann-Zaidins M, Touger-Decker R. Supply and management structures. In: Hermann-Zaidins M, Touger-Decker R, eds. *Nutrition Support in Home Health*. Rockville, MD: Aspen Publishers, Inc.; 1989:25–39.

15. Nelson JK, Mirtallo J, Evans-Stoner NJ. Considerations for home nutrition support. In: *A.S.P.E.N. Nutrition Support Practice Manual*. Silver Spring, MD: American Society for Parenteral and Enteral Nutrition; 1998:chap. 35:1–16.

16. Weckwerth J, Ireton-Jones C. Nutrition support in home care. In: Matarese LE, Gottschlich MM, eds. *Contemporary Nutrition Support Practice—A Clinical Guide*. Philadelphia, PA: WB Saunders Company; 1998:611–623.

17. Bloch AS. Preparing the patient for home enteral management. In: Hermann-Zaidins M, Touger-Decker R, eds. *Nutrition Support in Home Health*. Rockville, MD: Aspen Publishers, Inc.; 1989:89–100.

18. Evans MA, Czopek S. Home nutrition support materials. *Nutr Clin Pract* 1995;10:37–39.

19. Flesch R. *The Art of Readable Writing*. New York, NY: Harper & Row; 1974:176–179, 247–251.

20. Evans-Stoner N, Weckwerth J, eds. *Selected Reviews in Nutrition Support—Home Care Edition*. Silver Spring, MD: American Society for Parenteral and Enteral Nutrition; 1996.

21. Loewenhardt PM. Assuring successful home enteral feedings. *Home Health Nurse* 1989; 7:16–21.

22. Young CK, White S. Preparing patients for tube feeding at home. *Am J Nurs* 1992;94:46.

23. Skipper A, Rotman N. A survey of the role of the dietitian in preparing patients for home enteral feeding. *J Am Diet Assoc* 1990;90:939–944.
24. Silkroski M, Ericson M. Enteral nutrition challenges in home care. *Nutr Clin Pract* 1998; 13:163–166.
25. Joint Commission on Accreditation of Healthcare Organizations. *1996 Comprehensive Accreditation Manual for Long-Term Care.* Oakbrook, IL: Joint Commission on Accreditation of Healthcare Organizations; 1996.
26. Health Care Financing Administration. Enteral Feeding: Current Practices and Outcome Measures. Satellite Broadcast; March 24, 1997; Baltimore, MD.
27. Guignoz Y, Vellas B, Garry PJ. Mini-nutritional assessment: a practical assessment tool for grading the nutritional state of elderly patients. *Facts and Res Gerontol* 1994; 2:15–60.
28. Detsky AS, McLaughlin JR, Baker JP, et al. What is subjective global assessment of nutritional status? *J Parenter Enteral Nutr* 1987;11:8–11.
29. Posthauer ME, Russell C. Ensuring optimal nutrition in long-term care. *Nutr Clin Pract* 1997;12:247–255.
30. Thomas DR, Kamel HK, Morley JE. Nutritional deficiencies in long-term care, part III: OBRA regulations and administrative and legal issues. *Annals of Long-Term Care.* Special report/supplement. Plainsboro, NJ: Multimedia Healthcare/Freedom, LLC; 1999:23–31.
31. American Dietetic Association. Nutrition monitoring of the home parenteral and enteral patient. *J Am Diet Assoc* 1994;94:664–666.
32. Mayo TW. Forgoing artificial nutrition and hydration: legal and ethical considerations *Nutr Clin Pract* 1996;11:254–264.
33. Ahronheim JC, Moreno JD, Zuckerman C. *Ethics in Clinical Practice.* 2nd ed. Gaithersburg, MD: Aspen Publishers, Inc.; 2000.
34. *In re Quinlan*, 70 N.J. 10, 355 A.2d 647, *cert. denied*, 429 U.S. 922 (1976).
35. *Cruzan v. Harmon*, 760 S.W.2d 408 (Mo. 1988).
36. King D. Ethical issues of home nutrition support. In: Hermann-Zaidins M, Touger-Decker R, eds. *Nutrition Support in Home Health.* Rockville, MD: Aspen Publishers, Inc; 1989:229–240.

SUGGESTED READINGS

Ahronheim JC, Moreno JD, Zuckerman C. *Ethics in Clinical Practice.* 2nd ed. Gaithersburg, MD: Aspen Publishers, Inc.; 2000.

American Society for Parenteral and Enteral Nutrition (A.S.P.E.N.). Reimbursement issues in nutrition support. In: *The A.S.P.E.N. Nutrition Support Practice Manual.* Silver Spring, MD: American Society for Parenteral and Enteral Nutrition; 1998:1–40.

Committee on Nutrition Services for Medicare Beneficiaries, Food and Nutrition Board, Institute of Medicine. Nutrition services in post-acute, long-term care and in community-based programs. In: *The Role of Nutrition in Maintaining Health in the Nation's Elderly: Evaluating Coverage of Nutrition Services for the Medicare Population.* Washington, DC: National Academy Press; 2000:225–253.

Goff K. Enteral and parenteral nutrition transitioning from hospital to home. *Nurs Case Manag* 1998;3:67–74.

Gottschlich MM, Fuhrman P, Hammond K, Holcombe B, Seidner D (eds) *The Science and Practice of Nutrition Support: A Case Based Core Curriculum.* Dubuque, IA: Kendall/Hunt Publishing Company, 2001.

Joint Commission on Accreditation of Healthcare Organizations. *1997–1998 Comprehensive Accreditation Manual for Home Care*. Oakbrook Terrace, IL: Joint Commission on Accreditation of Healthcare Organizations; 1996. http://www.jcaho.org

McNamara E, Flood P, Kennedy NP. Home enteral tube feeding: A growing problem? *Ir Med Sci* 1999;168:246–247.

Mitchell SL, Kiely DK, Lipsitz LA. The risk factors and impact on survival of feeding tube placement in nursing home residents with severe cognitive impairment. *Arch Intern Med* 1997;157:327–332.

Rudberg MA, Egleston BL, Grant MD, et al. Effectiveness of feeding tubes in nursing home residents with swallowing disorders. *J Parenter Enteral Nutr* 2000;24:97–102.

Sanders H, Newall S, Norton B, et al. Gastrostomy feeding in the elderly after acute dysphasgic stroke. *J Nutr Health Aging* 2000;4:58–60.

Schneider SM, Pouget I, Staccini P, et al. Quality of life in long-term home enteral nutrition patients. *Clin Nutr* 2000;19:23–28.

Wilson MM. The management of dehydration in the nursing home. *J Nutr Health Aging* 1999;3:53–61.

RESOURCES

Oley Foundation
Albany Medical Center
214 Hun Memorial
Albany, NY 12208–3478
800–776–OLEY (6539)
http://www.wizvax.net/oleyfdn

Fiber Sources-Benefiber
Foodservice Resource
Novartis Nutrition
Minneapolis, MN 55440–0370
800–999–9978

Uni-Fiber
Niche Pharmaceuticals
200 North Oak Street
Roanoke, TX 76262
800–677–0355

HCFA and the Medicare and Medicaid Programs search page
http://www.hcfa.gov/search.htm

Library of Congress home page
http://www.loc.gov/

National Hospice and Palliative Care Organization
1700 Diagonal Road
Suite 300
Alexandria, VA 22313
703–243–5900
http://www.nho.org

Long-term Care Survey Monitor
www.opuscomm.com

Gerontological Society of America
1030 15th Street NW
Suite 250
Washington, D.C. 20005
202–842–1275
www.geron.org

National Association for Home Care
228 Seventh Street SE
Washington, D.C. 20003
202–547–7424
www.nahc.org

Standards of Home Health Nursing Practice
American Nurses' Association
2420 Pershing Road
Kansas City, MO 64108
Best Practice Network
www.best4health.org

11

Improving the Quality of Enteral Nutrition Care

MARCIA SILKROSKI

Many advances in the area of nutrition support have taken place in the last 30 years. Professionals committed to delivering quality care have spent numerous hours on research, observations, and documentation in an attempt to improve patient outcomes. This chapter reviews the evolution of quality assurance programs over the last few decades (see Exhibit 11–1), demonstrates how to use clinical pathways, discusses a quality improvement plan, and gives the reader a better understanding of the accreditation process offered by the Joint Commission on Accreditation of Healthcare Organizations.

INFLUENCE OF JOINT COMMISSION ON ACCREDITATION OF HEALTHCARE ORGANIZATIONS

Possibly the most recognized accrediting organization among health care professionals is the Joint Commission on Accreditation of Healthcare Organizations (JCAHO). The JCAHO has been in existence since 1951. Its development came about after World War II when the need for uniform standards for non-surgical specialties (e.g., medicine, nursing, pharmacy, and radiology), became evident.[1] Since this time, the JCAHO has been in the business of quality management in order to help patients to achieve the best possible outcome.

JCAHO is a private, nonprofit corporation that establishes standards for care provided by hospitals and health care organizations and audits those organizations regarding their adherence to those standards.[2] The JCAHO accredits more than 19,000 health care organizations in the United States and many other countries. Home care is the largest segment, followed by hospitals. Other eligi-

---

Exhibit 11–1 Fifty years of change to impact quality of care

1950s JCAH (Joint Commission on Accreditation of Hospitals) grew from the American College of Surgeons Hospital Standardization Program established in 1917.

1960s Medicare and Medicaid programs form as part of the Social Security Amendment.

1970s PSROs—Professional Standards Review Organizations developed to protect the monies allocated from the Social Security Act by pinpointing those services that are not considered medically appropriate.

1980s DRGs—Diagnosis Related Groups were introduced to hospitals, causing administrators to scrutinize costs and seek reimbursement through a prospective payment system. JCAHO—JCAH expands to include other "Healthcare Organizations."

1990s JCAHO rolls out the Agenda for Change originally developed in the 1980s.

2000s ORYX will undoubtedly take center stage within JCAHO.

ble health care organizations include long-term care facilities, health care networks, ambulatory care facilities, clinical laboratories, preferred provider organizations, and behavioral health care facilities. Health care organizations seek Joint Commission accreditation for many reasons (see Exhibit 11–2). The functions performed by JCAHO are shown in Exhibit 11–3.

JCAHO STANDARDS

Effective January 1995, the JCAHO specifically identified nutrition care standards to which all health care organizations would eventually be held accountable. These standards appear in each of its Accreditation Manuals[3–5] and are referred to as the Agenda for Change. The Agenda for Change project was originally drafted in 1987. These new standards are based on performance rather than the previous structure- and process-oriented standards.[6]

JCAHO standards address a health care organization's level of performance in specific areas. An example of the nutrition standards is shown in Exhibit 11–4.

The standards are detail-oriented and specify important functions relating to the care of individuals by health care providers.

The TX.4 nutrition standards, in the Care, Service, Treatment and Rehabilitation section, focus on multidisciplinary teams that determine a patient's care needs and deliver the nutritional care. Monitoring is also included in these standards.

Due in part to the participation in the National Nutrition Screening Initiative created by the American Academy of Family Physicians, the American Dietetic Association, and the National Council on Aging, JCAHO has mandated nutrition screening standards.[2] These standards were originally developed to raise awareness of health care professionals dealing with the elderly population, though they are used for a variety of institutionalized settings now. The JCAHO publishes examples of how to meet the standards. Therefore, in each manual, Joint Commission prints implementation examples that focus on "good practices" and evidence examples that demonstrate compliance of the standard via data collection. These examples are merely suggestions. Facilities are left to interpret the examples as they apply to their practices. Suggested readings and other educational resources are included at the end of each chapter.

For each standard, the Accreditation Manual for Hospitals (AMH) lists the intent or purpose and the scoring guideline. The scoring guideline is a descriptive tool used to assist the hospital in its efforts to comply with the standard. It was developed to reduce or eliminate surveyor variation in the evaluation process. The scoring process begins with a 1, indicating full compliance. Scores of 2 through 5 indicate some degree of non-compliance and require the surveyor to write a recommendation in the final accreditation report. An organization does not need to be in full compliance with *every* standard in order to be accredited, but it must demonstrate an overall compliance with the full set of applicable standards. The role of the surveyor is to find problems with existing

---

Exhibit 11–4 JCAHO TX.4 standards

TX.4   Each patient's nutrition care is planned.

TX.4.1   An interdisciplinary nutrition therapy plan is developed and periodically updated for patients at nutritional risk.

TX.4.1.1   When appropriate to the patient groups served by a unit, meals and snacks support program goals.

TX.4.2   Authorized individuals prescribe or order food and nutrition products in a timely manner.

TX.4.3   Responsibilities are assigned for all activities involved in safe and accurate provision of food and nutrition products.

TX.4.4   Food and nutrition products are distributed and administered in a safe, accurate, timely, and acceptable manner.

TX.4.5   Each patient's response to nutrition care is monitored.

TX.4.6   The nutrition care service meets patients' needs for special diets and accommodates altered diet schedules.

TX.4.7   Nutrition care practices are standardized throughout the organization.

care as well as to provide education and consultation so health care organizations can improve.

A future initiative within the Agenda for Change is to develop an Indicator Measurement System (IMSystem) for measurement of data. Also referred to as ORYX, the IMSystem is intended to measure the quality of performance over time. On a regular basis, organizations will feed data on certain recognized clinical indicators to a centralized point and to the Joint Commission. Eventually, this national reference database is to grow in size, in value, and in worth. Hospitals may then use it to benchmark their performance on national standards. This would allow the JCAHO to act as a clearinghouse for the best practice guidelines and serve as a link between hospitals having difficulty in a particular area to those who perform it well.

The JCAHO Department of Standards publishes quarterly updates to its manuals that show changes to its existing standards. All other manuals (home care, ambulatory care) are updated biannually.

HAZARD ANALYSIS CRITICAL CONTROL POINTS (HACCP)

The 1999 updates to the AMH included the Hazard Analysis and Critical Control Points (HACCP) program guidelines.[7] HACCP is a food safety system designed by the Food and Drug Administration to help identify foods and procedures that are most likely to cause foodborne illness. It outlines procedures that reduce the risk of foodborne outbreaks and procedures for monitoring to assure food safety. See Exhibit 11–5 for a description of Hazards and Critical Control Points.

The written HACCP system is an illustration of operational steps, hazards, critical control points, standards (criteria), types of monitoring, corrective actions

---

Exhibit 11–5 Examples of hazards and critical control points within HACCP plan

Hazards are:
- Micro-organisms that can grow during preparation, storage, and/or holding of prepared items
- Micro-organisms or toxins that survive heating
- Chemicals that can contaminate food or food-contact surfaces
- Physical objects that accidentally enter food

Critical Control Points are:
A practice or procedure that would
- Eliminate or remove a hazard from occurring
- Prevent a hazard from happening
- Lessen the risk that a hazard will take place

(if standards are not met), and records. Most of the guidelines identified within HACCP relate to food service. However, some pertain directly to the handling and administration of enteral feedings. See Table 11–1 for an example of an HACCP system for enteral nutrition.

The requirement to follow HACCP for tube feeding was a major change in the JCAHO standards. It is mentioned throughout the Food and Nutrition Section as well as the section for Infection Control. These requirements raised questions among professionals regarding the use of a closed versus an open system to provide safe enteral nutrition therapy. (See Chapter 5, Tube Feeding Administration, for a more complete description of these systems.)

CLOSED VERSUS OPEN SYSTEMS

The literature has justifiable arguments for both open and closed systems. Main issues of debate include nursing time to administer feedings, labor cost to prepare and administer feedings, cost of equipment/supplies, availability of formulas in closed containers, bacterial contamination, and waste of formula after allowed hang time.

Some researchers have shown a significant saving in nursing time, formula waste, and overall cost by utilizing the closed system.[8] A comprehensive study determined that it took approximately 14 minutes per patient per day to manage an open system as compared to approximately 2 minutes per patient per day for the closed system.[8] One long-term care facility showed no benefit to a closed system because nurses were providing precise bolus tube feedings to their relatively stable patient population.[9] Other studies have shown benefits (both clinical and economic) for the closed system in the more critical setting, despite the feedings being placed on hold frequently for testing, procedures, and therapies.[10–13]

A major concern among clinicians is for patients to receive the proper amount of tube feeding.[14] By utilizing an open system, formula is often wasted due to frequent discontinuation of feedings and short hang times. An advantage of the closed system is that patients often receive a greater amount of their prescribed tube feeding,[15] due to lengthy allowable hang times.

A criticism of the closed system is that there is no room for alteration of the feeding, and there is waste if the formula type is frequently changed. Additives are of concern (e.g., protein powders, medications, non-sterile blue dye) because they are a potential source of bacterial contamination.[13, 16,17] A closed system virtually eliminates that type of contamination because there is no break in the system. If necessary, protein powders can be diluted and administered via bolus method similar to medications, and blue dye is available from manufacturers in sterile single units. Other types of contamination are still possible, such as touch-contamination or contamination through rinsing and reusing enteral feeding bags,[18] but closed systems seem to significantly reduce the problem of contamination that is a potential source of nosocomial infections. Tube feedings are often started on very ill, malnourished patients (elderly, criti-

Table 11–1 HACCP system for enteral nutrition

NEW YORK-PRESBYTERIAN HOSPITAL
NEW YORK WEILL CORNELL CENTER
DEPARTMENT OF FOOD AND NUTRITION
HAZARD ANALYSIS CRITICAL CONTROL POINT (HACCP) PLAN FOR ENTERAL FEEDING AND ADMINISTRATION

Flow Process	Hazard	Concern (CCP or CP)	Control Criteria	Monitor Method (Procedure)	Action Plan (criteria failure)
Purchase	Contamination of enteral feeding products by chemical, microbiological or particulate matter; breakdown in quality control at point of production.	CP (CONTROL POINT)	Purchase from approved, inspected and certified vendors.	Monitor vendors for adherence to purchasing specifications. Inspect delivery upon receipt. Receive notification from vendors/FDA regarding quality control issues.	Reject delivery not adhering to specifications without exception. Follow food recall procedures to address quality control issues.
Receiving	Contamination of enteral feeding products by chemical, microbiological or particulate matter through improper receiving methods.	CP	Verify delivery based upon receiving criteria. Immediately remove received enteral feeding products for appropriate storage.	Monitor receiving process and vendor adherence to specifications for delivery. Document vendor problems on Vendor Receiving Report.	Coach/counsel employees in proper receiving techniques. If necessary, revise receiving procedures according to HACCP guidelines.
Storage	Contamination of enteral feeding products by chemical, microbiological or particulate matter due to improper storage and handling procedures.	CP	For liquid protein module, verify adherence to temperature standards for freezer units prior to thawing and refrigeration units during/after thawing. For MCT	Monitor temperatures in refrigeration/freezer units and dry storage areas. Monitor product expiration dates. Verify safety and sanitation process by conducting	Immediately remove enteral feeding products in affected refrigerator/freezer to a unit that is operating within standards; discard mixed or portioned product that has exceeded 2

continues

Table 11-1 continued

Flow Process	Hazard	Concern (CCP or CP)	Control Criteria	Monitor Method (Procedure)	Action Plan (criteria failure)
			module and all other products, verify the correct temperature for dry storage areas. Verify adherence to "first in first out" (FIFO), safety and sanitation standards in all storage areas. Remove dented cans from circulation.	monthly Safety and Sanitation Inspections.	hour limit of storage without temperature regulation. Shut down and repair refrigerators/freezers unable to maintain temperature standards. Remove products in affected dry storage areas to an area that meets temperature standard. Return to vendor/discard products that have exceeded expiration date as noted by the manufacturer. Return dented cans to vendor. Coach/counsel employees in monitoring and action procedures.
Thaw	Contamination of enteral feeding products due to inappropriate thawing and/or utilization of thawed item beyond specified time frame.	CCP (CRITICAL CONTROL POINT)	Thaw liquid protein module and Health Shakes completely using approved method of thawing under refrigeration only. Do not thaw at room temperature. Label each	Monitor thawing temperature. Do not use until completely thawed. Verify thawing schedule to enteral formula production schedule.	Thaw fully if frozen and reject items of questionable quality. Discard thawed items that have exceeded expiration date. Coach/counsel employees in proper thawing methods. If

necessary, revise thawing procedures according to HACCP guidelines.			

continues

Step	Code	Hazard	Controls	Verification
			unopened carton of liquid protein module with the date placed in the refrigerator for thawing. If unopened and unused after 5 days, the product is to be discarded. Health Shakes are labeled with an expiration date 12 days from transfer from freezer to thaw under refrigeration.	Verify cleaning and sanitizing process. Observe that separation of enteral feeding products and raw or processed food items and cleaning compounds is maintained. Verify adherence to enteral formula orders and recipes.	Discard questionable enteral formula ingredients. Reject ingredients not meeting acceptance criteria. Coach/counsel employees in proper enteral formula preparation methods. If necessary, revise enteral formula preparation procedures according to HACCP guidelines.
Preparation	CP	Introduction of microbes, chemicals or particulates by process and/or equipment cross contamination and/or employees.	Train employees in proper enteral feeding product handling techniques and sanitation. Wash hands prior to preparing feedings or modular components. Prepare according to enteral formula recipe. Use tap water for reconstituting Pediatric Vivonex and Ceralyte. See HACCP guidelines for Potable Water page ___. (Note: Distilled or sterile water is used in the preparation of enteral formulas upon		

Table 11–1 continued

Flow Process	Hazard	Concern (CCP or CP)	Control Criteria	Monitor Method (Procedure)	Action Plan (criteria failure)
			specific order only.) Clean and sanitize equipment and utensils prior to use. Protect enteral feeding products from cross contamination.		
Cold Holding	Spores germinate and microorganisms multiply at temperatures above 40°F.	CCP	Seal, label and date (date opened) opened cartons of liquid protein module used in EFPL. Store and hold under refrigeration of 40°F or less. Discard any open carton that has been unused after 48 hours of opening. Seal, label and date (date opened) opened bottles of MCT oil used in EFPL. Store and hold in dry storage (do not refrigerate). Discard any open bottle that has been unused after 3 months of opening. Seal, label: formula, rate of	Monitor refrigeration temperature and verify accuracy of temperature monitoring device. Conduct daily inventory of prepared or open enteral feeding products to verify expiration/discard procedures.	Monitor refrigeration temperature for 40°F or less. If temperature standards are not being met, immediately remove prepared or open enteral feeding products to refrigerator that maintains the required temperature. Coach/counsel employees in enteral feeding product monitoring methods. Discard formulas that have exceeded shelf life criteria.

continues

		CP		
administration, patient name, room # and date (current date prepared) all reconstituted mixed enteral formula and portioned protein, fat or carbohydrate modules. With the exception of unopened cans of enteral formula, MCT oil and powdered CHO module (which are stored at room temperature), store any mixed, reconstituted or portioned modules under refrigeration at 40°F or less until delivered to patient care units for administration. Verify temperature accuracy of refrigeration monitor. Inventory product to detect items at or near expiration.				Monitor timeliness of delivery of enteral feeding products to nursing units. Discard mixed or portioned product that has exceeded 2 hour limit of storage without temperature regulation. Coach/counsel
Delivery to Nursing Unit	Surviving microorganisms can grow in inadequately maintained mixed enteral feeding products. Spores that survived can begin to grow during the inade-	CP	After preparation, enteral feeding products will be stored on dinner meal service carts under refrigeration until delivered to	

Table 11-1 continued

Flow Process	Hazard	Concern (CCP or CP)	Control Criteria	Monitor Method (Procedure)	Action Plan (criteria failure)
	quate temperature delivery process. Chemical and particulates cannot be destroyed.		nursing units according to delivery schedule.		employees in enteral feeding product delivery procedures. If necessary, revise delivery procedures according to HACCP guidelines.
Cold Holding On Nursing Units	Surviving microorganism can grow in inadequately maintained mixed or open enteral feeding products. Spores can survive and begin to grow during the inadequate refrigeration holding process. Chemical and particulates cannot be destroyed.	CCP	Verify that all mixed enteral formulas, modular components and open containers of enteral feeding products are sealed, labeled as to contents, patient name, room # and dated. Store and hold mixed enteral feeding formulas and liquid protein module under refrigeration at 40°F or less in nourishment station refrigerators. Verify temperature accuracy of refrigeration monitor. Inventory product to detect items at or near expiration. All mixed enteral for-	Monitor refrigeration temperature and verify accuracy of temperature monitoring device. Conduct daily inventory of prepared or open enteral feeding products to verify expiration/discard procedures.	Monitor refrigeration temperature for 40°F or less. If temperature standards are not being met, immediately remove prepared, modular components or open enteral feeding products to a refrigerator that maintains the required temperature. Coach/counsel staff/employees in enteral feeding product monitoring methods. Discard formulas that have exceeded shelf life criteria.

	CCP			
		tainers of formula or containers of liquid protein module are discarded 24 hours after the production date.		
Enteral Feeding Administration	CCP	All enteral feeding products, at room temperature, can support microbial growth. Formula manipulation or using procedures that increase handling of formulas or administration systems increases the potential for contamination.	Wash hands prior to handling feedings and administration systems. Avoid touching any part of the container or administration system that will come in contact with the feeding. Inspect seals and reservoirs for damage prior to utilization. Avoid adding medications directly to the feeding; if necessary, flush tube after administration with tap water. Date/time each component of the system also indicating patient name and formula (on feeding bag). Limit hang time of feeding to 8 hours; if admixture, limit hang time to 4 hours. Empty feeding bags of product	Monitor staff for adherence to proper enteral feeding administration techniques.	Discard product that has exceeded limit for hang time. Coach/counsel staff on proper enteral formula administration procedures. If necessary, revise enteral formula administration procedures according to HACCP guidelines.

continues

Table 11-1 continued

FLOW PROCESS	HAZARD	CONCERN (CCP or CP)	CONTROL CRITERIA	MONITOR METHOD (Procedure)	ACTION PLAN (criteria failure)
			completely prior to pouring newly opened product into the bag. Flush bag with tap water before filling with additional formula. Use administration sets with Y-ports and drip chambers. Cap disconnected sets. Change administration sets and syringes used for flushing the tubes every 24 hours.		
Sanitize (On-going process through various stages of the system)	Destruction of microbes during the cleaning and sanitizing process. Introduction of microbes, chemicals or particulates by cross contamination and/or employees.	CP	Train employees in proper enteral feeding product handling techniques and sanitation. Clean and sanitize equipment and utensils prior to use. Protect products from contamination.	Verify cleaning and sanitizing process. Observe that separation of enteral feeding preparation and storage and sanitation processes is maintained.	Re-clean and re-sanitize all preparation equipment. Coach/counsel employees in proper sanitation procedures. Discard enteral feeding products contaminated during sanitation process. If necessary, revise sanitation procedures according to HACCP guidelines.

cally ill, post-transplant, or with cancer or HIV/AIDS). Immune-compromise is common among these patients; therefore, every effort to reduce the likelihood of contamination should be taken.

HACCP also addresses issues related to reconstituting formula from powder (e.g., Vivonex from Novartis, Minneapolis, MN), how long a "blended" tube feeding should be held with or without refrigeration, proper cleaning and sanitizing for blenders, and when to discard expired formula. Occasionally, hospitals mix 2 or more tube feeding products to create a new one. This practice is not often necessary due to the wide array of commercial formulas already available; it also increases the potential for contamination and waste. Additionally, such practice does not assure that patients are receiving and/or absorbing the special formula. One study attempted to track waste, and noted an exorbitant amount of "blended" formula delivered to the nursing floor only to be left in the refrigerator well beyond the expiration date.[8] Usually these specialty formulas are costly to prepare and deliver (in terms of labor), and store (refrigerate), when reviewing total expenses. The theme throughout the HACCP guidelines is that the less handling or manipulation, the safer the product will be and the better the outcome for the patient.

Overall, each facility is unique. The debate related to preference for closed versus open systems is likely to remain an issue for some time.[19] Manufacturers of commercial formulas will continue to meet the demands of patients and clinicians. In this era of cost-driven quality care, clinicians realize that the expense of providing enteral nutrition exceeds the cost of formula alone. The price of bags, sets, labor, and potential for waste and bacterial contamination should also be scrutinized. In cases where products must be limited due to space or cost, or to avoid prescription confusion, obtaining input from all disciplines related to formula selection is wise. Having a specific protocol for initiating and choosing formula also helps to manage costs and provide more consistent care.

CLINICAL PATHWAYS

Clinical pathways were created to provide clear standards or protocols for patient care and ultimately lead to cost efficiency. Clinical pathways are also described as critical pathways or care mapping. Those methods have been used since the 1970s by engineers managing projects in the construction field.[20] One medical director of a major commercial insurance company cites four benefits from using clinical "guidelines": better outcomes, faster patient recovery, reduced costs, and increased physician accountability.[21]

The goal of the clinical pathway is to provide standardized care 80% of the time for the best possible patient outcome in a particular population. Most clinical pathways are categorized by patient diagnosis (e.g., diabetes, cancer, AIDS) and further classified by scope (e.g., enteral nutrition, home care, preoperative care). Interventions or actions are then identified (e.g., education, nutrition care, medications, treatments). Next, outcomes are defined to give a directive for meeting goals. Finally, clinical pathways state when minimum documentation is to occur.[20]

A clinical pathway should be designed as a relevant and useful tool to perform a task on a consistent basis. If patients are not responding to treatment more than 20% of the time, then either the pathway should be altered or adapted to meet their needs or the staff should be better trained at managing the clinical pathway to get the desired results.

Comprehensive development of a clinical pathway should include a multidisciplinary team of clinicians and/or professionals. A team leader should be appointed and pathways should be reviewed and revised on a regular basis by the team. They should be maintained as a permanent part of the patient's medical record.[20]

Ireton-Jones et al. developed several clinical pathways for home care patients. Two examples are shown in Tables 11–2 and 11–3. Lykins also developed a pathway for tube feeding, which is shown in Table 11–4.[22]

Paper pathways have been the standard since their integration into health care, approximately 1983. The trend in many hospitals is to move in the direction of automated or computerized systems for all documentation. Computerized pathways are being adapted in several facilities. Computerization of the pathways offers many advantages to the staff, but requires a computer-savvy individual who has the ability to translate the written pathway detail into language that can be loaded into an automated system.[23,24]

QUALITY IMPROVEMENT PROGRAMS

Developing a quality improvement (QI) program requires knowledge of only a few basic principles. Many examples are available in the literature for how to develop such a program. The main concept is to study areas that are most important to the individual facility. Begin by reviewing the mission or purpose of the facility. Plan to identify and monitor the problems that relate to the provision of care. Once the data is gathered and analyzed, changes can be made based on the results. A key element to a successful QI program is having staff input in the planning stages. If the staff responsible for data collection understands the importance of quality patient care, the data-tracking and analyzing phase should proceed smoothly.

The Institute for Healthcare Improvement (IHI) in Boston, Massachusetts, posed 3 questions in its improvement model that Schneider et al. showed can be applied to nutrition support.[25] They developed the following questions to aid in achieving change.

1. What are we trying to accomplish?
2. How will we know that a change results in an improvement?
3. What changes can we make that will result in an improvement?

Table 11–2 Clinical pathway for home enteral monitoring

Home Enteral Monitoring

Dates							
Parameters	**Baseline**	**Day 3**	**Week 2**	**Week 3**	**Week 4**	**Week 6**	**Week 8**
Laboratory Studies	Chemical Profile, Mg, CBC, PT				Chemical Profile, Mg, Zn		
CNN Clinical Assessment							
1) Physical & Nutrition Assessment —Pt/therapy compliance	√	√ Phone Contact	√		√		
2) Quality of Life —SF-36	√				√		√
3) Karnofsky Functional Scale	√				√		√
Communications *Quarterly Summary*							

Dates							
Parameters	**Week 12**	**Month 4**	**Month 5**	**Month 6**	**Month 9**	**Month 12**	**Month 18**
Laboratory Studies	Chemical Profile, Mg, Fe			Chemical Profile, Mg, Fe		Chemical Profile, Mg, CBC, Fe	Chemical Profile, Fe
CNN Clinical Assessment							
1) Physical & Nutrition Assessment —Pt/therapy compliance	√			√		√	√
2) Quality of Life —SF-36				√		√ then every 6 months	
3) Karnofsky Functional Scale				√		√ then every 6 months	
Communications *Quarterly Summary*	√			√	√	√	

Home enteral monitoring portion of a sample human immunodeficiency virus clinical pathway for home nutrition support for adults.

The initial step to evoke change is developing an aim, and a measurable goal. An example of this follows:

Aim: Patients should receive the prescribed amount of tube feeding on a daily basis.

Goal: 100% of patients on tube feedings will receive the prescribed amount.

Table 11–3 Clinical pathway for transition from parenteral to enteral therapy

Transition from TPN to Enteral Therapy

Dates							
Parameters	**Week 1**	**Week 2**	**Week 3**	**Week 4**	**Week 5**	**Week 6**	**Week 8**
TPN Prescription	Progressively decrease days on TPN every 1–2 weeks				Discontinue TPN		
Laboratory Studies	Lytes, Mg, Phos, BUN/Creat	Lytes, Mg, Phos, BUN/Creat	Lytes, Mg, Phos, BUN/Creat	Lytes, Mg, Phos, BUN/Creat		Lytes, Mg, Phos, BUN/Creat	Lytes, Mg, Phos, BUN/Creat
CNN Clinical Assessment							
1) Physical & Nutrition Assessment —Pt/therapy compliance	√	√	√	√			√
2) Quality of Life —SF-36	√			√			√
3) Karnofsky Functional Scale	√			√			√

Transition from total parenteral nutrition (TPN) to enteral therapy portion of a sample human immunodeficiency virus clinical pathway for home nutrition support for adults.

Next, a tracking system is put in place to determine if improvement is truly occurring. The number of patients who do receive the prescribed amount of tube feeding versus those who do not would be recorded and compared with the goal. Any deviations from the full prescription would be considered not meeting the goal. Through a team approach, issues can be identified that impede meeting the goal, and a new aim or goal created to address the problems identified. Strategies for improving the aim often result, and standards such as the clinical pathways described earlier in this chapter may be developed.

CONCLUSION

Enteral feeding dates back to ancient Egyptian times; however, the products and methods used have evolved considerably.[26] As long as there are individuals with a functional gastrointestinal tract and no way to assimilate nutrients by mouth, tube feedings will likely exist well into the future. Many advances will likely take place in this time. It is speculated that more specialized formulas will be introduced, methods to determine exactly which nutrients are deficient and how to replete them will probably be discovered. Ways to administer the formula via a mini-pump or rapid infusion technique may be the trend in the next decade. Whatever the progression, one thing remains clear: the administration of enteral nutrition is an advanced practice not to be handled haphazardly. It is a necessary method of delivering high-quality nutrition support to a patient in need. It comes with advantages and disadvantages like every other treatment

Table 11–4 Clinical pathway for tube feeding

	Initiation Phase (I) (24–48 hours)	Intermediate Phase (II) (variable)	Transition Phase (III) (24 hours)
Criteria (A)	1) Malnourished patient with inadequate oral intake for the past 5 days 2) Patient with normal nutritional status, meeting <50% estimated needs orally for previous 7–10 days 3) Traumatized or severely catabolic patient unable to eat ≥ 50% estimated needs in 3–5 days, with functioning GI tract 4) Patient with condition or disease state that will prevent adequate po intake for greater than 5 days, with functioning GI tract	1) Assess for ability to meet needs orally or potential to increase oral intake via cyclic TF	1) Feeding tube is not removed until patient meeting ≥ 2/3 estimated nutrition needs
Access Device (B)	1) Nasogastric tube 2) Nasoduodenal tube 3) PEG or PEJ 4) Surgical gastrostomy or Jejunostomy	1) Tube remains patent and flushes easily 2) Transpyloric tube does not yield residual when aspirated each shift	
Lab Tests (C)	Baseline: 1) Panel 20	Routine: 1) Panel 10 weekly 2) Panel 20 weekly	
Proper Delivery of Appropriate Formula (D)	1) Proper dilution if >500 Mosmo/Kg H_2O 2) Initiate at slow rate of 10–25 cc/hr 3) Isotonic TF initiated at FS 4) Enteral product selected is indicated for patient's condition	1) Patient receiving full rate and strength of TF needed to meet estimated nutrition needs 2) Product changes are appropriate and indicated	
Tolerance Addressed (E)	1) Residuals checked and documented every 4 hours 2) Stool frequency and volume documented 3) Tube is patent and flushed with 50cc H_2O every shift and after each medication given down feeding tube	1) Residuals not greater than double the hourly TF rate or 100 cc's 2) Patient remains free of aspiration 3) Patient free of abdominal distention and cramping 4) Patient free of nausea or vomiting	

	Initiation Phase (I) (24–48 hours)	Intermediate Phase (II) (variable)	Transition Phase (III) (24 hours)
Desired Outcomes (F)	1) TF started within 48° of indentified needs 2) Patient meets 100% estimated needs within 48 hours of TF initiation 3) Fluid balance 4) Euglycemia	1) Patient meeting 100% estimated nutrition needs 2) Fluid balance 3) Euglycemia 4) Improvement in visceral proteins 5) Stability or improvement in body weight 6) Proper wound healing	1) Patient able to meet 2/3 estimated needs before TF D/C'd 2) Stability in body weight 3) Proper wound healing

option. Through continued efforts by dedicated professionals to provide quality nutrition care, enteral nutrition will remain a viable nutrition support option to improve a patient's quality of life.

REFERENCES:

1. Graham NO. *Quality Assurance in Hospitals.* Rockville, MD: Aspen Publishers, Inc.; 1990:3–13.
2. Patterson CH. Joint commission standards. *Nutritional assessment: The key to well-nourished outcomes.* Newark, DE: Dade Behring, Inc.; 1999:24–29.
3. Joint Commission on Accreditation of Healthcare Organizations. *1996 Accreditation Manual for Hospitals.* Oakbrook Terrace, IL: Joint Commission on Accreditation of Healthcare Organizations; 1995.
4. Joint Commission on Accreditation of Healthcare Organizations. *1997–1998 Comprehensive Accreditation Manual for Home Care.* Oakbrook Terrace, IL: Joint Commission on Accreditation of Healthcare Organizations; 1996.
5. Joint Commission on Accreditation of Healthcare Organizations. *1996 Accreditation Manual for Long Term Care.* Oakbrook Terrace, IL: Joint Commission on Accreditation of Healthcare Organizations; 1995.
6. Dougherty D, Bankhead R, Kushner R, Winkler M. Nutrition care given new importance in JCAHO standards. *Nutr Clin Pract* 1995;10:26–31.
7. Joint Commission on Accreditation of Healthcare Organizations. *Comprehensive Accreditation Manual for Hospitals: The Official Handbook.* CAMH Update 3, August 1999: IC20–IC21. Oakbrook Terrace, IL: Joint Commission on Accreditation of Healthcare Organizations.
8. Silkroski M, Allen F, Storm H. Tube feeding audit reveals hidden costs and risks of current practice. *Nutr Clin Pract* 1998;13:283–290.
9. Herlick S, Vogt C, Pangman V, Fallis W. Open vs. closed system of intermittent enteral feeding study in two long term care facilities. *JPEN* 2000;24:S10.
10. Inman KJ, Davidson BC, Sibbald WJ, Rutledge FS. Closed enteral systems in the intensive care unit: evaluating their economic impact. *Nutr Clin Pract* 1998;13:S42–S45.
11. Detinger B, Faucher K, Ostrom S, Schmidl M. Controlling bacterial contamination of an enteral formula through the use of a unique closed system: contamination, enteral formulas, closed system. *Nutrition* 1995;11:747–750.
12. Rupp M, Weseman R, Marion N, Iwen P. Evaluation of bacterial contamination of a sterile, non-air-dependent enteral feeding system in immunocompromised patients. *Nutr Clin Pract* 1999;14:135–137.
13. Wagner D, Elmore M, Knoll D. Evaluation of "closed" vs. "open" systems for the delivery of peptide-based enteral diets. *JPEN* 1994;18:453–457.
14. Abernathy G, Heizer W, Holcombe B, et al. Efficacy of tube feeding in supplying energy requirements of hospitalized patients. *JPEN* 1989;14:387–391.
15. Rees R, Ryan J, Attrill H, Silk D. Clinical evaluation of a two-liter prepackaged enteral diet delivery system: a controlled trial. *JPEN* 1988;12:274–277.
16. File T, Tan J, Thompson R, Stephens C, Thompson P. An outbreak of pseudomonas aeruginosa ventilator-associated respiratory infections due to contaminated food coloring dye—further evidence of the significance of gastric colonization preceding nosocomial pneumonia. *Infec Cont and Hosp Epidem* 1995;16:417–418.
17. Navajas M, Chacon D, Solvas J, Vargas R. Bacterial contamination of enteral feedings as a possible risk of nosocomial infection. *J Hosp Infect* 1992;21:111–120.

18. Kohn-Keeth C, Shott S, Olree K. The effects of rinsing enteral delivery sets on formula contamination. *Nutr Clin Pract* 1996;11:269–272.
19. Storm HM, Skipper AS. Closed system enteral feedings: point-counterpoint. *Nutr Clin Pract* 2000;15:193–200.
20. Ireton-Jones C, Orr M, Hennessy K. Clinical pathways in home nutrition support. *J Am Diet Assoc* 1997;97:1003–1007.
21. O'Malley S. Pathways: improving outcomes, not just "cookbook medicine." *Qual Lett Healthc Lead* 1997;9:12–14.
22. Lykins TC. Nutrition support clinical pathways. *Nutr Clin Pract* 1996;11:16–20.
23. Chu S, Cesnik B. Modeling computerized clinical pathways. *Medinfo* 1998;9:559–563.
24. Glassman KS, Kelly J. Facilitating care management through computerized clinical pathways. *Top Health Inf Manage* 1998;19:70–78.
25. Schneider PJ, Bothe A, Bisognago M. Improving the nutrition support process: assuring that more patients receive optimal nutrition support. *Nutr Clin Pract* 1999;14:221–226.
26. Hamaoui E. Assessing the nutrition support team. *JPEN* 1987;11:412.

SUGGESTED READINGS

American Society for Parenteral and Enteral Nutrition. *Clinical Pathways and Algorithms for Delivery of Parenteral and Enteral Nutrition Support in Adults.* Silver Spring, MD: American Society for Parenteral and Enteral Nutrition; 1997.

Borum ML, Lynn J, Zhong Z, et al. The effect of nutritional supplementation on survival in seriously ill hospitalized adults: An evaluation of the SUPPORT data. Study to understand prognoses and preference for outcomes and risks of treatments. *J Am Geriatr Soc* 2000;48:S33–S38.

Escott-Stump S, Krauss B, Pavlinac J, et al. Joint Commission on Accreditation of Healthcare Organizations: Friend, not foe. *J Am Diet Assoc* 2000;100:839–844.

Gottschlich MM, Fuhrman P, Hammond K, Holcombe B, Seidner D (eds) *The Science and Practice of Nutrition Support: A Case Based Core Curriculum.* Dubuque, IA: Kendall/Hunt Publishing Company, 2001.

Health care in transition: charting a course for nutrition support professionals. *Nutr Clin Pract* 1995;10(suppl).

Hennessy K, Orr M, Curtas S. Nutrition support nursing: a specialty practice: historical development. *Clin Nurse Specialist* 1990;4:67–70.

Heyland DK. Enteral and parenteral nutrition in the seriously ill, hospitalized patient: A critical review of the evidence. *J Nutr Health Aging* 2000;4:31–41.

Incorporating nutrition care into critical pathways for improved outcomes. Columbus, OH: Ross Laboratories, Division of Abbott Laboratories; September 1994.

RESOURCES

Joint Commission on Accreditation of Healthcare Organizations (JCAHO)
One Renaissance Boulevard
Oakbrook Terrace, IL 60181
630–792–5000
www.jcaho.org

Institute for Healthcare Improvement (IHI)
135 Francis Street
Boston, MA 02215
617–754–4800
www.ihi.org

Food and Drug Administration (FDA)
Office of Consumer Affairs
5600 Fishers Lane HFE-88
Rockville, MD 20857
301–443–3170

A

Glossary

Adenosine triphosphate—(ATP) a nucleotide occurring in all cells where it stores energy in the form of high-energy phosphate bonds.

Adapters—small devices either attached to or independent of the distal end of a feeding tube that allow the feeding tube to fit well with the administration tubing set and/or allow for tube flushing and medication administration.

Adjusted body weight—a calculation to estimate metabolically active tissue and therefore energy requirements for an obese person, using actual and ideal body weights.

Administration sets—tubing sets that connect the feeding bag or container to the feeding tube.

Advance directive—written instruction, by a coherent patient, for medical treatment in case of loss of mental capacity.

Alternate site care—any number of places where care might be offered to a patient (e.g., assisted living facilities, skilled nursing units, sub-acute care centers, in-home care).

Amino acids—organic compounds that are the basic building blocks that construct proteins.

Anabolism—constructive processes by which living cells convert simple substances to more complex compounds; opposite of catabolism.

Anorexia—chronic lack or loss of appetite for food.

Anorexia nervosa—a refusal to eat adequate food due to emotional states such as anxiety, anger, fear, or irritation. This psychological starvation occurs primarily in young women who have a disturbance in body image (perceiving themselves fatter than they actually are), and can lead to severe malnutrition.

Anthropometry—the science of measuring size, weights, and proportion of the human body.

Antioxidants—an agent that prevents oxidation thus preventing release of free radicals. Nutrient antioxidants include vitamins C, E, and beta-carotene.

Appetite—the desire for food.

Arginine—a semiessential amino acid that is believed to enhance immune function and wound healing.

Aspiration—the inhalation of food or liquid into the lungs, which may lead to pneumonia.

Bacterial translocation—endotoxin that should be contained in the gastrointestinal tract enters the portal system as a result of malabsorption and malnutrition.

Basal metabolic rate—(BMR) the energy needed to maintain life when the body is at complete rest after a 12-hour fast.

Bioelectrical impedence—(BIA) a method for estimating body fat using low-intensity electrical current.

Blenderized tube feeding—tube feeding formula made from blenderized foods.

Body mass index—(BMI) an assessment measurement tool using weight and height to determine nutrition status.

Bolus feeding administration—method of feeding in which a large volume of formula is given in a short period of time, usually through a large syringe.

Calibration—to determine the accuracy of an instrument, usually by measurement of its variation from a standard, to ascertain necessary correction factors.

Caloric density—the property expressed by the amount of calories per volume of formula. Example: 1 calorie/milliliter of formula.

Calorie—a unit of heat by which energy is measured; the amount of heat required to raise the temperature of 1 kilogram of water by 1 degree Celsius under standard conditions. Often expressed in kilocalories (kcals)—there are 1000 calories in a kcal.

Carbohydrate—a compound of carbon, hydrogen, and oxygen; an immediate energy source for the body, it includes sugars, starches, and fibers.

Case manager—an individual who arranges for certain areas of care for a given patient or case. Case managers may provide this care in the hospital or make arrangements for out-of-hospital care.

Casein—the principal protein of cow's milk; an intact protein polymer often found in tube feeding formulas.

Catabolism—a destructive process where a complex substance (tissue) is metabolically converted by living cells into smaller compounds. The opposite of anabolism.

Central venous access—insertion of an indwelling catheter into a central vein (subclavian, jugular) for the purpose of administering fluid and/or medications, and for the measurement of central venous pressure.

Certificate of Medical Necessity—(CMN) a form developed by the Health Care Financing Administration (HCFA) that a physician must complete in order to receive reimbursement for Nutrition Support Services from Medicare.

Clinical indicator—an instrument that measures a quantifiable aspect of nutrition care to guide professionals in monitoring and evaluating nutrition care quality and/or appropriateness.

Clinical pathway—a clinical guide or protocol to predict best possible patient outcome.

Closed system—a tube-feeding product where the container is pre-filled with formula so there is no break in the system, potentially giving less cause for bacterial contamination.

Continuous feeding administration—feeding administration method where formula is delivered in low volumes over 24 hours, usually using an enteral feeding pump.

Continuous quality improvement—(CQI) a systematic approach to assessing and improving the effectiveness and reliability of processes (nutrition care), using a scientific methodology and teamwork.

Cost-effectiveness—the comparison of the benefit or good to be achieved by a therapy to the monetary cost of that therapy.

Cyclic feeding administration—feeding administration method where formula is delivered continuously but over only a specified amount of time such as 10–18 hours.

Dehydration—body water depletion, which occurs whenever body output exceeds water input.

Dementia—irreversible loss of mental function.

Depletion—the reduction of stored nutrients (e.g., energy, fat, and protein).

Dextrose—a highly water-soluble form of glucose (carbohydrate); often used in IV solutions.

Diagnosis Related Groups—(DRG) the capitated rate allowed by insurance carriers according to patient diagnosis.

Diarrhea—stool output that is considered in excess of normal. Usually consists of loose or watery frequent stools.

Discharge planning—the process of gathering patient information in an effort to arrange for care after discharge.

Distension—the act of being stretched out or enlarged.

Drug-nutrient interaction—an event that occurs when a drug effect is altered by ingested nutrients or when a medication alters nutrient availability.

Dysphagia—physiological swallowing difficulty that can lead to severe nutritional compromise without treatment.

Electrolytes—salts that dissolve in water and dissociate into ions.

Elemental—tube feeding formula type that is made up of basic nutrient units such as amino acids, short or medium chain triglycerides, and monosaccharides. This type of formula is considered easier to digest and absorb than polymeric formulas.

Energy—the ability to do work; derived from the diet, energy is expressed in calories.

Enteral—into the stomach or intestine; a term used to describe tube feedings.

Enteral access devices—tubes placed into the GI tract for the delivery of enteral formula and medications.

Enteral nutrition—nutrition provided into the gastrointestinal tract.

Enteral pump—infusion pump designed specifically for delivery of enteral formula into an enteral feeding access.

Fasting—abstention from food for a period of time.

Fat—term that can be used to describe adipose tissue of the body or all lipids—specifically triglycerides.

Fecal matter—body waste, discharged from the intestine. Also called stool, excreta, or excrement.

Feeding containers or bags—enteral formula administration receptacles that hold feeding and attach to administration tubing for delivery. Some are collapsible, some are rigid.

Fiber—that portion of ingested foodstuffs that cannot be broken down by intestinal enzymes and therefore passes through the colon undigested.

Food safety—a term used to describe the handling procedures, sanitation, and freshness of food.

Foodborne illness—an outbreak or illness that occurs after the consumption of a contaminated food source (e.g., salmonella poisoning).

Flushing—process of pushing water through the feeding tube in order to clear it of formula or medications and/or restore patency.

Formula—tube feeding solution that is most often commercially prepared and provides a complete liquid diet for those patients on enteral nutrition.

Frame size—an estimated size of a person's bones; used in assessing body weight.

Fructooligosaccharide—a carbohydrate-fiber source that is not digested in the GI tract but fermented by bacteria in the colon.

Gastrostomy tube—enteral access device that is placed either endoscopically, surgically, or radiologically with the tip of the tube positioned in the stomach. This tube is considered for long-term enteral feeding.

Glucose—a monosaccharide (simple sugar) found in carbohydrate foods; the chief source of energy for living organisms; found in normal blood circulation.

Glutamine—a conditionally essential amino acid that has been found to be the preferred fuel for the enterocytes, macrophages, and lymphocytes.

Gravity controlled—administration method of infusing tube feeding formula with the assistance of gravity and not with the use of an enteral feeding pump. This method is often used with intermittent gastric feedings.

Half-life—the time in which the radioactivity usually associated with a particular isotope is reduced by half through radioactive decay.

Hazard Analysis Critical Control Points—(HACCP) a food safety system designed by the Food and Drug Administration (FDA) to help identify foods and procedures that are most likely to cause foodborne illness.

Health Care Financing Administration—(HCFA) an agency within the Department of Health and Human Services (HHS) that administers the Medicare program.

Height—a measure of a person's length or stature.

Hemodynamic monitoring—continuous monitoring of the movement of blood and the pressures being exerted in the veins, arteries, and chambers of the heart.

Home care—medical care provided to patients in their homes.

Hospice—a community of professional and nonprofessional people, supplemented by volunteer services, that provides palliative and supportive care for terminally ill persons in the last stages of life and their families.

Hypercatabolic—a metabolic state where the patient is breaking down more protein and excreting more nitrogen than he or she is retaining.

Hypermetabolic—a metabolic state where the energy expenditure of the patient is significantly higher than baseline and the patient requires much more nutrition than normal. This usually occurs with severe stress, sepsis, or trauma.

Hypertonic or hyperosmolar—a property of a tube feeding formula where the osmolality (particles per volume of solute) is greater than 300 mOsm.

Iatrogenic—usually an adverse condition resulting from the activity of a physician, surgeon, or hospital service.

Ideal body weight—(IBW) a predicted weight where a person is said to be in proportion to height and consistent with the "healthiest" weight according to standards; may also be expressed as ideal body weight range (IBWR).

Ileocecal valve—the sphincter muscle separating the small and large intestines.

Indicators—prospectively determined measures used as normative standards within a quality assurance process. The American Society for Parenteral and Enteral Nutrition (A.S.P.E.N.) outlines 3 indicators; Clinical, Process, and Outcome Indicators.

Indirect calorimetry—the measurement of expired and inspired gas volumes and concentrations to arrive at energy expenditure within 4% accuracy.

Insurance claim—written documentation of a patient's diagnosis and/or treatment submitted to his or her insurance company for payment or reimbursement.

Intermittent feeding administration—a feeding administration method where a larger volume of formula is delivered over about 30 minutes and is given at set intervals throughout the day. It is usually given via the gravity method and allows the patient increased mobility.

Isotonic—tube feeding formula osmolality of about 300 mOsm, which is equivalent to the body fluid osmolality.

Jejunostomy tube—enteral access device that is placed either endoscopically, surgically, or radiologically with the tip of the tube positioned in the jejunum. This tube is considered for long-term enteral feeding.

Joint Commission on Accreditation of Healthcare Organizations—(JCAHO) private, nonprofit corporation that establishes standards of care provided by hospitals and health care organizations and audits those organizations regarding their adherence to those standards.

Kilocalorie—(kcal) large calorie; see calorie.

Kilogram—(kg) a unit of mass (weight) of the metric system; 1000 grams equals 1 kilogram.

Krebs cycle—the series of metabolic reactions in which acetyl Coenzyme A (CoA) is oxidized into 2 molecules of carbon dioxide and a free CoA, with the release of energy; also known as the tricarboxylic acid cycle (TCA).

Kwashiorkor—malnutrition related to protein depletion over a short period of time.

Lactose—a disaccharide composed of 2 simple sugars, glucose and galactose; commonly known as milk sugar.

Living will—part of an advance directive that specifies those interventions not desired by the patient under certain conditions (e.g., mechanical ventilation, blood transfusion, and resuscitation).

Long-chain triglycerides—(LCT) saturated lipid source that has 14–24 carbon fatty acid chains. This is one of the primary sources of fat in tube feeding formulas.

Low profile feeding device—a skin level enteral feeding device used for patients who would benefit from not having a tube extend out of their abdomen.

Malabsorption—impaired intestinal absorption of nutrients.

Malnutrition—poor nourishment resulting either from improper dietary intake or a defect in metabolism that prevents absorption of nutrients.

Marasmic-Kwashiorkor—result of chronic starvation combined with a metabolic stress such as sepsis.

Marasmus—protein-calorie malnutrition resulting from a chronically poor intake of protein, energy, vitamins, and minerals, but usually with retention of appetite and mental alertness.

Mastication—the act of chewing.

Medicaid—state agency with organized programs to financially assist people with medical conditions; can be sole source of medical coverage, or a supplement to another plan.

Medicare—federally funded program of the Social Security Administration designed to provide medical payment to all individuals over the age of 65. Incapacitated, younger individuals may qualify for Medicare coverage when other reimbursement options are exhausted.

Medication suspension—liquid dosage form with solids suspended in liquids; usually requires shaking.

Medium chain triglycerides—(MCT) saturated lipid source that has 6–12 carbon fatty acid chains. This is one of the primary sources of fat in many tube feeding formulas for patients with malabsorption or impaired fat digestion.

Metabolism—the sum total of all the chemical reactions that go on in the body.

Meter—basic unit of linear measure of the metric system; equals 39.371 inches.

Micronutrient—nutrients required by the body in very small quantities such as vitamins and trace elements.

Mineral—any naturally occurring nonorganic homogeneous solid substances. There are at least 19 minerals circulating in the body—13 are essential to health and should be provided by the diet.

Minimum Data Set—(MDS) a set of basic assessment forms developed by the Health Care Financing Administration (HCFA) to be completed on every resident in a long-term care or sub-acute care facility.

Modality—a method of application.

Modular formula—a formula made by combining several prepared mixtures or modules.

Morbidity—the condition of being deceased; the ratio of sick to well persons in a community.

Mortality—the quality of being mortal; the death rate or ratio of total number of deaths to the total number of the population.

Nasoenteric tube—a feeding tube that is placed through the nose with its distal end in either the stomach or small intestine.

Nitrogen—a chemical element; a gas constituting about four-fifths of common air; soluble in blood and body fluids; occurs naturally in all proteins and amino acids.

Nitrogen balance—the state of the body in regard to the rate of protein intake and protein utilization.

Nomogram—a graph with several scales arranged so that a straightedge laid on the graph intersects the scales at related values of the variables; the values of any two variables can be used to find the values of the others.

Nosocomial infection—infection acquired while in the hospital.

Nutrient—a substance obtained from food and used in the body to promote growth, maintenance, or repair of body tissues; proteins, carbohydrates, fats, vitamins, minerals, trace elements, and water.

Nutrition assessment—a comprehensive evaluation of factors that influence or reflect nutrition status; its tools include histories, physical examinations, anthropometric measures, and biochemical analysis.

Nutrition screening—the use of preliminary nutrition assessment techniques to identify people who are malnourished or are at risk for malnutrition.

Nutrition support—provision of specially formulated and/or delivered parenteral or enteral nutrients to maintain or restore optimal nutrition status.

Nutritional status—condition of patient as determined by nutritional assessment.

Obesity—a chronic disease characterized by excessive body fat in relation to lean body tissue.

Oley Foundation—established in 1983, The Oley Foundation for Home Parenteral & Enteral Nutrition conducts research and education to provide a support network for those sustained on home nutrition support therapies.

Oligomeric—formulas that contain small nutrient units such as oligosaccharides, peptides, and short and medium-chain triglycerides. Often called semielemental formulas.

Open system—an enteral formula that is poured into a container every few hours and administered to a patient. Hang times vary, but the general guideline is not to hang an open system longer than 4 hours due to risk of bacterial contamination. Opposite of Closed System.

Osmolality—property expressed by number of particles per volume of solute.

Outcome indicator—an instrument that looks at the results of practitioner's activities, including complications, adverse events, short-term results of specific procedures and treatments, and long-term status of patient's health and functioning.

Overfeeding—a form of malnutrition in that it provides excessive nutriture to a person sufficient to cause disease or complication of health.

Parenteral nutrition—(PN) nutrients provided directly into the venous system.

Peptide—the constituent parts of protein; yields, 2 or more amino acids upon hydrolysis.

Peripheral parenteral nutrition—(PPN) nutrients delivered intravenously into a peripheral vein, usually the hand or forearm.

Polymeric—formulas that contain large nutrient units such as polysaccharides, intact protein, and long-chain triglycerides.

Portal circulation—the circulation of blood through larger vessels from the capillaries of one organ to those of another; specifically from the gastrointestinal tract (GI) and spleen to the portal vein in the liver.

Practice guideline—systematically developed statement to assist practitioner and patient decisions about appropriate health care for specific circumstances. Statements suggesting the proper indications for doing a procedure or treatment or the proper management for specific clinical problems.

Prealbumin—carries thyroxine and facilitates the transport of retinol-binding protein; a sensitive biochemical marker of visceral protein status; 2-day half-life; also known as thyroxine-binding prealbumin or transthyretin.

Prefilled containers—Commercially available feeding bags that are filled with formula at the manufacturing site and then spiked at the bedside with an administration set.

Pressure necrosis—tissue breakdown that occurs from tube pressure on nares or around insertion site, generally associated with poor stabilization techniques.

Process indicator—an instrument that assesses data concerning functions carried out by practitioners, including assessment, treatment, treatment planning, technical aspects of performing treatment, management of complications, and indications for treatments and procedures.

Protein—large, organic compound made up of amino acids and joined by peptides; essential to structure and function of cell walls, various membranes, connective tissue, and muscles of the body.

Protein-energy malnutrition—(PEM) a defiency of protein and food energy; the world's most widespread malnutrition problem.

Pump controlled—administration method in which formula is infused using an enteral pump, which assures accurate volume delivery.

Quality assessment—the measurement of the technical and interpersonal aspects of health care and services and the outcomes of the care and service; provides information that may be used in CQI activities.

Quality assurance—the certification of continuous, optimal, effective, and efficient health and nutrition care in an effort to improve patient outcomes.

Refeeding syndrome—a set of physiological and metabolic complications associated with reintroducing adequate nutrition too rapidly for a person with severe protein-calorie malnutrition.

Reimbursement—receiving preapproved financial assistance from an agency to help pay for medical costs.

Repletion—to reestablish nutritional stores.

Residuals—that amount of tube feeding remaining upon aspiration of stomach contents; used to determine how quickly a patient is tolerating tube feeding formula or if there is a problem with peristalsis.

Resting metabolic rate—(RMR) amount of energy expended 2 hours post-absorption of a meal under conditions of rest and thermal neutrality; approximately 10% higher than basal metabolic rate (BMR).

Serum albumin—a plasma protein synthesized in the liver, responsible for colloidal osmotic pressure; also a transport protein for fatty acids, bilirubin, many drugs, and hormones. A decrease in serum albumin may occur with metabolic stresses such as liver disease, malnutrition, severe burns, and kidney failure.

Skinfold calipers—a measurement device used in a nutrition assessment to measure subcutaneous fat at a particular site; 3 sites or more can often be used to estimate total body fat; common areas to measure are the triceps, subscapular, biceps, and chest.

Somatic—pertaining to or characteristic of the body.

Sorbitol—a carbohydrate, often added to medications, that may cause gastrointestinal distress.

Soy polysaccharide—this fiber is primarily insoluble and is the most prevalent fiber source in fiber-containing formulas. It may prevent constipation and diarrhea.

Soy protein isolates—primary protein from the soybean that is used in soy-based formulas.

Starvation—continuous deprivation of food and its morbid effects.

Subjective data—data obtained in a nutrition assessment that is perceived only by the affected individual and not by the examiner.

Subjective Global Assessment—(SGA) a type of assessment tool developed by Detsky and colleagues that involves rating the final results in 3 categories of nutritional state.

Total parenteral nutrition—the intravenous delivery of all nutrients via a central catheter (see central venous access).

Transitional feeding—progression from one mode of feeding to another, while continuously administering estimated nutrient requirements.

Transthyretin—(see prealbumin).

Tube clogging—occlusion of tube often caused by medications, viscous formulas, or insufficient flushing.

Tube displacement—accidental removal or movement of feeding tube wherein tip of tube is not in GI tract where it was originally placed.

Tube feeding—(TF) providing a nutrient solution via a tube into the stomach or intestines; enteral nutrition.

Usual body weight—(UBW) body weight most frequently obtained over a specified period of time.

Villi—fingerlike projections of the cellular membrane that line the small intestine and are primarily responsible for absorption of nutrients.

Vitamin—an organic substance found in foods and essential in small quantities for growth, health, and the preservation of life.

Wasting—a term used to describe the effects of starvation; refers to protein and energy malnutrition.

Weight—heaviness; the degree to which a body is drawn toward the earth by gravity; used in nutrition assessment to determine nutritional status.

Whey—the watery part of milk remaining after separation of the casein.

B

Patient Education Resources

American Society for Parenteral and Enteral Nutrition

What is Enteral Nutrition? Pamphlet.

Overview of enteral feeding. Available 50 fliers for $30 ASPEN members/$45 non-members

www.nutritioncare.org

Phone: 1–800–727–8972, ext. 1234, ext. 1140, or ext. 1219 (outside the US)

FAX: 1–800–220–3499

Bard Inventional Products

C. R. Bard Inc.

129 Concord Road

Billerica, MA 01821

1–800–225–1332

www.bardinterventional.com

- Patient Care Wall Charts and Booklets
  Fastrac Gastric Access Port Guidelines for Patient Care
  Fastrac Gastric Access Port Patient Information
  Use and Care of Bard PEG and Button Feeding Devices
  The Bard Button Replacement Gastrostomy Device Guidelines for Patient Care
  Gauderer Genie System Guidelines for Patient Care
- Patient Care Videotapes
  The Bard Button Replacement Gastrostomy Device Guidelines for Patient Care
  Bard Guidewire System & Ponsky "Pull" PEG Guidelines for Patient Care

Kendall Healthcare Products Company

15 Hampshire St.

Mansfield, MA 02048

1–800–962–9888 ask for enteral marketing

www.kendallhq.com

Informational products such as:

- *Home Tube-Feeding: Practical Tips & Techniques*
- *Care and Maintenance of your Entristar Skin Level Gastrostomy*
- *Kangaroo Feeding Pump Instruction Cards*
- *Kangaroo Feeding Pump Video Instructions*
- *Coloring Book: Feeding Time with Roo and Joe*

Mayo Clinic

Gastrostomy Button Sticker (TM), MC1456–10

MIC-KEY Tube Feeding Stickers, MC1456–0

Nasal Tube Sticker, MC1456–07

Needle Catheter Jejunostomy (NCJ) Sticker, MC1456–02

Percutaneous Endoscopic Gastrostomy (PEG) Sticker, MC1456–04

Percutaneous Endoscopic Gastrostomy With Jejunal Extension (PEG-J) Sticker, MC1456–05

Replacement Gastrostomy Sticker, MC1456–08

Straight Catheter Sticker, MC1456–03

Straight Catheter With Balloon Sticker, MC1456–06
Surgical Jejunostomy Tube Sticker, MC1456–12
Transgastric Jejunal Sticker, MC1456–11
Tube Feeding at Home, MC1456 Pamphlet
Tube Feeding at Home for Infants, Children, and Teenagers, MC1456–01 Pamphlet

Mead Johnson Nutritionals

A Bristol-Myers Squibb Company
400 West Lloyd Expressway
Evansville, IN 47721
1–800–457–3550
www.meadjohnson.com/products/index/html
Consumer information on nutritional formulas such as Isocal.

Nestlé Clinical Nutrition

Three Parkway North, Suite 500
PO Box 760
Deerfield, IL 60015–0760
1–800–422–ASK2 for consumers to call

Oley Foundation

Provides an Information Clearinghouse for consumers dependent upon home parenteral
and enteral nutrition. Oley staff and volunteers may be able to help with such topics
as: care of feeding tube and skin at the ostomy/wound site, traveling with enteral
nutrition, therapy complications, patient/family support groups/insurance issues, and
more. Contact at 1–800–776–OLEY or (518) 262–5079 or visit the Web site at
www.oley.org.

Ross Products/Division of Abbott Laboratories

625 Cleveland Avenue
Columbus, OH 43215
1–800–544–7495
www.ross.com
- Booklets:
  Tube Feeding at Home: For Nasogastric, Nasoduodenal, or Nasojejunal Tube Feeding 1996
  Tube Feeding at Home: For Gastrostomy or Jejunostomy Tube Feeding 1996
- Video:
  Tube Feeding: A Matter of Nutrition

C

Patient Information

All people need enough food and nutrients to fight illness, heal wounds, and gain back the weight and strength they may have lost. Sometimes with an illness, you may have a decrease in appetite, inability to swallow, or a blockage of your gastrointestinal tract. In this case, your doctor may suggest and prescribe a tube feeding. This tube feeding will provide you with liquid nutrition (formula) that will help you recover. You may need this for only a short time while you are in the hospital or for a longer time.

WHAT TYPE OF TUBE WILL I NEED?

There are several types of tubes available. Those that are in for only a short time are placed through the nose and down into the stomach or upper small intestine. If you need a tube for a longer time, you can have one placed directly into your stomach or intestine through your belly. That type of tube will be less noticeable to others.

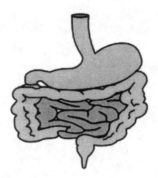

HOW OFTEN DO I NEED THESE FEEDINGS?

Some people need to have these feedings throughout the day and night. Others will need a certain volume of formula every 3 to 6 hours, similar to a meal schedule. Your doctor, other health care providers, yourself, and your caregivers will work out a feeding schedule that works best for you and the type of tube that you have.

WILL I ALSO BE ABLE TO EAT BY MOUTH?

You may be able to eat with this tube if your illness and swallowing ability allow it. Your doctor will discuss this with you. If allowed to eat, you should have no problem eating while the tube is in place.

HOW WILL I LEARN TO HANDLE THIS?

Generally in the hospital, a dietitian and/or nurse will begin teaching you and your caregivers how to handle these feedings. You may also have home care nurses continue with the instruction and answer all of your questions until you feel comfortable with the procedures.

WHAT WILL I NEED TO LEARN?

You and your caregivers will learn how to give you the feeding formula, how to flush and care for the tube, and to watch for any problems. You will be given your nurse's and doctor's contact information to call if you have any problems.

Most patients who need this type of feeding do well with it and feel stronger receiving the nutrition they need.

List of Sources

CHAPTER 1

Exhibit 1–1 Reprinted with permission from D. Kovacevich, et al., Nutrition Risk Classification: A Reproducible and Valid Tool for Nurses, *Nutrition in Clinical Practice,* Vol. 12, p. 22, © 1997, American Society For Parenteral & Enteral Nutrition.

Exhibit 1–2 Reprinted with permission from A.S. Detsky, What is Subjective Global Assessment of Nutritional Status?, *Journal of Parenteral and Enteral Nutrition,* Vol. 11, pp. 8–14, © 1987, American Society For Parenteral & Enteral Nutrition.

Figure 1–1 Reprinted with permission from J.L. Rombeau, et al., *Atlas of Nutritional Support Techniques,* © 1989, Lippincott Williams & Wilkins.

Figure 1–2 Reprinted with permission from J.L. Rombeau, et al., *Atlas of Nutritional Support Techniques,* © 1989, Lippincott Williams & Wilkins.

Figure 1–4 Reprinted with permission from J.L. Rombeau, et al., *Atlas of Nutritional Support Techniques,* © 1989, Lippincott Williams & Wilkins.

Figure 1–5 Reprinted with permission from J.L. Rombeau, et al., *Atlas of Nutritional Support Techniques,* © 1989, Lippincott Williams & Wilkins.

Figure 1–6 Reprinted with permission from J.L. Rombeau, et al., *Atlas of Nutritional Support Techniques,* © 1989, Lippincott Williams & Wilkins.

Figure 1–7 Reprinted with permission from J.L. Rombeau, et al., *Atlas of Nutritional Support Techniques,* © 1989, Lippincott Williams & Wilkins.

Figure 1–8 Reprinted with permission from *The Body Test,* material of the Dietitians of Canada.

Figure 1–9 Adapted with permission from M.A. Brunnstrom, *Clinical Kinesiology,* 3rd Edition, © 1981, F.A. Davis.

Figure 1–10 Reprinted with permission from Krause and Mahan, eds., *Food, Nutrition and Diet Therapy, 7th Edition,* p. 209, © 1984, W.B. Saunders Company.

Figure 1–11 Reprinted with permission from J.L. Rombeau, et al., *Atlas of Nutritional Support Techniques,* © 1989, Lippincott Williams & Wilkins.

Figure 1–12 Reprinted with permission from G. Rainey-McDonald, R.L. Holliday, and B.A. Wells, Nomograms for Predicting Resting Energy Expenditure of Hospitalized Patients, *Journal of Parenteral and Enteral Nutrition,* Vol. 6, No. 1, pp. 59–60, © 1982, American Society For Parenteral & Enteral Nutrition.

Table 1–1 Reprinted with permission from J. Rindal, Metabolic Nurse Clinician, Department of Surgery, University of Minnesota, Minneapolis, MN, © 1996.

Table 1–2 From HANES I - Anthropometry, Goniometry, Skeletal Age, Bone Density, and Cortical Thickness, Ages 1–74, *National Health and Nutrition Examination Survey, 1971–1975,* National Center for Health Statistics. Reprinted with permission from Metropolitan Life Insurance Company.

Table 1–3   Reprinted with permission from *1979 Build Study,* Society of Actuaries and Association of Life Insurance Medical Directors of America, © 1980, Metropolitan Life Insurance Company.

Table 1–4   Adapted with permission from K.M. Teasley-Strawburg and J.D. Anderson, Assessment, Prevalence and Clinical Significance of Malnutrition, in *Pharmacotherapy: A Pathophysiological Approach, 3rd Edition,* J.T. DiPiro, et al., eds., © 1999, McGraw-Hill Companies; and E.P. Shronts and K.P. Hammond, Nutrition Assessment, in *1998 A.S.P.E.N. Nutrition Support Practice Manual,* © 1998, American Society For Parenteral & Enteral Nutrition.

CHAPTER 2

Exhibit 2–1 Adapted with permission from P.A. Guenter, et al., Delivery Systems and Administration of Enteral Nutrition, in *Enteral and Tube Feeding, 3rd Edition,* J.L. Rombeau and R.H. Rolandelli, eds., p. 242, © 1997, W.B. Saunders Company.

Figure 2–1   Adapted with permission from A.S.P.E.N. Board of Directors, *Guidelines for the Use of Parenteral and Enteral Nutrition in Adult and Pediatric Patients and Journal of Parenteral and Enteral Nutrition,* Vol. 17, Supplement 4, p. 7SA, © 1993, American Society For Parenteral & Enteral Nutrition.

CHAPTER 3

Exhibit 3–1   Adapted with permission from P.A. Guenter, et al., Delivery Systems and Administration of Enteral Nutrition, in *Enteral and Tube Feeding, 3rd Edition,* J.L. Rombeau and R.H. Rolandelli, eds., pp. 240–267, © 1997, W.B. Saunders Company.

Figure 3–1   Adapted with permission from P.A. Guenter, et al., Delivery Systems and Administration of Enteral Nutrition, in *Enteral and Tube Feeding, 3rd Edition,* J.L. Rombeau and R.H. Rolandelli, eds., © 1997, W.B. Saunders Company.

Figure 3–2   Permission to reprint from CORPAK MedSystems, Wheeling, IL.

Figure 3–3   Reprinted with permission from P.A. Guenter, et al., Delivery Systems and Administration of Enteral Nutrition, in *Enteral and Tube Feeding, 3rd Edition,* J.L. Rombeau and R.H. Rolandelli, eds., © 1997, W.B. Saunders Company.

Figure 3–4   Reprinted with permission from J.L. Rombeau, et al., *Atlas of Nutritional Support Techniques,* © 1989, Lippincott Williams & Wilkins.

Figure 3–5   Courtesy of Ross Products Division, Abbott Laboratories, Inc., Columbus, OH.

Figure 3–6   Courtesy of Ross Products Division, Abbott Laboratories, Inc., Columbus, OH.

Figure 3–7   Reprinted with permission from J.L. Rombeau, et al., *Atlas of Nutritional Support Techniques,* © 1989, Lippincott Williams & Wilkins.

Figure 3–8 Reprinted with permission from J.L. Rombeau, et al., *Atlas of Nutritional Support Techniques,* © 1989, Lippincott Williams & Wilkins.

Figure 3–9 Courtesy of Ross Products Division, Abbott Laboratories, Inc., Columbus, OH.

Figure 3–10 Reprinted with permission from J.L. Rombeau, et al., *Atlas of Nutritional Support Techniques,* © 1989, Lippincott Williams & Wilkins.

Figure 3–11 Reprinted with permission from J.L. Rombeau, et al., *Atlas of Nutritional Support Techniques,* © 1989, Lippincott Williams & Wilkins.

Table 3–1 Adapted with permission from C.A. Monturo, Enteral Access Device Selection, N*utrition in Clinical Practice,* Vol. 5, pp. 207–213, © 1990, American Society For Parenteral & Enteral Nutrition.

CHAPTER 4

Figure 4–1 Reprinted with permission from J.L. Rombeau, et al., *Atlas of Nutritional Support Techniques,* © 1989, Lippincott Williams & Wilkins.

Figure 4–2 Courtesy of Hollister Incorporated, Libertyville, IL.

Figure 4–3a Permission to reprint from CORPAK MedSystems, Wheeling, IL.

Figure 4–3b Permission to reprint from CORPAK MedSystems, Wheeling, IL.

Figure 4–4 Courtesy of ZEVEX, Inc., Salty Lake City, UT.

Figure 4–5 Courtesy of Ross Products Division, Abbott Laboratories, Inc., Columbus, OH.

Figure 4–6 Courtesy of Hollister Incorporated, Libertyville, IL.

Figure 4–7 Reprinted with permission from B. Heximer, Pressure Necrosis: Implications and Interventions for Peg Tubes, *Nutrition in Clinical Practice,* Vol. 12, pp. 256–258, © 1997, American Society For Parenteral & Enteral Nutrition.

CHAPTER 5

Exhibit 5–5 Adapted with permission from P.A. Guenter, et al., Delivery Systems and Administration of Enteral Nutrition, in *Enteral and Tube Feeding, 3rd Edition,* J.L. Rombeau and R.H. Rolandelli, eds., © 1997, W.B. Saunders Company.

Figure 5–2 Courtesy of Ross Products Division, Abbott Laboratories, Inc., Columbus, OH.

Figure 5–3 Courtesy of Kendall Healthcare Products, Mansfield, MA.

Figure 5–4 Courtesy of Ross Products Division, Abbott Laboratories, Inc., Columbus, OH.

Table 5–1 Reprinted with permission from P.A. Guenter, et al., Delivery Systems and Administration of Enteral Nutrition, in *Enteral and Tube Feeding, 3rd Edition,* J.L. Rombeau and R.H. Rolandelli, eds., © 1997, W.B. Saunders Company.

Table 5–5 Adapted with permission from K.T. Ideno, Enteral Nutrition, in *Nutrition Support Dietetics Core Curriculum, 2nd Edition,* MM. Gottschlich,

L.E. Matarese, and E.P. Shronts, eds., p. 102, © 1993, American Society For Parenteral & Enteral Nutrition.

CHAPTER 6

Figure 6–1   Copyright © Nestle Clinical Nutrition, Deerfield, IL.

Table 6–1   Adapted with permission from D.R. Johnson and M.S. Nyffeler, Drug-nutrient Considerations for Enteral Nutrition, in *The A.S.P.E.N. Nutrition Support Practice Manual,* R. Merritt, ed., © 1998, American Society For Parenteral & Enteral Nutrition.

Table 6–2   Adapted with permission from D.R. Johnson and M.S. Nyffeler, Drug-nutrient Considerations for Enteral Nutrition, in *The A.S.P.E.N. Nutrition Support Practice Manual,* R. Merritt, ed., © 1998, American Society For Parenteral & Enteral Nutrition.

CHAPTER 7

Exhibit 7–1   Adapted with permission from L. Lord, L. Trumbore, and G. Zaloga, Enteral Nutrition Implementation and Management, in *The A.S.P.E.N. Nutrition Support Practice Manual,* R. Merritt, ed., © 1998, American Society For Parenteral & Enteral Nutrition.

Exhibit 7–2   Copyright, © 1995, Peggi Guenter, Ph.D., RN, CHSN, All rights reserved. 135 Winchester Road, Merion Station, PA 19066.

Exhibit 7–3   Copyright, © 1995, Peggi Guenter, Ph.D., RN, CHSN, All rights reserved. 135 Winchester Road, Merion Station, PA 19066.

Figure 7–1   Permission to reprint from CORPAK MedSystems, Wheeling, IL.

Figure 7–2   Permission to reprint from CORPAK MedSystems, Wheeling, IL.

Table 7–1   Adapted with permission from P.A. Guenter, et al., Delivery Systems and Administration of Enteral Nutrition, in *Enteral and Tube Feeding, 3rd Edition,* J.L. Rombeau and R.H. Rolandelli, eds., © 1997, W.B. Saunders Company.

Table 7–2   Reprinted with permission from E.H. Frankel, To Add or Not to Add Blue Dye to Tube Feeding, That is the Question, *A.S.P.E.N. 24th Clinical Congress Proceedings,* p. 289, © 2000, American Society For Parenteral & Enteral Nutrition.

CHAPTER 8

Figure 8–2   Reprinted with permission from S.M. Hunt and J.L. Groff, eds., *Advanced Nutrition and Human Metabolism,* p. 87, © 1990, NTC/Contemporary Publishing Company.

CHAPTER 9

Figure 9–3   Courtesy of The Children's Mercy Hospital and Clinics, Kansas City, MO.

Figure 9–4 Courtesy of The Children's Mercy Hospital and Clinics, Kansas City, MO.

Figure 9–5 Courtesy of Dana Barry, Certified Pediatric Nurse Practitioner, The Children's Mercy Hospital and Clinics, Kansas City, MO.

Figure 9–6 Courtesy of The Children's Mercy Hospital and Clinics, Kansas City, MO.

Table 9–2 Adapted with permission from *Recommended Dietary Allowances: 10th Edition.* Copyright 1989 by the National Academy of Sciences. Courtesy of the National Academy Press, Washington, DC.

Table 9–3 Adapted with permission from *Energy and Protein Requirements: Report of a Joint FAO/WHO/UNU Expert Consultation,* pp. 71, 178, © 1985, World Health Organization.

Table 9–3 Adapted with permission from C.P. Page, T.C. Hardin, and G. Melnick, eds., *Nutritional Assessment and Support - A Primer, 2nd Edition,* p. 32, © 1994, Lippincott Williams & Wilkins.

Table 9–4 Adapted with permission from K.B. Johnson, et al., eds., *The Harriet Lane Handbook,* pp. 164–165, © 1993, Mosby-Yearbook, Inc.

CHAPTER 10

Figure 10–1 Reprinted from Health Care Financing Administration, U.S. Department of Health and Human Services.

Figure 10–2 Reprinted from Health Care Financing Administration, U.S. Department of Health and Human Services.

Figure 10–3 Reprinted with permission of Briggs Corporation, Des Moines, Iowa 50306. (800) 247–2343.

Figure 10–4 Reprinted with permission of Briggs Corporation, Des Moines, Iowa 50306. (800) 247–2343.

Table 10–1 Reprinted from Durable Medical Equipment Regional Carrier (DMERC), Supplier Manual, Region B, 1994, Health Care Financing Administration, U.S. Department of Health and Human Services.

CHAPTER 11

Exhibit 11–4 © Joint Commission: *Comprehensive Accreditation Manual for Hospitals.* Oakbrook Terrace, IL: Joint Commission on Accreditation of Healthcare Organizations, 1999–2000. Reprinted with permission.

Table 11–1 Reprinted with permission from *Hazard Analysis Critical Control Point (HACCP) Plan for Enteral Feeding and Administration,* © 1999, New York Presbyterian Hospital, New York Cornell Medical Center.

Table 11–2 Courtesy of Coram Healthcare Corporation, Denver, CO.

Table 11–3 Courtesy of Coram Healthcare Corporation, Denver, CO.

Table 11–4 Reprinted with permission from T.C. Lykins, Nutrition Support Clinical Pathways, *Nutrition in Clinical Practice,* Vol. 11, p. 19, © 1996, American Society For Parenteral & Enteral Nutrition.

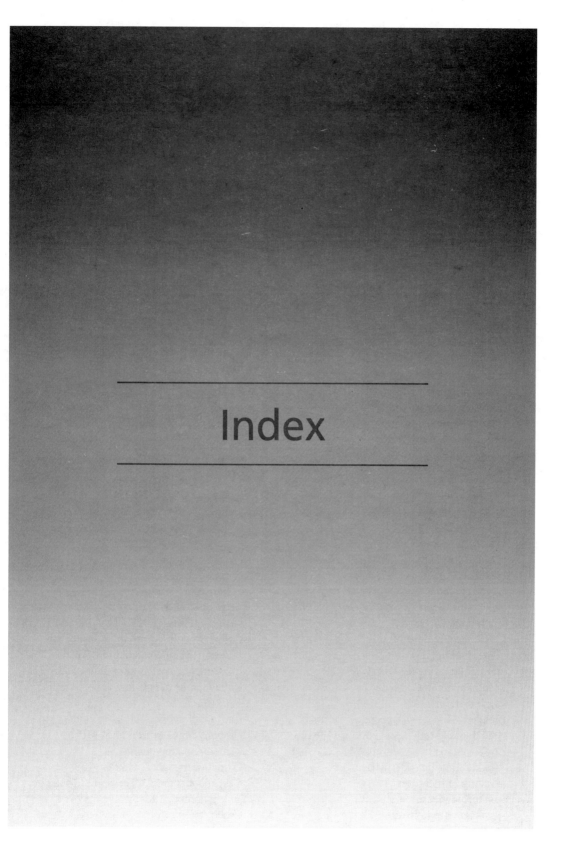

Index

Casein
  casein-based hydrolysate infant formulas,
    150–151
  in feeding formulas, 42
Certificate of Medical Necessity, 192–195
Chemically defined formulas, characteristics
    of, 43
Choice dm, 45
Ciprofloxacin, interaction with food, 102
Citrotein, 133
Clear liquid diet, 131
Clinical pathways
  example of, 234–236
  goals of, 231–232
Clog-Zapper, 111, 112, 113
Closed delivery system, 88–89
  versus open systems, 222, 231
Clostridium difficile, and diarrhea, 116
Complications
  aspiration, 113–114
  gastrointestinal complications, 115–117
  injury to surrounding tissues, 112
  long-term tube use, 63
  metabolic complications, 117–119
  nasogastric feeding tubes, 53, 163–164
  pediatric patients and gastrostomy tubes,
    165, 170, 172–174
  pediatric patients and jejunostomy tubes,
    174, 181–182
  tube displacement, 108–110
  tube injury, 110
  tube occlusion, 110–111
Constipation, 116–117
  causes of, 116
  pediatric patients, 182
  prevention/treatment of, 42, 116–117
Containers (feeding bags), 87–88
  bacterial growth prevention, 88
Continuous feeding
  method, 83–84
  pediatric patients, 177–178, 178
  protocol for, 85
ConvaTec, 77
Corn syrup, in feeding formulas, 41
Cornstarch, in feeding formulas, 41
Cow's milk, infant formulas, 149, 151, 152
Critcare HN, 43
Crucial, 46
Cruzan decision, 211
Cyclic feeding, 84–85

D

Declogger, 111
Dehydration
  causes of, 117
  signs in children, 181
  treatment of, 117
Deliver 2.0, 43
DiabetiSource, 45
Diarrhea, 115–116
  causes of, 115
  definition of, 115
  and fiber in formulas, 42
  and hypertonic formulas, 85
  and medication administration, 97–98
  nursing measures, 115–116
  pediatric patients, 182
  treatment of, 116
Diet history, 5, 8
  calorie counts method, 8
  food frequency model, 5, 8
  pediatric patient, 140–143
  24-hour recall, 5
  usual intake method, 8
Direct calorimetry, energy expenditure cal-
    culation, 25
Discharge planning
  case management assessment, 190–191
  and health care team, 198–199
  reimbursement, 191–198
  See also Home care; Institutional settings
Documentation
  home care, 203–204
  Medicare, 192–195
Dressing, insertion site, 73–74
Drug-nutrient interactions, 100–102
  carbidopa-levodopa, 102
  ciprofloxacin, 102
  phenytoin, 100–101
  warfarin, 101–102
Dysphagia, 129–130
  causes of, 129, 130
  thickening fluids for patients, 130

E

Education
  child gastrostomy tubes, 166–169
  child nasogastric tube feeding, 156–159
  home care, 200–202
  institutional settings, 205

Education—*continued*
  patient education resources, 254–255
  pediatric jejunostomy tubes, 175–176
Elbow breadth, frame measure, 13–14
Electrolyte/mineral abnormalities, 118–119
Elemental formulas
  characteristics of, 43
  infant formulas, 151
  pediatric formulas, 153, 154
Energy expenditure. See Calorie require-
    ments assessment
Ensure, 133
Ensure Plus, 133
Enteral nutrition
  clinical decision-making algorithm
    about, 39
  contraindications for, 40
  feeding process, steps in, 38–39
  formulas, 40–46
  indications for, 38, 40
  compared to parenteral nutrition, 38
Enteral pumps, 89–90
  alarm system, 89
  automatic flush pump, 89–90, 91
  manufacturers of, 90
  pros/cons of, 89

F

Fats
  adding to formulas, 46
  of formulas, 41
Feeding access devices
  gastrostomy tubes, 56–58
  jejunostomy tubes, 58–63
  nasogastric feeding tubes, 52–56
  skin-level feeding device, 61, 63
Feeding administration methods
  bolus method, 82
  continuous feeding, 83–84, 85
  cyclic feeding, 84–85
  decision-making algorithm, 83
  intermittent method, 82–83, 84
  modular administration, 87
  patient monitoring, 90–91
  progression/assessment of feeding, 86–87
  starter regimen, 85–86
Feeding delivery devices
  containers (feeding bags), 87–88
  enteral pumps, 89–90
  open versus closed system, 88–89

Fiber
  for diarrhea, 116
  fiber source products, 202
  of formulas, 42
Fibronectin, assessment of level, 24
Fick equation, energy expenditure
    calculation, 26
Fish oils (omega-3 fatty acids), in feeding
    formulas, 41, 46
Flesch Reading Ease Score, 201
Flexiflo Quantum Pump, 90
Fluid overload, signs of, 181
Fluid retention, conditions related to, 181
Fluids
  dehydration treatment, 117
  requirements, calculation of, 30–31
  thickening for patients, 130
Flushing
  automatic flush pump, 89–90, 91
  flush fluids, 111, 167, 174
  nasogastric feeding tubes, 70–71, 72
  pediatric gastrostomy tubes, 167
  pediatric jejunostomy tubes, 174
  pediatric NGT, 162
  tube occlusion problem, 111–112
Food frequency model, 5, 8
Formulas, 40–46
  calorically dense formulas, 43
  carbohydrates, 41
  chemically defined formulas, 43
  drug-nutrient interactions, 100–102
  fats, 41
  fiber, 42
  glucose intolerance formulas, 45
  guidelines for selection, 44
  hepatic dysfunction formulas, 45
  high-protein formulas, 43
  homemade, 40
  immune enhancing formulas, 45–46
  modular supplements, 46
  pediatric formulas, 152–155
  polymeric formulas, 43
  protein, 42
  pulmonary formulas, 45
  renal formulas, 43, 45
  water content, 42
  wound-healing formulas, 46
Frame size measures, 13–14
  elbow breadth, 13–14
  wrist circumference, 13

change in tube feeding, proof of, 192
Medicare Waiver, 198
regional breakdown, 195, 198
Medication administration
crushing medication, 99–100
dilution with water, 99
drug-nutrient interactions, 97, 100–102
forms of medication, 97–98
goal in, 96
medications to avoid via tube, 100
and nurse expertise, 96
osmolality of liquid medications, 98
pediatric gastrostomy tubes, 169–170
pediatric jejunostomy tubes, 177
sorbitol in medications, 97–98, 99
steps in administration, 102–103
Megace, 133
Metabolic complications, 117–119
dehydration, 117
electolyte/mineral abnormalities, 118–119
hyperglycemia, 117–118
refeeding syndrome, 118–119
signs of, 129
Metropolitan Life Insurance Tables, limitations of, 16
Microlipid, 46
Micronutrients, in feeding formulas, 42
Mineral abnormalities, 118–119
Minerals, in feeding formulas, 42
Mini-Nutritional Assessment tool, 204
Minimum Data Set (MDS), 204
Moducal, 46
Modular supplements
administration of, 87
pediatric patients, 151–152, 153
types of, 46
Mouth care, and nasogastric tube, 70

N

Nasogastric feeding tubes, 52–56
clogged tubes, handling of, 162, 164
complications of, 53, 163–164
features of tubes, 52, 54–55
feeding problems, development of, 163
flushing tube, 162
flushing/irrigation of, 70–71, 72
home care, 162–163
measurement of tube for placement, 160–161

and otitis media/sinusitis, 163
patient care, 70–71
placement in adolescent, 160
placement in adult patient, 53–54, 56
placement in infant, 159
placement in toddler, 159
securing from patient removal, 70
securing tube, 70, 71
tube placement management, 161–162
Nasogastric feeding tubes and pediatric patient, 155–164
indications for, 156
parent education, 156–159
size of tube, 156
Nepro, 45
Nitrogen balance
calculation of, 30
meaning of, 30
Nocturnal feeding method
method, 84–85
pediatric jejunostomy tubes, 179–180
pediatric patients, 179–180
Nomograms, energy expenditure calculation, 28, 29
NovaSource Pulmonary, 45
Novasource Renal, 45
NuBasics, 133
Nutren 1.0, 43
Nutren 1.5, 43
NutriHep, 45
Nutrisource Protein, 46
Nutrition assessment, 3–8
institutional settings, 204–308
pediatric patients, 140–145
Nutrition prescription, 24–31
calorie requirements assessment, 24–28
fluid requirements, 30–31
nitrogen balance, 30
protein requirements assessment, 28
Nutrition screening
admission nutrition screening tool, 4
diet history, 5, 8
pediatric patients, 140–144
physical assessment for malnourished, 6–8
Subjective Global Assessment (SGA), 5, 9
NutriVent, 45
Nutrsource Carbohydrate, 46
Nutrsource Lipid, 46

O

Oils, in feeding formulas, 41, 45
Omnibus Budget Reconciliation Act of
    1987, 205
Open delivery system, 88–89
    versus closed systems, 222, 231
Optimental, 46
Order sets/protocols, 92
Osmolality, liquid medications, 98
Otitis media, children on nasogastric feeding
    tubes, 163
Overfeeding problem
    negative effects of, 127
    and transitional feeding, 126–127
Oxepa, 45

P

Parenteral nutrition, compared to enteral
    nutrition, 38
Patient assessment
    anthropometrics, 8–21
    assessment team, 2
    biochemical assessment, 21–24
    for malnutrition, 2–3
    nutrition assessment, 3–8
    nutrition prescription, 24–31
Patient care
    dressing insertion site, 73–74
    replacement of tube, 77–78
    skin breakdown problem, 75–77
Patient monitoring, 90–91
    daily inspection for migration, 74
    home care/institutional settings, 205, 209
    laboratory monitoring, 90–91
    pediatric patients, 180–181
    during progression of feeding, 86–87
    of residuals, 86
    of stool output, 86
    tolerance assessment, 90
    during transitional phase, 133–134
Patient Self-Determination Act, 211
Pectin, in feeding formulas, 42
Pediatric formulas, 152–155
    blenderized formulas, 154
    elemental formulas, 153, 154
    hydrolyzed whey, 153, 154
    soy based formulas, 154
Pediatric patients
    assessment of, 140–145
    bolus feeding, 178–179

breast milk, 147–149
    care of feeding system, 183
    complications, 181–182
    continuous feeding, 178
    formula selection, 154–155
    gastrostomy tubes, 164–174
    gravity feeding, 178
    infant formula, 149–152
    initiation of feedings, 180
    jejunostomy tubes, 174–177
    modulars for, 151–152, 153
    nasogastric feeding tubes, 155–164
    nocturnal feeding, 179–180
    nutrient imbalance, signs of, 146
    nutrient requirements estimation,
        145, 147
    patient monitoring, 180–181
    pediatric formulas, 152–155
    progression of feedings, 180
    psycosocial issues, 184
    short and long term goals, 147
    transition feeding, 183–184
PEG Cleaning Brush, 111
Peptamen, 43
Perative, 43
Percent ideal body weight, 16–17
Percent usual weight, 17
Percent weight change, 18
Peripheral parenteral nutrition (PPN)
    discontinuation of, 131
    nature of, 124
    time limitations for, 124
Phenytoin, interaction with food, 100–101
Physical assessment
    anthropometrics, 8–21
    for malnutrition, 6–8
Pneumonia, aspiration pneumonia, 113
Polycose, 46
Polymeric formulas, characteristics of, 43
Portagen, 151
Prealbumin, assessment of level, 23
Promix, 46
ProMod, 46
Promote, 43, 46
Protain XL, 46
Protein
    protein requirements assessment, 28
    protein status, biochemical assessment,
        21–24
Protein-energy malnutrition (PEM), features
    of, 3

Protein and formulas, 42
   protein hydrolysate formulas, 150
   protein modular supplements, 46
Psycosocial issues, pediatric patients, 184
Pulmocare, 45
Pulmonary formulas, characteristics of, 45

Q

Quality of care
   clinical pathways, 231–232
   and Hazard Analysis and Critical Control
      Points (HACCP), 221–222
   and Joint Commission on Accreditation of
      Healthcare Organizations (JCAHO),
      218–221
   open versus closed systems, 222, 231
   quality improvement programs, 232–234

R

Recommended Dietary Allowances (RDAs),
   pediatric patients, 147
Recumbent method, height measure, 12–13
Refeeding syndrome, 118–119
   causes of, 127
   persons at risk for, 127
   prevention of, 127
   and transitional feeding, 127
Reimbursement, 191–198
   commercial insurance companies, 191
   Medicare, 191–198
Renal formulas, characteristics of, 43, 45
Renalcal, 45
Replacement of tube, 77–78
   conditions for replacement, 77, 110
   procedure in, 78
   replacement devices, 77
Replete, 43, 46
Residuals, monitoring of, 86, 182
Resource, 133
Resource Utilization Groups (RUG–III), 205
Respalor, 45
Resting metabolic rate (RMR), meaning
   of, 24
Retinol binding protein (RBP), assessment
   of level, 23

S

Self-administration of feedings, 82
Similac Lactose-free, 149

Sinusitis, children on nasogastric feeding
   tubes, 163
Skeleton in the Hospital Closet, The
   (Butterworth), 2
Skin breakdown, 75–77
   causes of, 76
   prevention of, 76–77
Skin care
   drainage at G-tube site, 172
   dressing insertion site, 73–74
   granulation tissue, 77, 172–173
   pediatric gastrostomy tube, 165, 172
   skin assessment tool, 171
Skin-level feeding device, 61, 63
Skinfold measurements, 20
   pediatric patients, 143–144
Somatomedin C, assessment of level, 24
Sorbitol, in liquid medication, 97–98, 99
Soy-based formulas
   infant formula, 149–150
   pediatric formulas, 154
   soy polysaccharide in, 42
Stamm gastrostomy, 58, 60
Starvation, malnutrition, 2–3
Stomadhesive wafers, 77
Stool output
   monitoring, 86
   Stool Output Assessment Tool, 118
Subjective Global Assessment (SGA),
   5, 9, 204
Sustacal, 133
Swallowing difficulty, dysphagia,
   129–130

T

Thickening agents, for liquids, 130
ThickenUp, 130
Total energy expenditure (TEE), meaning
   of, 25
Total iron-binding capacity (TIBC), transferrin levels, 24
Total parenteral nutrition (TPN)
   access devices, 124
   and bacterial translocation, 128–129
   causes of, 129
   indications for, 124, 128
   transition to oral feeding, 131
Transferrin, assessment of level, 23–24
Transition feeding, pediatric patients,
   183–184

Transitional feeding
  appetite stimulation agents, 133
  assessment of patient for, 125–126
  clear liquid diet, 131
  decision-making algorithm, 125
  definition of, 124
  full liquid diet, 131, 132
  and GI function, 130–131
  method, 84–85
  monitoring of, 133–134
  overfeeding problem, 126–127
  and refeeding syndrome, 127
  with tube feedings, 131–132
Traumacal, 43
Triglycerides
  in feeding formulas, 41
  in infant formulas, 150, 151
Tube displacement, 108–110
  causes of, 108–109
  daily inspection for migration, 74
  and pediatric patient, 161–162, 163
  prevention of, 109–110
Tube injury, 110
  causes of, 110
  prevention of, 110
  and replacement of tube, 77–78, 110
Tube occlusion, 110–111
  causes of, 111
  declogging devices, 111–112
  pediatric NGT, 162, 164
  prevention of, 111
  See also Flushing
24-hour recall, 5
Two-Cal HN, 43